Health and Hygiene in Chinese East Asia

Health and Hygiene in Chinese East Asia

Policies and Publics in the Long Twentieth Century

Edited by Angela Ki Che Leung
and Charlotte Furth

Duke University Press   Durham and London   2010

Printed in the United States of America on acid-free paper ∞
Typeset in Charis by Tseng Information Systems, Inc.
Library of Congress Cataloging-in-Publication data appear
on the last printed page of this book.

Duke University Press gratefully acknowledges the support of the
Chiang Ching-Kuo Foundation for International Scholarly Exchange,
which provided funds toward the production of this book.

Contents

Acknowledgments, vii

INTRODUCTION
   Hygienic Modernity in Chinese East Asia, 1
Charlotte Furth

Part I. Tradition and Transition

The Evolution of the Idea of *Chuanran* Contagion
   in Imperial China, 25
Angela Ki Che Leung

The Treatment of Night Soil and Waste in Modern China, 51
Yu Xinzhong

Sovereignty and the Microscope:
   Constituting Notifiable Infectious Disease and Containing
   the Manchurian Plague (1910–11), 73
Sean Hsiang-lin Lei

Part II. Colonial Health and Hygiene

Eating Well in China:
   Diet and Hygiene in Nineteenth-Century Treaty Ports, 109
Shang-Jen Li

Vampires in Plagueland:
   The Multiple Meanings of *Weisheng* in Manchuria, 132
Ruth Rogaski

Have Someone Cut the Umbilical Cord:
  Women's Birthing Networks, Knowledge, and Skills
  in Colonial Taiwan, 160
Wu Chia-Ling

Part III. Campaigns for Epidemic Control

A Forgotten War:
  Malaria Eradication in Taiwan, 1905–65, 183
Lin Yi-ping and Liu Shiyung

The Elimination of Schistosomiasis in Jiaxing and Haining Counties,
  1948–58: Public Health as Political Movement, 204
Li Yushang

Conceptual Blind Spots, Media Blindfolds:
  The Case of SARS and Traditional Chinese Medicine, 228
Marta E. Hanson

Governing Germs from Outside and Within Borders:
  Controlling 2003 SARS Risk in Taiwan, 255
Tseng Yen-fen and Wu Chia-Ling

AFTERWORD
  Biomedicine in Chinese East Asia:
  From Semicolonial to Postcolonial?, 273
Warwick Anderson

Timeline, 279

Glossary, 283

Bibliography, 287

Contributors, 323

Index, 327

Acknowledgments

This volume is the result of a group project that began in 2002 and has been generously supported by the Academia Sinica of Taipei, Taiwan. Angela Ki Che Leung, then a research fellow at the Sun Yat-sen Institute for Social Sciences and Philosophy, was the project organizer, while Sean Hsiang-lin Lei, Shang-Jen Li, Yi-ping Lin, Liu Shiyung, Ruth Rogaski, Wen-shan Yang, and Chia-Ling Wu served as core members. The group held two conferences on the concepts and practices of health and hygiene in modern Chinese societies at the Academia Sinica of Taipei, Taiwan, in 2003 and 2004 with the participation of other scholars, including Chia-feng Chang, Mei-hsia Chen, Charlotte Furth, Mark Harrison, Iijima Wataru, Pui-tak Lee, Li Yushang, Yen-fen Tseng, and Yu Xinzhong. Warwick Anderson came to Taiwan and gave a talk to the group shortly after the 2004 conference. For the sake of coherence, eleven papers (including the one contributed by Marta Hanson, which was not part of the conference agenda) were selected to be published as a volume.

The contributors to this volume have benefited greatly from the comments of the two anonymous readers of the manuscript, and those of the discussants at the two conferences: Che-chia Chang, Chih-Jou Chen, Chung-lin Ch'iu, Ping-yi Chu, Fan Yen-chiou [Fan Yanqiu], Fu Daiwei, Jen-der Lee, T'sui-jung Liu, Robert T.-H. Lü, Sung-chiao Shen, John Shepherd, Jen-to Yao, and Arthur Wolf.

The publication of this volume has received generous financial support from the Research Center for Humanities and Social Sciences (formerly the Sun Yat-sen Institute for Social Sciences and Philosophy) of the Academia Sinica. The center continues to host the research group on the history of health and hygiene.

Between 2002 and 2006, Pearl Huang took care of all administrative matters connected with the research project and the preparation of the volume.

Sophie Lu has continued the work since 2006. Sabine Wilms of Happy Goat Productions served ably as technical editor, ensuring conformity in English style, format, romanization, and bibliographical entries from the diverse contributors. Last but not least, Reynolds Smith and Sharon Torian of Duke University Press have given full editorial support to the volume, and Pamela Morrison and Rebecca Fowler have provided our manuscript with the most meticulous copyediting care during the final stages of its publication.

Introduction

Hygienic Modernity in Chinese East Asia

Charlotte Furth

The chapters in this volume are about the intersections of power, culture, and science that have gone into the struggle to overcome disease and improve people's health in some Chinese regions of East Asia over the course of the "long" twentieth century—since the late Qing reforms gathered momentum in the 1860s. Part of the volume adds to the story that has been told of colonial medicine—but the geographical focus here shifts from the British Empire to two East Asian empires, those of the waning Qing dynasty in China (1644–1911) and the new empire of Japan (1895–1945), and to the republican and communist regimes that followed these empires in Taiwan and mainland China, respectively. The diverse and very specific geographical focuses of these chapters view China from the perspective of a variety of regions far from the centers of Chinese state power. The chapters by Sean Hsiang-lin Lei and Ruth Rogaski look primarily at Manchuria under Qing and Japanese rule. Marta Hanson's narrative moves to the far southern Pearl River delta, while three others (by Yu Xinzhong, Shang-Jen Li, and Li Yushang) that deal with mainland topics in fact are rooted in the regionally specific experience of Jiangnan, in the lower Yangzi delta. Three chapters (by Wu Chia-Ling, Lin Yi-ping and Liu Shiyung, and Tseng Yen-fen and Wu Chia-Ling) deal with the island of Taiwan under Japanese rule and under American patronage after the Second World War. Moreover, even though in the West the history of sanitary science has mostly been written around urban experience, none of these chapters tell the story of a major modern city. Instead, they locate much of their action in the countryside, along a continuum of medium to small towns and villages. The most important metropole, offstage but influencing the action, is Tokyo, the capital of the Japanese Empire. The very different regimes of empire engaged here—dynastic or colonial—do not produce an overarching narrative of imperialism as the shaper of colonial medicine; nor do the various localities examined easily stand in for China as a whole.

Rather, as a group these chapters suggest that a critical history of public health—commonly analyzed as a state- and nation-building project, during both the colonial and post-colonial eras—is richer when we can trace global genealogies of scientific practices in interaction with highly local situations. When chapters show us outbreaks of disease—plague, malaria, SARS (severe acute respiratory syndrome)—as environmental phenomena in motion, we are driven to follow paths that elude the logic of either imperial colony or nation-state, drawing in both international and local players across a variety of regimes that successively governed portions of the Chinese cultural sphere. Each case is embedded in a local situation and a local power grid, yet reveals transnational and international influences and interventions, whether we are dealing with midwives in colonial Taipei, the night-soil economy in treaty-port Shanghai, the plague fighters of the period 1910–19 in Manchuria, or the successive Japanese, American, and international projects for malaria control in Taiwan.

In fact the perspectives that have shaped this picture of several regionally discrete Chinas, each rooted in local conditions, are themselves the product of the situated knowledge of the core group of contributors, seven of whom live and work in Taiwan. (The other two Chinese contributors are from the People's Republic of China, and only two besides myself are native English-speaking Americans.) Conceived and developed by a working group from the Academia Sinica in Taipei, this volume assembles for the first time for an Anglophone audience the voices of a group of Chinese specialists reflecting together upon their own culture's pre-modern and modern medical history. The regional Chinese geographies that emerge in these pages are selective and partly the result of happenstance (there is nothing from central, southwest, or northwest China, or from Hong Kong or Singapore). But what is here reflects the intellectual networks of a group of cosmopolitan provincials whose work upends conventional understandings of center and periphery without, however, reifying any purely local knowledge of Taiwan alone. These chapters reflect the possibly unique circumstances of Taiwan—outside the framework of the normative nation-state system, yet prosperous and technically advanced, serving as a crossroad of the knowledge systems of both the East Asian and North Atlantic spheres.

At that crossroad, modern scholarship on the history of Chinese medicine and science has been nurtured for over fifty years. Taiwan's intellectual elite, politically marginalized as refugees from communism or as former colonials of the island, nevertheless built upon Chinese and Japanese state and public identifications of science with modernity that go back to the nineteenth century. As Anglophone intellectual influence and patronage increased after the Second World War, the study of Chinese science in Taiwan was nourished by the inspirational Science and Civilisation series by Joseph Needham and his Chinese collaborators that took shape in the mid-twentieth century.[1] The Taipei-based Academia Sinica carried forward the "Enlightenment" modern scholarship[2] of the pre-communist twentieth century, absorbed the perspectives of Anglo-American social history and cultural studies movements, and in the last decade has branched out into science and technology studies (STS)—a project that rejects the humanist-positivist divide to bring multidisciplinary perspectives to bear upon institutions and movements at the intersection of science and society.

This intellectual trajectory lies behind the present volume's historical perspective upon the science and politics of public health policymaking and action over the course of 150 years. Part of the background is a deep history of medicine in Chinese civilization. Not only do Chinese scholars today have access to an impressive 2,000-year-old archive, but they have produced a relatively well-studied modern history of classical medicine written in their own language and not merely derived from pioneering investigations from the first world. Researchers based on Taiwan, including contributors to this volume, have written on an array of fruitful topics: about the relations between medicine and the imperial state, medieval medicine and gender, ancient religion and healing; about Chinese responses to the early modern Western sciences introduced by the Jesuits, and the sociology of medical practitioners, as well as culturally informed epidemiological histories of specific diseases including smallpox and leprosy. Accordingly these researchers see the introduction of Western biomedicine and the project of hygienic modernity against a historical background that cannot be confined to narratives of resistance or accommodation, or captured by treating indigenous patterns of belief and practice simply as folk traditions.

At the same time, because the world seen from this perspective may be largely Sinophone, but cannot be identified with any one state or political regime, it encourages the recognition of both the universalism of modernizing claims for the scientific transformation of medicine and the embeddedness of actual practices in diverse local conditions. Such a perspective also helps us to move beyond the discourse of medicine and nation, mediated by the experience of imperialism, which has so far dominated the English-language scholarship of colonial medicine.

Here there is a visible contrast between the directions taken by Chinese scholarship and the dominant portrait of Indian colonial medicine framed by South Asia's history under British rule. Concerning India, the discourse of colonial medicine has been shaped by British scholars interested both in colonial power relations and in the important role that natural history in the field and tropical medicine played in the evolution of cosmopolitan science in the nineteenth and twentieth centuries.[3] But the heterogeneous subcontinent lacked an easily accessible indigenous archive, and the British rulers of India were uninterested in native technological development. Among Indians, before the 1950s, modernizing local elites were more likely to study law and the humanities than science. Congress Party nationalists initially admired Japanese scientific precocity but did not imitate it.[4] Although in China the intellectually iconoclastic May Fourth movement of 1919 established "Mr. Science" as an icon of modern identity for almost all educated Chinese, in India the pursuit of science and medicine remained relatively undeveloped. As David Arnold has noted, medicine and public health had a low priority as a British tool of empire, and Indian elites also remained lukewarm about sanitary policies likely to be controversial among the populace.[5] Indian intellectuals interested in the history of science lamented that South Asia had no Joseph Needham to inspire their field.[6]

When, after independence, South Asian scholars found a critical voice with which to examine their own modern history, they focused on the class and cultural hierarchies that imperialism had left behind, making their signature subaltern studies movement an investigation into the cultural politics of identity. Their interventions created the concept of the postcolonial as a critical perspective on modern subjectivity, on lasting colonized states of mind rather than a simple period of time. If Indian postcolonial studies aimed to provincialize Europe—reimagining indigenous civilizations and claiming an alternative modernity—science was a particularly difficult field for such an endeavor. Both Indian and Chinese scholarship were hobbled by the problem of derivative discourse—that is, the search for an authentic indigenous science judged by scientistic standards.[7] Narratives about the plurality of sciences, the achievements of indigenous technologies, or the social networks that sustained local techno-practices all too easily merged into a story of scientific backwardness. Still, as Deepak Kumar has said, this crisis of colonial identity in China was "quick and sharp" in the early twentieth century, rather than long drawn out as in India.[8] Even down to the end of the nineteenth century, Chinese scholars were aggressive in claiming a scientific genealogy "on their own terms," while throughout the twentieth century, the cosmopolitan authority of modern science appealed to Marxists and liberals, and communists and nationalists, alike. Significantly, imperial Japan as well as the hegemonic West offered models.[9] The Chinese association of scientific achievement with successful modernity continues to have strong nationalist overtones in the PRC today, as anyone who saw the opening ceremonies of the 2008 Olympics in Beijing will attest.

This complex East Asian legacy—including modern Chinese traditions of Enlightenment scholarship and the experience of Japanese colonialism—has played a role in the perspectives on science studies that shape the Taiwan-based scholarship in this volume. In pursuing the social study of medicine here, contributors do not avoid the story of colonial medicine, but they do so without the baggage of either nationalist identity politics or subaltern consciousness. They bracket it between their mother civilization's medical history on the one hand, and, on the other hand, some regionally specific flows of the globally circulating technological practices we call modern public health.

The chapters are organized into three sections, roughly chronological in order. However, the chapters intersect thematically in ways that disrupt chronology and blur distinctions between tradition and modernity, while showing interactions between colonial, national, and transnational power centers. As narratives concerned with change through time, some chapters look back to indigenous Chinese knowledge and practices surrounding disease and cleanliness in the late imperial period (the Ming and Qing dynasties), and others move forward to the 2003 SARS outbreak that pitted institutions of multiple Chinese states against a rapidly moving public health crisis that could not be managed within conventional political boundaries. Across this broad time scale, the chapters that touch on indigenous Chinese medicine and hygiene show both persistence and transformation in ways that complicate the notion of a sharp divide between medical tradition and modern biomedicine. In addition, although the chronological grouping of specific chapters suggests such a conventional transition between imperial and modern China (marked by the revolution of 1911) as well as a break between colonial and postcolonial eras (divided by the end of the Second World War), the contents of the chapters are connected in ways that blur these classifications. In the first section, "Tradition and Transition," the chapters by Leung, Yu, and Lei center on ideas of cleanliness and contagion in successive epidemiological settings in late imperial China. But these chapters exhibit links to treaty-port models of modern hygiene and to both medical and public health approaches to epidemics from the plague in the early twentieth century to the outbreak of SARS in the early twenty-first century.

The middle section, "Colonial Health and Hygiene," groups stories of Taiwan and Manchuria under Japanese rule, and of treaty-port Shanghai. The Shanghai story links back to Yu's discussion of late imperial practices surrounding the night-soil economy in the first section, while Japanese public health projects in Manchuria in the 1930s may usefully be linked to the campaign against plague in the last decade of the Qing Empire.

The third section, "Campaigns for Epidemic Control," shifts perspective to public health as a transnational phenomenon. As rapidly moving, borderless outbreaks, modern epidemics like plague, cholera, and smallpox have been natural subjects for pioneering work in the global history of health and disease. In this volume, case studies of public health projects aimed at curbing epidemics use Chinese sources but are well suited to understanding scientific knowledge and practice as globally circulating, adapting to both technological change and different regimes of power. The section leads off with Lin and Liu's narrative of both prewar and postwar campaigns against malaria on Taiwan, where readers will certainly be led to question the distinction between colonial rule and postcolonial dependency. It continues with Li Yushang's account of the Maoist campaign against schistosomiasis in the mid-twentieth century, and two chapters on SARS. In none of these chapters does the postcolonial identify easily with the national. Rather, these chapters call attention both to local, regionally specific health problems, and to the transnational dimensions of public health crises in the second half of the twentieth century. Politically, the discussions of malaria and SARS invite comparison with Lei's earlier account of the role of non-Chinese international players in the plague-fighting campaigns of the late Qing Empire. As history of science, they show how technical strategies evolve and change, always under political and social constraints. In sum, each case study—shaped by local social and technical systems, political resources, and available scientific understandings—takes its place in a critical historical genealogy of modern public health movements which deployed a variety of state and international levers of power as they seesawed between utopian goals and coercive means.

Tradition and Transition

"Hygienic modernity" refers to the term *weisheng* (*eisei* in Japanese), less as a translation than as a pointer to the changing conceptualizations of this classical Chinese phrase as it was applied to projects for sanitary reform and disease control in and around the old Chinese middle kingdom from the late nineteenth century through the twentieth. As analyzed by Ruth Rogaski in her seminal book on the topic,[10] the term *weisheng* for centuries reminded Chinese of health regimens that were the responsibility of the individual — regimens that couched medical advice in the language of prevention more than in that of cure, and gave moral and even religious underpinnings to moderation in diet and conduct. Hygienic modernity was born when *weisheng* was given a public meaning, first as part of Meiji Japan's modernizing sanitary movement (*eisei*, in Japanese), and later throughout the Chinese cultural sphere. In time, *weisheng* came to designate both the ideals of public health as entitlements justifying the exercise of modern state power, and the bureaucratic institutions charged with carrying out public health policy. But the chapters here analyze sophisticated preexisting ideas, cultural habits, and forms of social and political agency in ways that complicate this picture of a traditional *weisheng* of personal hygiene being transformed into a modern *weisheng* of public health institutions.

For example, Yu looks at what described a clean city street in Qing dynasty Jiangnan as an early public health issue, showing how cleanliness was achieved through a combination of commercial and community management of night soil. Wu shows us some of the reasons for the resiliency of the network of local, lay midwives in colonial Taiwan in the face of a Japanese campaign to replace them with experts in so-called scientific motherhood. Shang-Jen Li finds British residents of treaty-port Shanghai who came to appreciate the logic of local Chinese regimens for healthy living. Hanson's chapter on the role of traditional Chinese medicine in the medical management of the SARS epidemic in Guangzhou reminds us that classical Chinese medicine did not simply fade away under the assault of biomedical reforms. Rather, it underwent a twentieth-century transformation that, in concert with PRC state sponsorship, has made its modern hybrid form of TCM (traditional Chinese medicine) into an established sector of the health-care system.

Leung elaborates the important theme of the conceptual plasticity of pre-modern China's inherited language of health and disease. Her chapter shows that in both learned medicine and popular culture, *chuanran*, the key classical Chinese term for disease transmission through polluting agents, suggested several implicit models of contagion or contamination using the metaphor of something dyed or stained. This idea coexisted with an evolving learned medical discourse that had a basically configurationist approach to the etiology of disease, basing it on people's bodily constitutions in interaction with seasonal cycles and local environments. The most sophisticated forms of this configurationism were worked out in doctrines about febrile diseases, identified as Cold Damage (*shanghan*) and Warm disease (*wenbing*).

European medical history teaches that the broad idea of contagion—involving human contact with some sort of polluting agent—has been a historical concept of disease transmission that ordinary people intuitively acted upon, even as learned medical discourse struggled to come up with satisfactory theories of disease etiology. Leung shows that discussions of similar issues in the Chinese medical literature occurred even before the twelfth century. Here configurationist (environmental) and contagionist (polluting agent) models of disease etiology could not easily be teased apart. If Ming and Qing learned medical orthodoxy built upon the venerable tradition of Cold Damage disorders, in which fevers were attributed to damage from the *qi* (breath, air, energy) of unseasonable manifestations of seasonal cold and wind, epidemic fevers—when large numbers of people got sick at the same time—led leading experts to posit more elaborate configurationist models of long-term climate cycles. Beginning in the seventeenth century, many doctors shifted to a more regional focus, locating the source of disease in the *qi* of particular local environments. These latter configurationist doctrines sound very like miasma theories: as polluting agents, the *qi* of swampy southern microclimates, or the filth that came from human neglect—rotten organic matter, corpses, or trash heaps—were all *chuanran*. Such interpretations of contagion existed side by side with understandings of some serious chronic disease patterns (such as *xulao*, or "consumption," identified with modern tuberculosis, and *mafeng*, or "numb wind," identified with leprosy) as transmitted from person to person directly, either though heredity or sexual intercourse.

In sum, Leung argues that preexisting understandings of *chuanran* prepared Chinese to some extent for the novel views of contagion brought into China by late-nineteenth-century biomedical germ theory; but at the same time, the understandings confined the Chinese perception of contagion to certain traditional categories of chronic disease. This effectively excluded new forms of epidemics from consideration. Therefore, when Chinese of the late Qing read the English "germ"—itself a popular hybrid term—as *chong* (vermin), they were riffing on old ideas of the transmission of consumption (*xulao, feilao, shilao*) by invisible worms passed along from the bodies of those who died of the disease—a notion that easily inflected early-twentieth-century understandings of tuberculosis.[11] As the chapter by Sean Hsiang-lin Lei points out, the real novelty of the medical discourse surrounding the Manchurian pneumonic plague crisis of 1911 lay not in the realization that a disease might be catching (*ranbing*), but in the construction of a whole new etiological disease category (infectious disease, or *chuanranbing*). Since an infectious disease was defined as one transmitted by a miscroscopic pathogen, this disease category depended upon germ theory. Moreover, this new category drew a sharp distinction between acute and chronic disorders, something more blurred in classical medical teachings.

However, the resilience of the learned medical traditions of etiology based on constitutions and environments shows in the way both TCM experts and citizens of China responded to the SARS crisis. Lei tells us that in Manchuria in 1912, physicians trained in classical medical doctrines died treating plague victims because they refused to accept germ theory—much less the innovative model of respiratory transmission promoted by Wu Lien-teh (Wu Liande), the bio-medically trained doctor in charge of public health measures. But Hanson shows that in Guangzhou in 2003, TCM herbal formulas were widely used both as prophylaxis by the general public and in hospital treatment of victims. Bypassing the issue of contagion or infection and sticking to their perennial criticism of germ theory as reductionistic, TCM physicians claimed familiarity with SARS as a recognizable kind of southeastern regional disease outbreak, following the pattern of Warm disease disorder—a purely indigenous nineteenth-century revision of Cold Damage disease doctrine. In hospital treatment in Guangzhou, the TCM physicians used established formulas that targeted each of the four stages of progress of disease as defined by Warm disease doctrine—without, however, rejecting the practices of isolating patients or aseptic management of the hospital environment. The Manchurian plague experience may have empowered bio-medical critics of Chinese medicine to an unprecedented extent, but over the long term, supporters of Chinese medicine took refuge in the view that plague was a new and uniquely deadly disease not seen before in China. A century later TCM came out of the SARS experience with its credibility intact, confirming its current partnership with biomedicine in the PRC's unique state-supported system of integrated Chinese and Western medicine (*Zhong xi yi jiehe*).

In Yu's fascinating chapter, we learn that a clean street in a Jiangnan city between the sixteenth and nineteenth centuries depended upon the commoditization of night soil, in which urban excrement was gathered and sold to farmers for fertilizer. In this environment a household's latrine was a source of profit, and a network of dung gatherers (at the bottom), neighborhood night soil contractors (in the middle), and boatmen plying the waters between cities and countryside maintained a trade that was understood as supporting both urban commerce and agricultural production. Rubbish collection was a supplementary and less smoothly functioning business: a certain amount of waste management was organized by local merchants with shops on major commercial streets, and more occasionally it was subsidized as a community service—by official or gentry task forces that undertook particular projects, such as dredging watercourses. Jiangnan elites were aware of the aesthetics involved and often criticized the stench and filth of northern cities—even Beijing, the capital city—compared to their own home region, which was warm and wet enough to support the night soil trade year-round.

When Shanghai opened up as a British-controlled treaty port in 1852, the new foreign concession's Municipal Council adapted this existing system for the territory under its governance. Soon recognizing the economic value of night soil, the Council attempted to make night soil contractors into municipal employees and to use profits from the agricultural trade to make its sanitation department self-supporting. What changed, gradually, was more a conceptual framework than a technological system, as urban sanitation was rationalized in terms of public health, while rules proliferated to foster a modern hygienic aesthetic by curbing odors and confining the labor of collection to nighttime hours. This hybrid local system helped keep groundwater cleaner, and as a result Chinese cities—as well as Japanese ones—were slow to install sewage treatment plants or encourage the use of flush toilets. The benefits to agriculture remained, although the costs of new sanitary workers, equipment, and surveillance meant that for the ultimate consumer, the peasant, fertilizer costs went up.

After the crisis of the Sino-Japanese war in 1894–95, Chinese nationalist elites broadened their horizons beyond Shanghai-style urban order to look to Japan as a model. As city after city in China established municipal sanitation services in the last fifteen years of Qing rule, Japanese-style hygiene police, supervised by public security forces, ushered in regimes of hygienic modernity that were both nationalist and colonial. Nonetheless, the substrata of older patterns of urban organization remain visible, if only historians know how to look for them.

Colonial Health and Hygiene

The question of whether China became a Western colony after the opium wars of the 1840s and 1850s is still debated. Some scholars see the coastal treaty ports, the military incursions that created them, and the institutional and cultural innovations they stimulated as the key to understanding China's path to modernity.[12] Others, perhaps a larger number, focus on the much broader urban and rural heartlands of China, and the agency of reformist elites and regional and central governments in defending Chinese sovereignty and instigating nationalist revolution. Mao Zedong's famous formula describing his struggling nation—"semifeudal, semicolonial"—remains relevant, calling attention to the limited geographical range of the coastal treaty ports and the foreign-controlled railway lines that branched out from them, as well as to the vast countryside beyond, where the majority of the population lived.

This semicolonial world of the British-dominated treaty ports is evoked in the chapter by Shang-Jen Li here, but also by the work of Yu Xinzhong in the previous section. Among the treaty ports, Shanghai particularly was a laboratory for new urban systems of control, surveillance, and aesthetics. British missionaries, merchants, and diplomats represented China as a tropical environment debilitating to Western residents, and the privileged European powers pushed for action against epidemic diseases that threatened their own citizens' well-being and, by extension, that of the native Chinese. Li's chapter shows how British residents rationalized food preferences brought from home as they dealt with the anxieties of expatriate life—invoking familiar themes of mid-nineteenth-century discourse on tropical medicine about the health effects of climates, constitutions, races, and civilizations. Yu shows how the Shanghai International Settlement became a symbol of hygienic modernity, even as its infant bureaucracies built upon traditional patterns of sanitary management based on the economics of night soil.

But the chapters by Rogaski and Wu in this section, and the one by Lin and Liu in the third section of the volume, shift the focus to imperial Japan. Beginning in 1874, Meiji Japan adopted Western medicine, especially as practiced in Germany, as the basis for its reformed medical system. Biomedical laboratory research by European-trained Japanese scientists advanced quickly, led by the Institute of Infectious Diseases (Denzenbyō Kenkyusho, later incorporated into Tokyo University), established by Kitasato Shibasaburo in the tradition of the germ theory of Robert Koch, his teacher. According to the Japanese scholar Iijima Wataru, imperial expansion shaped research agendas even before the First World War. In the 1920s, after the creation of the Greater East Asia Co-Prosperity Sphere (*Dai-tō-a Kyōeikenhe*), the study of southern medicine (*nanho igaku*) was developed for tropical areas and expansion medicine (*kaitogu igaku*) for temperate continental regions.[13] Both the research on tropical parasites in the tradition of southern medicine and the exploration of northern endemics in expansion medicine were closely linked to local public health reforms in various Japanese colonies, including Taiwan and Manchuria.

Iijima implies that the most sophisticated modern medical researchers who studied or worked with Kitasato Shibasaburo focused their energies on Japan's colonies partly because the epidemiological management of the Japanese home islands was controlled by a rival organization (the Tokyo Medical School). But from a more global perspective, we can see how these Japanese medical researchers, like British colonial scientists, used their nation's colonies as field laboratories for research controlled from the metropolitan center. Expansion medicine was about fostering Japanese settlements in Manchuria, and so focused on understanding how Japanese might best adapt to the Manchurian environment, but—as Rogaski shows—the perception of that environment as a wilderness made the researchers see the local people who were the objects of rural hygiene projects as primitive creatures at one with the natural environment.

Yet from the point of view of Japanese relations with the West, we can also see the asymmetrical character of Japanese scientific networks exemplified by Kitasato. His contributions to the Koch laboratory were unremarked in Europe,[14] but they built his position as a leader in Tokyo, so that he embodied the diagnostic achievements of germ theory when sent to Hong Kong to fight the plague epidemic of 1894–95 there. In this way, beginning in the 1890s, Japanese-controlled regions on the periphery of the East Asian continental heartland—Taiwan and Manchuria—became laboratories where new hygienic practices were introduced to Chinese people. The Meiji government, from 1868 onward committed to westernization of the Japanese archipelago, brought the zeal of a convert and the autocratic impulses of a self-confident paternalism to its agenda for creating a model modern empire able to rival and even surpass those of the Western powers. The chapters in this volume on the Taiwanese case show how the blueprints originating in Bismarckian Germany prompted reforms implemented in Japan, which were then adapted for Taiwan, the planned model Japanese colony. In contrast to the looser strategies of indirect rule practiced by the British in the vast Indian subcontinent, Japanese governance of Taiwan achieved a penetration of local society possibly unequaled anywhere else in the colonial world.

The chapters here on Japanese malaria control and on the reform of midwifery in Taiwan are both framed by this fine grid of Japanese governmental supervision. A key institution was the imported Japanese sanitary police, responsible for both the island-wide household registration system that included records of all births, and the enforcement of sanitary regulations in the villages—which contributed to the multi-pronged strategy for the control of malaria analyzed here by Lin and Liu. Initiated in 1905, even before state-mandated collection of population statistics in Japan itself, this household registration system is praised today by historical demographers as one of the most thorough in the world for its time.[15] Further, as colonial educational institutions spread, locally trained physicians and other health professionals found career opportunities in clinical and research medical science—so successfully that modern medical doctors came to constitute a significant proportion of the island's educated elite.[16] The antimalaria drive described by Lin and Liu was just one example of a colonial policy of sanitary reform, education, and surveillance that reached a large proportion of an apparently compliant population.

By comparison, in Manchuria, Japanese rule was always in the hands of the military, though indirect before 1932 and after 1937 overwhelmed by the Sino-Japanese and the world wars. In Rogaski's chapter here, hygienic modernity came first of all in the form of scientific investigation. The vast land of Manchuria, imagined as a still-untamed frontier, was a laboratory for Japan's modern scientists from many disciplines: archaeology, linguistics, and anthropology, as well as the expansion medicine discussed above. However, although the military-run South Manchurian Railway Company's civilian research arm produced remarkable scholarship, Rogaski shows that the legacy of Japanese scientific medicine in Manchuria has been symbolized by the notorious hospital of Military Medical Unit 731, dedicated to biological warfare—where lethal wartime experiments on human subjects were conducted. In Manchuria colonial policies of hygienic modernity have come to be remembered in the context of a violent military occupation. Modern nationalist ideology and anti-Japanese passion still dominate PRC discourse about today's three northeastern provinces (i.e., Manchuria) during the first half of the twentieth century. Indeed, Rogaski shows that local Chinese responses to coercive Japanese vaccination campaigns to control plague and other epidemic diseases fit patterns recorded in other colonial settings like India: distrust, panic, and rumors about the colonizers' supposedly malevolent intent.[17] At the same time, she blurs the distinction between colonizer and colonized by showing us that in the two decades of semi-colonial rule before 1932, Chinese biomedically trained experts, including Wu Lien-teh's ongoing plague prevention organization, were partners with Japanese scientists in Manchuria, embracing common strategies and goals.

In the study of colonial medicine in India, centered on the British Empire, public health was first analyzed in terms of state projects of surveillance and control, animated by imperial ideologies of race, gender, and civilization. Since the cultural turn of the 1970s and 1980s, the emphasis has shifted to the theme of the subjectivity of the colonized "other." The achievement of the subaltern studies movement among South Asianists from the Indian subcontinent was to go beyond a straightforward rhetoric of nationalist resistance and empowerment and probe the complex identity formations produced by the fact that, for English-speaking and educated South Asians, the categories and languages of analysis for understanding modernity were themselves a product of colonialism.

The chapters here on the Taiwan case reveal the contours of the Japanese state's colonial project, but do not connect either accommodation (in the case of malaria eradication) or resistance (of birthing women) with anti-colonial politics or nationalist identity formation. Their work pretty much bypasses subaltern studies models of interpretation altogether. The ambivalence—the benevolence and promise as well as the coercion and submission—entailed by Japanese-mandated hygienic modernity do emerge from the Taiwan materials. Lin and Liu give the colonial medical project of the first half of the twentieth century credit for laying the groundwork for its postcolonial sequel in the Republic of China in the 1950s and 1960s, under the auspices of the American sponsored and funded World Health Organization (WHO). When the island was declared free of malaria in 1965, it was a story of genuine medical progress in the eyes of the Taiwanese people, who had by and large complied with public health interventions from a variety of regimes over the years. In Lin and Liu's retrospective, the focus is on the nexus of power and politics that guided the choice of anti-malarial strategies in both colonial and postcolonial settings—a nexus that in their analysis involved issues of cost, available technologies, administrative infrastructure, and current scientific understandings. Public health emerges not as a primary site of either colonial or postcolonial state building, but as a local instantiation of more globally diffused health policy projects.

It is interesting that in this volume the most detailed narrative of local resistance to the Japanese project of hygienic modernity comes from a study of women's health. Although Japanese policy on Taiwan aimed to reform midwifery along the Meiji model, Wu found and interviewed elderly survivors of female networks that were relatively indifferent to propaganda for scientific childbirth. In dismantling the Japanese version of a widespread colonial stereotype of ignorant mothers and unhygienic native midwives,[18] Wu argues for the medical rationality of some established lay obstetrical practices, like the use of alum and sesame oil to dress the umbilical cord, and also for the receptivity of midwives to simple aseptic measures, like sterilizing scissors or knives with boiling water. She suggests that the modest gains in infant survival under Japanese colonialism owed more to the improvement of public sanitation in the cities than to scientific health education of mothers or midwives. And her main conclusion is that female social networks determined women's choices of attendants at their home births, while, ironically, biomedical teachings about childbirth increased women's perception of risk. Thus we are left not with a colonized identity or a derivative discourse of modernity, but with women whose comfort with their purely local traditions of obstetrics was based on gender, class, and kinship solidarities and connected to a shared belief that childbirth is natural and normal.

In writing about colonial medicine and public health in Taiwan, these scholars bypass themes of colonial identity to return the reader to the science itself and the complex social and technical systems through which it operates. Their work suggests that in Taiwan neither medical tradition nor medical science was mobilized by the local population to serve anticolonial ends. To be trained as a modern midwife, or as a doctor supporting research and clinical work on malaria, was a route to a modern professional identity, valued for its social prestige and its humanistic aura independent of politics. These authors write about the colonial medicine of Taiwan as social scientists and historians whose critical perspectives are directed at the politics and culture of public health policies and campaigns themselves.

Recently some scholars have questioned the usefulness of the very category of colonial medicine. With particular reference to the experience of the British Empire, they point to the fact that in India the overwhelming majority of modern medical specialists and providers were local people, including many operating outside formal colonial bureaucratic institutions; and they reject cultural theories of hegemonic discourse propounded by the largely South Asian proponents of subaltern studies. Japanese hygienic modernity in Taiwan may be a better case study for such an interpretation: policies of assimilation and "Japanization" contrast with British colonial policies that maintained caste-like hierarchies of race.[19] Japanese policies in Taiwan achieved a consensus supporting public health as a social good shared by colonized and colonizers alike—argued for by the fact that after the early 1920s travel between the island and the Japanese mainland was unrestricted, on the ground that both populations could be considered "healthy."[20]

Beyond the issue of comparative colonialisms, medical history itself may be better understood when we frame the colonial in a larger historical trajectory. Looked at over the history of the twentieth century, legitimating ideologies of modern medical science must be imagined as plural, given the power of indigenous, traditional health practices to continue to be embedded in people's daily life. In addition, for the colonized in Taiwan, a career as a medical scientist provided an attractive modern identity, even though the cultural resources for such a path were not evenly distributed across the island landscape. Chinese people's attachment to indigenous practices and beliefs, and their aspirations to participate in a global culture of modern science, took a specific local color in colonial situations, but they both survived the colonial era and continue to interact today.

Campaigns for Epidemic Control

Chapters in the present volume deal with four case studies of public health campaigns in Chinese East Asia: against plague in Manchuria (1911–12), malaria in Taiwan (from 1910 into the 1980s), schistosomiasis in the lower Yangzi delta (1948–58), and SARS in South China, Taiwan, and Singapore (2003). Three of these four are local responses to diseases that have challenged modern public health systems around the globe. Only one—against malaria—was directed by a colonial regime, and even here Lin and Liu compare and contrast Japanese malaria policies before the Second World War with those of the Republic of China in cooperation with the World Health Organization in the postwar years. Two—against plague and schistosomiasis—were sponsored by Chinese governments that saw success as critical to the popular legitimacy, national sovereignty, and international prestige of their respective regimes. Two—against plague and SARS—were manifestations of a global health crisis that mobilized international organizations as well as individual states.

Looking at all four of these movements together, the issues of colonial medicine are less important than longer-term patterns of public health policymaking and action. One sees common goals and strategies pursued by a variety of East Asian regimes, whether empire or nation, communist or capitalist, democratic or authoritarian. One way to analyze these commonalities is to look for an international style of public health campaigns that emerges in the twentieth century—the age when technologies based on germ theory first became available for widespread use. Such an approach will emphasize the globalizing thrust of modern public health regimes, increasingly underwritten by international organizations dominated by the more powerful global political players. It may also draw upon Foucauldian notions of modern state governmentality, where public health campaigns based on an Enlightenment ideology of health as an entitlement serve to propagate, legitimate, and consolidate power, and eventually to inform the subjectivity of citizens themselves.

These public health movements are marked by coercion and utopianism, a campaign style of politics, the intrusion of the state into private domains ordinarily left alone, and appeals to the authority of science to justify policy. Outsiders may suspect a will to power in public health bureaucracies and their governmental sponsors, whose actions in public health emergencies legitimizes state power in other dimensions of national life. Workers within public health bureaucracies are more likely to see themselves as be-leaguered humanitarian professionals, probably underfunded and certainly constrained by politically driven policymakers as well as ignorant or pan-icky citizens. When they dealt with emergencies, more than in their every-day work of disease prevention and health education, public health pro-fessionals captured public attention with militant rhetoric, metaphors of battle, and utopian promises of a disease-free future.

However, each of these four public health movements had its local his-torical context and style of implementation, and commonalities were not evenly distributed among them. The campaign against pneumonic plague in late Qing Manchuria was a pioneering one, and beyond the goal of saving lives was a desire to demonstrate the hitherto underappreciated power of Western medicine against the claims of the indigenous Chinese medical establishment. This demonstration effect was important for the Qing state's newly fledged nationalist credentials in the spotlight of critical interna-tional scrutiny—and threatened action—by the dominant European powers and Japan. As a campaign reflecting on China's national reputation and prestige, the fight against plague in Manchuria most closely resembles the antischistosomiasis campaign in the People's Republic in the 1950s. As a response to a potentially borderless global health emergency, it bears com-parison with the fight against SARS almost exactly one hundred years later. In the case of SARS, what is striking is the greater reach of WHO as an inter-national organization operating outside the direct sphere of the nation-state system. In 2003 it was more difficult, if not impossible, for any of the various Chinas of the Nanyang region to make nationalist claims about the success-ful resolution of the crisis.

The PRC's battle against schistosomiasis and the Japanese colonial anti-malaria campaigns were directed against debilitating chronic diseases rather than acute epidemics. Both involved labor-intensive mobilizations at the grass-roots level. But although the Japanese network of community health stations and the Communist Party's leadership of peasant villagers were both shaped by cost considerations, and both reached rural popula-tions, the Maoist campaign was the self-consciously populist one, its politi-cal agenda more trumpeted and its paternalism more disguised.

A striking contrast is the incremental pragmatism of the Japanese orga-nization—with its emphasis on both prevention and cure, mosquito control and treatment of sufferers from the disease—and the PRC's radical goal of eradication and its mass campaign style of action. Maoist propaganda rhetorically evoked images of an acute epidemic, comparing snail eradication to the control of plague rats, and evoking the traditional community ritual of "bidding farewell to the plague god" in Warm disease (*wenyi*) outbreaks. Neither biomedical nor TCM doctors would have agreed with this reclassification of the chronic disorder of schistosomiasis as an epidemic emergency.

Ironically, in its utopian aspirations and its ability to mobilize large populations for its realization, the Maoist schistosomiasis campaign is more comparable not with Japanese antimalaria strategies, but with the postcolonial American-inspired war on Taiwan's malaria-carrying mosquitoes with islandwide DDT sprayings. We are accustomed to think of the manufactured emergencies of the 1950s public health campaigns in mainland China as the product of a uniquely Maoist campaign style of politics. However, looking at them side by side with a Taiwanese campaign encouraged by highly respected international aid groups and the UN health establishment invites critical reflections on global patterns of public health projects in the age of germ theory. Public health movements involve political and social mobilizations; policy always involves choices; and the human fears and hopes aroused by health and disease become a resource that both constrains and legitimizes drastic action.

With malaria, Lin and Liu offer a historical perspective; with SARS, Tseng and Wu offer a contemporary one on public health campaigns. Both chapters call for awareness that, even in the hands of experts, public health policies are driven by judgments that are partially subjective. This is true whether the actors are agents of a colonial power making decisions affecting the colonized inferior, or agents of a democratic government forced to decide how far personal freedoms may be repressed for the collective good. With hindsight, both Li Yushang and Lin and Liu point to the negative side effects of these campaigns and, along with their very real successes, to their long-term failure to attain their sweeping goals. The authors show that politically strategic decision making, the labeling of "side effects," and the paradoxes of unintended consequences are central to a critical history of public health regimes. Historical perspectives on SARS also encourage us to consider this paradox: SARS found public health professionals operating in a moral economy of risk, in which people claimed the right to safety; while in spite of the high-tech, twenty-first-century speed of expert analysis and decision making about the epidemic, medicine had to fall back on one of the oldest and crudest of control measures, quarantine.

But public health is not just about epidemic crises. The vast majority of twentieth-century public health bureaucracies were engaged in the mundane activities of education, prevention, and monitoring. In passing, our essayists illustrate this fact with their discussions of childbirth education and marsh drainage in Taiwan, the enforcement of sanitary ordinances concerning night soil in Shanghai, and vaccination drives in Manchuria. But it is the campaigns—mobilizations in response to acute emergencies—that capture public attention. The media give such cases more attention, and scholarship follows suit. Successful interventions such as occurred in the plague and SARS outbreaks discussed here have been the best public testimony for the potential of public health, and the most compelling legitimizers of its power. In cases of chronic disease, it has been far more difficult to claim that public health interventions—rather than long-term, less-well-understood changes in society, economy, and technology—have been responsible for improvements in people's well-being. As scholars, we need to be critically aware of our participation in this image of public health as driven by crisis, of its special twentieth-century relevance in the age of germ theory, and of the interests served by such an image.

For finally, it is on the daily level that hygienic modernity has penetrated most deeply in Chinese East Asia. This may not have supplied enough ideological traction to ensure an orderly response to an epidemic crisis like SARS (here Tseng and Wu contrast Singapore's discipline with Taipei's confusion and Beijing's cover-up). However, the chapters in this volume have traced some of the paths by which the more quotidian disciplines of public health have over the course of the twentieth century become part of Chinese normality. However locally inflected, such disciplines have gained much of their authority from their global circulation.

NOTES

1. The series Science and Civilisation in China began publication in 1954, and has continued since Needham's death in 1995. Originally planned as seven volumes, the series has ballooned to 22 separate published titles to date, with five more pending. See http://www.nri.org.uk/science.html.

2. This term, popularized by Hu Shi, was used to characterize the intellectual and social reform movements of the years immediately after the overthrow of the imperial system, roughly 1915–27.

3. A good overview is Arnold, *Science, Technology and Medicine in Colonial India*, part of *The New Cambridge History of India*.

4. Sen, "The Character of the Introduction of Western Science in India during the Eighteenth and the Nineteenth Centuries," in Habib and Raina, eds., *Social History of Science in Colonial India*, 69–82. See also Kumar, *Science and the Raj*, 212, 225–26.

5. See Harrison, *Public Health in British India*, 228–34. See also Arnold, *Science, Technology and Medicine in Colonial India*.

6. For an overview, see Raina, *Images and Contexts*. Indian engagements with Joseph Needham and the so-called Needham question about the nondevelopment of science in Asia are discussed in Habib and Raina, eds., *Situating the History of Science*.

7. The landmark study here is Chatterjee's 1986 book, *Nationalist Thought and the Colonial World*.

8. Kumar, *Science and the Raj*, 226.

9. This has been argued by Elman in *On Their Own Terms* and in *A Cultural History of Modern Science in China*.

10. Rogaski, *Hygienic Modernity*.

11. Andrews, "Tuberculosis and the Assimilation of Germ Theory in China, 1895–1937."

12. For recent articulations of this position, see Hevia, *English Lessons*, and L. Liu, *The Clash of Empires*.

13. Iijima, "Infectious and Parasitic Disease Studies in Taiwan, Manchuria and Korea under the Japanese Empire."

14. For Kitasato's career in Europe and his failure to be nominated for a Nobel Prize, see Bartholomew, "Japanese Nobel Candidates in the First Half of the Twentieth Century," 243–53.

15. Yang and Hsieh, "Infant Mortality in Colonial Taiwan 1905-1945."

16. See Lo, *Doctors within Borders*, 90–94, 117–31.

17. See Arnold, *Colonizing the Body*, 141–44, 211–26.

18. For efforts to reform midwifery in British India, see Arnold, *Science, Technology, and Medicine in Colonial India*, 89–91.

19. Kumar, *Science and the Raj*, 222–27, 231–36.

20. Lo, *Doctors within Borders*, 95–96.

Part I

Tradition and Transition

The Evolution of the Idea of
Chuanran Contagion in Imperial China

Angela Ki Che Leung

During the last years of Qing imperial rule, when Western medicine and notions of public health were being introduced in China, intellectuals and the political elite tended to accuse Chinese society of ignorance about proper behavior related to the avoidance of diseases. Such accusations usually became particularly severe during epidemics. The ordinary Chinese were typically blamed for being superstitious, filthy, and ignorant of germs and of the danger of the spread of diseases—in other words, totally lacking basic scientific knowledge of health and hygiene.

An article from February 14, 1911, in *Dagong Bao*, a major newspaper published in Tianjin, compared the Chinese people, oblivious as they were to the great danger of the epidemic of pneumonic plague devastating Manchuria, to ignorant children playing around a well, unaware of their imminent danger of falling in. In his contribution to this volume, Sean Hsiang-lin Lei draws our attention to an important remark in the same year by Xi Liang (1853–1917), governor general of the region: "In the beginning [of the outbreak], our bureaucrats, local gentry, and medical practitioners did not believe that epidemics [*yi*] could spread by contagion [*chuanran*]."[1]

The above two public remarks suggest that Chinese identified the plague as a manifestation of the indigenous medical category of *yi* or *wenyi* (epidemics), which was not contagious. This consensus reflected long-standing orthodox medical teachings about febrile diseases. The oldest umbrella category for these conditions was *shanghan* (Cold Damage). Built into *shanghan* doctrine were configurationist assumptions that outbreaks affecting many people at the same time were triggered by something in the environment: unseasonable weather, perhaps, or malign local *qi* (breath, energy). Epidemics were simply extreme variants of this pattern.

Elite writers noticed that the pneumonic plague epidemic in Manchuria—a consequence of increasing global traffic—was totally new to the Chinese.[2] Moreover, for the Chinese authors, this newness seemed to explain popular ignorance. Nevertheless, this does not mean that the idea that some diseases could spread by contagion (*chuanran*) was unknown in China before 1900.

For a Chinese person before 1900, what exactly did it mean for a disease to involve *chuanran*? In the twentieth century, the term quickly became the standard translation for the biomedical notion of "contagion" as "the communication of disease from one person to another by bodily contact."[3] But *chuanran* was actually an old word, used as early as the tenth century to express complex and ambiguous concepts about the spread of disease from person to person. Its root *ran*—literally, to dye—is part of ancient compound words (i.e., words made up of two or more characters) that convey notions such as transmission, infection, or even contagion. However, it is unlikely that a Chinese in the first years of the twentieth century talking about *chuanran* had in mind our biomedically inflected concept of a disease transmitted from person to person via a microscopic organism. Older ideas of *chuanran* specific to the Chinese context may have escaped our notice because today we take this modern meaning for granted. Such attitudes reveal the particular Chinese conceptualization of the *chuanran* (literally, transmission by dyeing) mode of the spread of diseases before the language of Western biomedicine came to dominate Chinese public discourse later on in the twentieth century.

The purpose of this essay, therefore, is not to study the history of the concept of contagion as defined by Western biomedicine in traditional Chinese society, but to trace the evolution of the term *chuanran* and its changing meanings, in comparison with other terms with the root *ran*. By so doing, we hope to gain a better understanding of the traditional Chinese idea of the communicability of diseases, indispensable for our assessment of the reception in China of the modern Western idea of contagion.

Contagion versus Chuanran

Even in Europe, contagion as the transmission of diseases from person to person is a modern notion. It is generally agreed that there was no clear idea of contagion by contact up to the Middle Ages.[4] Some historians believe that the Western idea of diseases' being communicable from one person to another came from Arabic medicine in the twelfth century and was largely related to nonepidemic diseases.[5] As late as the sixteenth century, when Girolamo Fracastoro published an important book on contagion, in which he further developed the idea of "seeds" of contagion, the mechanism and channels of contagion remained ambiguous.[6] Ambiguities about contagion continued well into the nineteenth century. As Margaret Pelling has convincingly emphasized, the modern idea of contagion inherited a story involving "striking contrast, between the germ theorists, and the sanitarians who were miasmatists and believed that smells caused diseases . . . The concepts of contagion, infection and miasma accumulated layers of connotation over time, and effectively became not single concepts but many."[7] The contrast has been largely simplified in modern literature on the history of medical thought.

Pelling points out, for example, that it is too simplistic to say that the idea of contagion was monopolized by the scientifically minded bacteriologists and that the so-called miasmatists were anti-contagionists. In fact, the two groups had some broadly similar ideas about contagion. The transmission of poison by water or air, for instance, was accepted by both, but the miasmatists were unclear on the process by which the poison could travel from the sick to the healthy.[8] For an influential doctor such as Max Josef von Pettenkofer, who was not a germ theorist, cholera and typhoid did not spread directly from one individual to another, but by water and air infected by germs that had become toxic in the soil after leaving the bodies of the sick.[9] Therefore the similarities and differences between the miasmatists and bacteriologists on the question of germs and contagion were complex and subtle in the mid-nineteenth century, when Western Europe experienced its first attacks of cholera.

This observation is also shared by François Delaporte in regard to the 1832 cholera epidemic in France.[10] In 1870, a discussion published in the *British and Foreign Medico-Chirurgical Review* on current theories of contagion admitted that "considerable obscurity still surrounds the whole question of the nature, origin and prevention of contagion."[11] Contagion is therefore a difficult concept to trace and clarify before the nineteenth century, even in Western societies. It was the gradual domination of germ theory from the late nineteenth century onward that finally shaped our modern understanding of contagion.

Chuanran, the Chinese term used by Xi Liang and other political and cultural elite writers around the beginning of the twentieth century, was equally ambiguous when used to express the spread of diseases. Between the tenth century and the end of the nineteenth, it was commonly used both as a verb and as a noun, but not as an adjective. It was used interchangeably with other terms with the root *ran*—such as *xiangran* (mutual dyeing), *ranyi* (exchange by dyeing), and *ganran* (affect by dyeing)—to express the spread of diseases during epidemics as well as the transmission of nonepidemic diseases. This illustrates the complexity and flexibility of the idea contained in the character *ran*. By the late imperial period, *chuanran* was clearly the most popular term to express the idea of the spread of diseases, including notions of contagion and infection.

Ran is a very old Chinese word, its first known meaning being to dye, implying tainting, staining, or changing color. It is interesting to note that the English word "infection" also originates from a root meaning "to put or dip into something," "leading to *inficere* and *infectio*, staining or dyeing." The same is true also of the nouns "contagion" and "miasma," "which derives from the Greek verb *miaino*, a counterpart to the Latin *inficere*. Impurity is therefore a basic element in all three concepts."[12] Similarly, the first Chinese concepts for the spread of diseases were also derived from the idea of tainting or dyeing, implying the polluting of an originally pure object after it comes into contact with a polluting source. The process of *ran* could also imply an implicit transformation of the nature of the polluted object after prolonged contact with the contaminating source.

Early Connotations of Ran

As already pointed out by Barbara Volkmar, *ran* is the key Chinese term related to the concept of the communication of diseases.[13] Today Chinese still use *ran* as a verb to describe catching a disease: *ranbing* literally means to become tainted with a disease. This term implies two processes—namely, a healthy person's coming into contact with a polluting source, and the subsequent corruption of the originally healthy body. However, *ran* was initially not used in any medical context. It should therefore be useful if we first trace the use of the word in ancient Chinese, for a better appreciation of the original use of *ran* as an expression of contamination.

Dyeing was an important undertaking in ancient China, especially the dyeing of raw white silk into different colors, a task that was entrusted only to specialists in the Western Zhou court (roughly the eleventh to eighth centuries BCE).[14] Later on, *ran*, always in the form of a verb, was used metaphorically, meaning to contaminate, especially in the context of bad customs and mores. The *Shang shu* (meaning "book of history," compiled around the fourth century BCE) already used *ran* to mean the corrupting of customs by external influence.[15] Such a usage was fairly common in ancient texts, mostly in the negative sense, but sometimes in the neutral or even positive sense, meaning customs were or could be *ran* (changed or improved) by external influences.[16] This usage of *ran* became very common in ancient classics and historical writings, often in combination with *jian* (to immerse): *jianran* literally means to take up new color after prolonged immersion. According to the philosopher Mozi, this process caused a "change in the nature" of a person.[17]

One of the first appearances of *ran* in the sense of disease spreading appears in the *San guo zhi* (History of the three kingdoms) from the third century CE. In the extreme south of China, where "water and earth" were saturated with "poisonous qi," soldiers and ordinary people traveling in and out of the region would "certainly develop illnesses and contaminate each other" (*zhuan xiang wu ran*).[18] The spread of disease is here linked to the concept of ubiquitous poisonous air and the large number of people exposed to such environmental influences. A similar term also appears in the *Zhouhou beiji fang* (Handy recipes for urgent uses), a famous contemporaneous medical text by Ge Hong (283–343). In this text, a dozen recipes, many of which are more ritual than herbal, are said to be effective in stopping *wenbing* (Warm Disease—that is, illnesses that are caught in the cold season but that develop only during the warm season), so that patients with such conditions would not *xiangran zhuo* (contaminate and affect each other). Judging from the fact that these recipes treated not only the patients themselves, but also members of the household and even the residence, we might conjecture that the idea of the spread of disease was linked essentially with contaminated bad air within the area of the household. The word *zhuo* is of particular interest here, as it emphasizes the effect of "being affected," implying some fundamental change in the healthy body after the tainting process. *Zhuo* would later on be used rather frequently with *ran* (*ranzhuo*) to express a serious case of disease-causing contamination.[19]

It is important to emphasize that phrases containing *ran* to convey the spread of disease did not appear in the earliest medical classics. Indeed, those works were mostly concerned with the cosmic relations between the individual body and the environment. Discussions on the body as a vehicle for disease transmission appear in the literature only after the third century CE.

In the following paragraphs, I attempt to show that there is a historical development of the terms incorporating *ran* toward more specific modes of disease transmission after their first appearance. I would, first of all, suggest the following chronology: The idea of the spread of disease by contamination emerged around the third century CE, evidenced by the fact that the first terms containing *ran* in this sense are found in this period. The idea began as a vague and complex notion. Its content became richer by the seventh century, when the major modes of disease transmission were described and more or less fixed. From the tenth century on, and particularly after the twelfth century, with the emergence and popularization of the term *chuanran*, contamination by personal contact with the sick gained increasing attention. This concept of transmission was developed fully and in more concrete terms in the late imperial period. I would like to begin this discussion with Chao Yuanfang's classic, *Zhubing yuan hou lun* (On the origins and symptoms of all diseases), an important text compiled in 610 CE, in which the basic modes of disease transmission were described in detail.[20]

Modes of Disease Transmission from the Seventh to the Twelfth Centuries

Chao Yuanfang's classic provides the fullest account of the main modes of disease transmission within the specific social and religious context of the early seventh century. We can distinguish three major modes of transmission that were expressed by terms containing *ran* and also *yi* (exchange) in this important text.

Transmission by Contamination and Switching (Answering Question 1015)

First, we find *jianran* (dye by immersion; also in the reverse order as *ranjian*). This term already occurs in ancient nonmedical texts to express the notion that prolonged contact with a polluting source provoked a change in the nature of a person. By contrast, Chao used the term to describe contamination within the body. Several disorders were characterized by the gradual growth of diseased parts inside the body that finally affected surrounding healthy parts, leading to more serious and distinct pathological conditions. The disorder called *zheng*, for instance, was initially caused by depletion of the viscera and bowels, leading to indigestion. The internal congestion "after prolonged and deep imbuing" later on coagulated into a solid and immovable block, finally turning into a *zheng* (concretion). Another example is excessive skin or a polyp growing on the eye, which was explained as the result of "prolonged tainting and immersion" of the corner of the eye with hot *qi* rising from the Liver. The symptom of "great heat" (*zhuangre*) in children was explained by conflicting cold and hot *qi* inside the intestines and stomach that "emerge after prolonged tainting and immersion."[21]

One can conjecture from these cases that *jianran* in such disorders referred to contamination of the healthy parts of the body by an originally smaller, sick part that had developed a pathology, after a period of "immersion." In a way, *jianran* is comparable to what we now understand as infection—that is, a kind of internal contamination causing a fundamental deterioration of the concerned body part, showing symptoms different from the original malaise.[22] The original disorder thus underwent a radical transformation after prolonged imbuing and became something quite different and more serious for the patient.

The second mode of *ran* as disease transmission discussed in Chao's text is expressed by the term *xiangran* (mutual contamination) or its variations, such as *zhuan xiangran yi* and *xiangran yi*. *Xiangran* was perhaps the most frequently used term for contamination in the medieval period—meaning, mostly, contamination by sickly *qi* that existed in a specific locality or was generated by patients. Most of the time, the term referred to tainting by bad, pathogenic *qi* in the atmosphere. Chao specifically saw unseasonable (*shi*) or perverse (*guaili*) *qi* as causing illnesses that would "contaminate and exchange [hosts]" (*xiangran yi*).[23] Warm Diseases (*wenbing*) would also emit a pathogenic *qi* (*bingqi*) that would shift, contaminate, and exchange hosts, in a two-stage process: annihilating first the entire family (*miemen*), and then outsiders.[24] Unlike the *shanghan* (Cold Damage) disorders caused by cold and discussed by Zhang Ji during the Han dynasty,[25] warm diseases and disorders caused by unseasonable *qi* would "affect by dyeing/contaminating" (*ranzhuo*)[26] and were thus more dangerous. Similar observations were also made by other major doctors of the period, such as Sun Simiao.[27] The key polluting element involved in the *xiangran* mode of transmission was the pathogenic *qi* that affected people under its influence. The presence of such *qi* was a necessary condition for the secondary person-to-person transmission that affected first family members and then outsiders.

The third mode—expressed by the terms *ranyi* (exchange by dyeing), *zhuyi* (exchange by pouring), and their variations—involved the specific

transmission of disorders directly from one person to another. Chao Yuanfang was one of the first medical authors to articulate the ancient idea of *zhu*
(outpouring, pouring) fully in medical terms.[28] Chao defined *zhu* as follows:
"Zhu [pouring] . . . implied [first] the *zhu* [stationing] of an illness [inside
the patient] that will be [later on] poured and exchanged [*zhuyi*] to a person close by after the patient's death."[29] One of the main pathogens believed
to be transmitted in this way was the one that caused consumption (*lao* or
zhai).

In the eighth century, the medical author Wang Tao described consumption suffered by children, called *gan* (infantile depletion) or sometimes *wugu*
(innocence), as a kind of *chuanshi* (corpse transmission), meaning a disorder caused by an outpouring of pathogens emerging from corpses: "Infants and children who suffer from *chuanzhu* [outpour transmission] [of
this disorder] are many."[30]

Among the several types of *zhu* disorders described by Chao, it would
be interesting to single out the magical transmission of *gu* (bug toxin) that
entered the body of the cursed patient with the ultimate intention of killing
him or her. After the death of the victim, the pathogen, called a *chong* (bug),
would pour into a nearby person and "contaminate and affect" (*ranzhuo*)
him or her.[31] This case deserves special attention as it implies the existence
of vicious bugs inside the body of the affected person. These ancient religious or magical connotations remained a prominent feature of *zhu* as described in medieval medical classics.[32]

A significant development in the seventh century in the medical ideas of
disease transmission was the new usage of the word *chuan*, the classic mode
of transference of a pathogen within a body.[33] *Chuan* was now used to describe the flowing of a pathogen from one body, dead or sick, to another,
healthy body, as in the above-mentioned *chuanshi* or in *fulian*, which described the flow of the (originally) static pathogen in sequence, as a result
of which a series of victims, usually from the same lineage, were killed by
the same pathogen as it flowed from one body to another.[34] This process did
not involve tainting or corruption after prolonged contact with a polluting
source. The word *chuan*, when combined with *zhu* (*chuanzhu*, meaning outpouring transmission) or *shi* (*chuanshi*, meaning corpse transmission), obtained this new meaning of the transmission of a pathogen from one body to
another. The influence of Buddhist and Daoist ideas of shared guilt or collective responsibility of the lineage on the medical expression of transmission
was marked in this period.[35]

Chao Yuanfang discussed another new medical idea related to *zhu*: If a weak person lived close in space to a patient with *zhu* disease, the *qi* would flow and shift, and the previously healthy person would contract the illness by "contamination and exchange" (*ranyi*) even when the latter was still alive. The fact that such an outpouring, called *sheng zhu* (*zhu* of the living) involved a process of contamination by a living patient further clarified the subtle difference that still existed between *chuan* transmission and *ran* (dyeing or contamination): The *zhu* transmission of the same disorder from one living body to another was essentially a *ran* process, in which contact between the two bodies caused contamination or some radical change in the originally healthy body. However, the *zhu* transmission of the same pathogen from a corpse to a living body was a *chuan* process, in which the pathogen simply left the dead body and traveled into another living body. Despite this difference, a key point is that the illness thus exchanged in both cases was still identical to the one suffered by the original patient or dead person,[36] while this was not specified in the above cases of *xiangran* (thus implying that the *xiangran* mode of transmission might include the spread of different disorders under the same perverse *qi*). In other words, the idea of the transmission of the same disorder was emphasized in the cases of *zhuyi*, *chuanzhu*, or *chuanshi*.

The descriptions of transmission modes involving *zhu*, *chuan*, and *ran* in Chao's classic show that in the seventh century, lines between *zhu* and *chuan* transmission and *ran* contamination began to blur. One should note particularly the new usage of the term *chuan* to express transmission of diseases from one body to another. This connotation prepares us for its eventual combination with the term *ran* (contamination) to create a new conception of disease spreading from one body to another—namely, *chuanran*.

Moreover, we can detect another characteristic of the *ranyi* or *zhuyi* mode of disease spreading: it sometimes involved a contaminating agent. One example in Chao's text is found in his discussion of the transmission of bad body smell (*huchou*; literally, a bad smell like that of a wild fox). According to Chao, inharmonious blood (*xue*) and *qi* caused a bad smell in the armpit: "This *qi* can contaminate, exchange [hosts], and affect others. Children who have this condition usually contract it from their wet nurses who have it in the first place."[37] In other words, breast milk, as the essence of blood and *qi*, was considered the agent of transmission of this disorder from the wet nurse to the infant. Sun Simiao summarized the two causes of this disorder as follows: "There are those who have this by heavens [*tiansheng*;

i.e., innately] and those who were contaminated [*ran*] by others to become smelly. It is hard to cure the former and easy to cure the latter."[38] The danger of bad milk, as the result of bad blood, would be further developed in the late imperial period.[39]

Finally, a subcategory of the third mode of person-to-person transmission by *yi* (exchange) was explained for the first time in these seventh-century texts—namely, exchange of disorders through sexual intercourse between a man and a woman. The term *yinyang yi* (exchange between *yin* and *yang*) first appeared in the Han classic on Cold Damage disorders, *Shanghan lun*, with descriptions of symptoms without any explanation.[40] Chao Yuanfang was one of the first to give this term a concrete interpretation: if a man or a woman had sexual intercourse before being completely cured of a Cold Damage disorder, Warm Disease, or unseasonable *qi* disorder (i.e., a disorder caused by the environment or weather), the person's sexual partner would fall ill. The reason the mechanism was called exchange was provided by Chao: "When *yin* and *yang* interact, the poison [dormant inside the original patient] will be activated and *duzhuo* [transfer and affect] the other person, like an exchange [*huanyi*]." This exchange occurred only during sexual intercourse between a man and a woman, not between partners of the same sex.[41] Sun also admitted that "the illness of a woman could be 'exchanged' to the man, and that of the man to the woman."[42] According to the *Shanghan lun* and the authors of the Sui and Tang texts, the illness thus exchanged was not similar to the original one and had its own specific symptoms.

Leaving aside the first mode of *jianran* that implied some kind of infection inside an individual body, the other two modes for the spread of diseases expressed by the terms *ran* and *yi* discussed above seem to allow us to draw the following conclusions, even though many points remain ambiguous or inconsistent: First, contamination was most damaging and widespread when there was a noxious *qi* affecting an entire locality. This would in turn provoke mutual contamination among people. Second, the exchange of a disease from an individual to another, not necessarily during an epidemic, was conceptualized in this period as involving two stages: the disorder would first be transferred to family members and then to outsiders. This two-stage transmission was systematic in the person-to-person *zhuyi* or *ranyi* mode and was only occasionally evoked in the *xiangran* mode, where an epidemic was implied. Third, it is unclear whether contamination in the *xiangran* mode caused disorders of the same symptoms, but the essential characteristic of the *zhuyi*, *chuanzhu*, or *chuanshi* mode was that the disorder thus transmitted was the same. Fourth, two specific channels of person-to-person ran contamination were specified in this medieval period: breast-feeding and sexual intercourse. An identical disorder was transmitted through the first channel, whereas the second would generate different disorders.

The Emergence of the Term *Chuanran*

Between the seventh and twelfth centuries, the term *chuanran* appeared both in literary and medical texts to describe the spread of diseases. One of the earliest examples is found in *Ji shen lu* (Records of the deities), by the early Song literatus Xu Xuan (917–92). In chapter three, Xu mentioned that the consumption of a fisherman's daughter was transmitted (*chuanran*) from one person to another, killing several people.[43] In the famous Song collection of occult anecdotes—*Yijian zhi* (Record of Yijian), by Hong Mai (1123–1202)—the family of a woman suffering from consumption avoided her for fear of *chuanran*.[44] A third early example is found in Chen Fu's *Nong shu* (Book on agriculture, ca. 1131–49) in which the author stressed that just as human diseases such as Wind disorders, consumption, and foot disorders could *chuanran*, peasants should keep healthy animals separate from sick ones.[45] A striking common feature of the above early records of *chuanran* is that the term referred predominantly to what we consider today as chronic disorders, especially consumption, believed to be transmitted by the ancient mode of *zhu* or *chuanzhu* mentioned above, often involving transmission by bugs flying out from corpses, affecting their family members. The term *chuanran* in these early cases was apparently not used to describe the spread of acute diseases.

The idea that consumption could be transmitted to others was very probably introduced by Daoist liturgists in the twelfth century. Lu Shizhong's ritual handbook revealed an emerging idea of disease transmission in relation to consumption, perceived to be transmitted by bugs. The text described rituals to prevent contagion by clothing, bedclothes, the bed, and utensils, or by entering the house of the patient or sharing food. Things used by the sick or deceased were believed to be impregnated with corrupt *qi* or polluting bug toxin (*gu*).[46] While disease transmission by bug toxin, as found in medical texts from the Sui and Tang dynasties, was typically described as occurring within a household, this Southern Song Daoist text recognized contagion irrespective of family relationship. Michel Strickmann considered this text a departure from the Daoist tradition that a chain of disease transmission was a consequence of shared guilt or genetic predisposition within a lineage. From then on, anyone in proximity to the sick or the dead was liable to *chuanran* contagion.[47] Such contagion was no longer uniquely a moral cause of disease; rather, it could simply be a consequence of carelessness.

One of the first medical authors to use the term *chuanran* was Zhang Gao (1149–1227), who mentioned two recipes to treat consumption and prevent the disorder from spreading.[48] Chen Yan, the author of the important medical text *San yin fang* (On the three causes of diseases, 1174) considered the common skin disorder ringworm as transmissible by physical contact with the sick even though its main cause was the stagnation of Blood and *qi* on the skin.[49] He was also the first to consider the *dafeng lai* disorder (big-wind scabies, an ancient disease now considered a kind of leprosy) as transmissible by contact. "Transmission through blood and *qi*," according to Chen, was not due to the retribution of sins from a former life, but to "carelessness."[50]

Chuanran by sexual intercourse began to be discussed in the twelfth century. We have seen how Chao Yuanfang and other seventh- and eighth-century doctors explained the "*yinyang* exchange" of Cold Damage, unseasonable *qi*, or Warm Disease through sexual intercourse, as a mechanism integral to a cosmic process involving a man (*yang*) and a woman (*yin*). In the twelfth century, this mechanism was conceived as yet another form of *ran* contamination. Cheng Wuji of the northern Jin (Jurchen) dynasty—who in 1156 wrote an authoritative commentary on the *Shanghan lun* (Treatise on cold damage)—explained the *yinyang* exchange as follows: "Residual poison [from the patient] contaminates the other person [*xiangran*] and affects [him or her] like an exchange [during sexual intercourse]."[51] The exchange was thus a contamination, a *ran* contagion. Cheng might have been influenced by the imperial medical encyclopedia compiled around 1111–17, *Shengji zonglu*, in which the same exchange was explained as an "exchange by contamination" (*ranyi*) whereby "the disorder of the man was transmitted [*chuan*] to the woman, or that of the woman to the man."[52] This particular disorder, which originally had belonged to the larger category of Cold Damage disorders, was gradually conceptualized as a mode of contamination through sexual intercourse. It was not only an exchange but also a *chuan* transference and a *ran* contamination.

Despite the first appearances of *chuanran* being applicable mainly to chronic diseases, the term seems to gradually have obtained a broader meaning, becoming applicable also to the spread of diseases during epidemics of acute disorders and, from the twelfth century onward, replacing the much older term *xiangran*. The popular use of the term *chuanran* can be seen in the much-quoted debate on the fear of contagion during epidemics by two important twelfth-century Confucian scholars. Both Cheng Jiong and Zhu Xi condemned the practice of abandoning one's relatives during epidemics for fear of *chuanran*, which was a common practice (*li su*) at the time. Even though Cheng and Zhu approached the debate differently,[53] their views reflected current ideas on the spread of epidemics as revealed in Chen Fu's *Nong shu*, mentioned earlier. In this text, Chen claimed that while diseases such as consumption and Wind disorders could mutually *chuanran*, the spread of epidemics was in fact due to the "steaming and smoking" of vicious *qi*.[54] Without making a conscious distinction between chronic and acute diseases, doctors of the time did differentiate among various modes of transmission for different diseases.

We could conclude from the descriptions in these twelfth-century texts that doctors and society had grown increasingly interested in the question of contamination or the transmission of medical disorders by physical contact with the sick. However, during epidemics and for certain chronic diseases, *chuanran* was still considered as one of the many causes of illness, not the only or even the main cause. For epidemics, classic configurationist explanations of pathogenic *qi*—the pollution of the environment by filth, bad weather, or social injustice, or vicious demons' generating perverse pathogenic *qi* and contaminating people in a locality with weak constitutions or morals—remained widely accepted, and the spread of disorders remained a *ran* process. Mutual contamination among inhabitants within a single locality was only a secondary cause. Finally, there was a growing interest in transmission by sexual intercourse. The above ideas on the spread of diseases by *chuanran* or *xiangran* were well established in Chinese medical texts by the twelfth century. In the subsequent Ming and Qing dynasties, doctors and scholars enriched the concept of *chuanran* by providing concrete details on the process of transmission.

The Ming-Qing Period (Fourteenth to Nineteenth Centuries)

Developments in the conceptualization of the spread of disease in the late imperial period included the following. First, doctors in the Ming and Qing dynasties provided many more concrete details about *ran* contamination. Second, *chuanran* clearly became the dominant term used to talk about the spread of disease from person to person, and it was increasingly used to mean transmission by physical contact, either direct or indirect, with the sick. Third, two lines of medical reasoning emerged. In one, *chuanran* was identified—with increasingly concrete details—with chronic diseases transmitted through intimate contact; in the other, medical innovators began to apply the concept to acute outbreaks of what we today would think of as epidemics.

In Ming and Qing medical texts about certain chronic diseases, three different paths of transmission by contact were described: by direct or indirect physical contact with the sick, by hereditary transmission, and by transmission through sexual intercourse. One of the first doctors to write on the first type of transmission was Gong Tingxian, a palace doctor of the early sixteenth century who authored several influential medical texts. His descriptions of the transmission of leprosy (*mafeng*) were reminiscent of the above-mentioned twelfth-century Daoist liturgical text, but couched in medical terms: "If careless while traveling, it could be transmitted [*chuanran*] in toilets, in living quarters, or by bedding and clothes."[55] The term "careless while traveling" reiterating ideas from Chen Yan's twelfth-century passage on consumption mentioned above, probably means "men carelessly seeking sexual pleasure during their travels." The consequence would be contagion by sexual intercourse or contact with materials contaminated by the sick as listed above. The second type of transmission by contact was hereditary transmission. As mentioned earlier, the medieval religious belief of shared guilt within a lineage was behind the notions of *zhuyi* (outpouring exchange), *ranyi* (exchange by dyeing), and *chuanshi* (corpse transmission), in which a disorder poured from a dead patient into a healthy person—usually the patient's progeny or a close relative—as in the case of consumption. The idea of hereditary transmission of disease in the late imperial period basically developed from these notions. Gong explained another cause for leprosy: "[The disorder could be] transmitted to others from ancestors or parents [to descendants], from husbands and wives, or other members of the family."[56]

The third type of transmission by physical contact was through sexual intercourse. We have already traced the development of the ancient idea of *yinyang* exchange that had developed into transmission by contamination through sexual intercourse during the Song dynasty. Sexual transmission was discussed in the late imperial period mostly in the context of a new disease called *yangmei chuang* (bayberry sores) or Guangdong sores, as it was believed to have originated in Guangdong province. Modern historians of medicine usually identify this disease as syphilis, which was first recorded in southern China during the first decade of the sixteenth century.[57]

Li Shizhen, the author of the great classical pharmacopeia *Bencao gangmu* (1579–93), was among the first to provide a detailed account of this disease:

> Bayberry sores are not recorded in the old recipes, and there were no patients with it. The disease has begun recently in the southeastern region and spread all over. It is because the southeastern region is low and warm. There are mountains with miasma that evaporates under the heat. People like to eat spicy and hot food. Men and women are lascivious and immoral. Dampness and heat accumulate deeply and form a pathogenic agent. This causes the development of noxious sores that are contagious to other people [*huxiang chuanran*]. Spreading from the south to the north, the disease is now everywhere. But then all those who fall victims are lascivious people.[58]

The spread of the disease through sex is clearly expressed in this passage, even though Li also emphasized the other causes of the disorder, especially the perverse climatic and environmental conditions and the unhealthy dietary regimen in the south.

The same idea was repeated by Chen Sicheng, who authored the first book devoted entirely to the disease, titled *Meichuang milu* (Secret record of rotten sores) and published in 1632: "Recently, customs have deteriorated, and numerous are those who indulge themselves in brothels and do not take precaution while doing so . . . Before they realize [that they are infected], they have already transmitted [the disease] to their wives and concubines or to their pretty boy servants. In earlier times, there were few medical books to correct this, which explains the uncontrolled transmission and contamination."[59] One should note here that the reason why leprosy was considered highly contagious in late imperial China was probably the fact that it was frequently confused with Guangdong sores.[60] In other words, the appearance of the new disease of Guangdong sores might have modified the etiological discussions of an old disease that had deceptively similar external symptoms, and enforced the idea of sexual transmission as a major channel of transmission.

Nevertheless, sexual transmission was still considered part of a general mode of transmission within a lineage. The belief that members of the same household had similar physical traits and lifestyles, making them more vulnerable to the transmission of diseases, remained strong. In religious terms, transmission was a consequence of shared guilt. For Guangdong sores, for instance, Chen considered *chuanran* to occur not only between husband and wife: "The disorder is not only transmitted through sexual intercourse . . . The disease can be transmitted [by the husband] to the wife or concubine. Even if the wife or concubine does not fall ill, the disease could be shifted (*yi*) to children, nephews, and grandchildren."[61] The 1742 imperial compendium *Yizong jinjian* provided a similar account of the transmission of leprosy: "One cause is transmission [*chuanran*] through the contact with a patient, or from parents, between husband and wife, or other family members."[62]

Despite the growing interest in the notion of *chuanran* as person-to-person transmission of disease in the late imperial period, there were still voices expressing reservations. While discussing the possible modes of transmitting *mafeng*, the early Ming palace doctor Liu Chun (1358–1418) expressed his doubts: "As for the question of *chuanran*, it may be possible. However, even though within the same family, there is mutual transmission [*xiangchuan*] through blood and channels, eating and drinking [in the same place], sharing the same habitat and temperament [*qiwei*], there should be no contamination [*ran*] if internal heat has not accumulated deeply into a toxin."[63] Although he accepted the possibility of mutual contamination within the same household because members shared similar physical traits, habits, and living space, he did not see this as a normal channel of transmission and reluctantly conceded that it was possible only if the internal accumulated poison had reached an extraordinary degree. This difficulty of accepting person-to-person transmission can still be detected in later texts. Xiao Xiaoting—the author of an important work on leprosy, *Fengmen quanshu*, with a preface dated 1796—wrote: "Some would say that [since] the *qi* and blood of a person each follows its own vessels, how could [any pathogen] be transmitted from one [person] to another?" Being himself convinced of the contagiousness of the disease, he tried to convince his readers by using an analogy: "Do they not realize that even scabies can be transmitted and contaminate others, to say nothing of leprosy?"[64] Liu and Xiao showed the difficulties of accepting *chuanran* when the vital Blood and *qi* of a person were believed to circulate in a closed system, corresponding to and interacting only with the cosmos.

The idea that *chuanran* contamination could be a factor in the spread of epidemic diseases began to be discussed in the seventeenth century.[65] The development was epitomized in the seventeenth century by an important work on epidemics authored by Wu Youxing (mid-seventeenth century), a native of the lower Yangzi region. For Wu, abnormal weather was only one of several factors that provoked noxious epidemic *qi*. He coined the term *zaqi* (impure *qi*) to express a kind of pollution-generating epidemic: *zaqi* "could originate from towns or from rural settlements . . . The so-called *zaqi* . . . actually is the breath emanating from the earth of a locality [*fangtu zhi qi*]. Such and such a *qi* will cause such and such a disorder."[66] Epidemic *qi*, therefore, was mostly earthly, linked to the specific material conditions of a locality, causing all victims to suffer from a similar disorder. This idea of epidemic *qi*, not unlike that of miasma in contemporaneous Europe, was often associated with dampness of the earth and with foul matter.[67] A combination of filth and dampness, when steaming from the soil and mixing with unseasonable *qi*, generated epidemics. Disease-causing filth was believed to steam and become a poisonous and infectious haze when the weather turned warm and humid. Zhang Lu, a late Ming doctor in the south (mid-seventeenth century), attributed *shiyi* (seasonal epidemics, specific in time and locality) to the emanation of filthy dampness from the earth, triggered by unseasonable, impure *qi*.[68]

One particular contribution of some southern Ming and Qing doctors to the idea that environmental pollution provoked epidemic *qi* was the emphasis on dead organic matter.[69] Death, to them, was the most dangerous and polluting element. Zhou Yangjun, an important early Qing doctor, was emphatic about the deadly polluting effect of corpses:

Because of the shallow burial of flesh and bones, *qi* emanating from corpses amasses in the earth, ascends and descends with [the *qi* of] heaven and earth, and drifts everywhere. People [under the influence of] this *qi* have no escape and will be infected with illness and die. This then aggravates seasonal pathogenic *qi* or corpse *qi*. It spreads and [people] get contaminated and recontaminated after prolonged immersion [in that *qi*; *fu xiang jianran*]. After a while, the *qi* becomes more deadly. Therefore epidemics always follow wars. Not only are people weakened by being under the influence of the *qi*, it is also that the accumulated filthy *qi* has reached an extreme level . . . The most venomous and filthy *qi* on earth produces epidemics.[70]

In other words, medical texts by many seventeenth-century southern doctors stressed that miasmatic *qi* emerging from the earth of a locality polluted by filth, dampness, and especially death was more devastating than the climatic *qi* causing Cold Damage disorders described in early medical classics. This harmful, earthly *qi* was, moreover, believed to enter the victim's body through the nostrils and the mouth. Wu explained that seasonal epidemics (*shiyi*), caused by special impure, epidemic breaths (*zaqi, liqi*), contaminated people "through the mouth and the nostrils . . . [whereas noncontaminating] Cold Damage pathogens enter [through] tiny pores [*haoqiao*] into the circulation vessels [*jing*] where they flow from one [vessel] to another. The effect of Cold Damage is immediate, whereas the contaminated victim of seasonal epidemics manifests symptoms only after a period of time." He also noted: "The mouth and the nostrils communicate directly with heaven. Received *qi* can come from heaven or from *chuanran*."[71] Wu's idea of *chuanran* was therefore closely associated with local epidemics, where victims were infected by a seasonal external pathogen through the upper respiratory system. Consistent with the configurationist explanation (related to cosmological or environmental patterns such as *yin* and *yang*, the five phases that constituted the basis of Chinese thought, and the six pathogenic *qi*) of epidemics, Wu's inventiveness rested in his singling out local epidemics from the general classic category of Cold Damage disorders, highlighting the infectiousness of the specific epidemic *qi*. It is from this tradition that TCM experts in China drew inspiration for explaining and treating SARS in the spring of 2003.[72]

In brief, the ideas of *chuanran* and contamination underwent interesting changes in the Ming-Qing period, although the basic modes of transmission remained largely unchanged since the seventh century. To explain the contaminating nature of epidemics, increasingly concrete elements such as filth caused by dead organic matter, in addition to dampness and warmth, were stressed. Local, earthly impure *qi* was now considered more dangerous than unseasonable atmospheric *qi*. For nonepidemic diseases, contamination and transmission were also described in more concrete terms, referring to mechanisms for indirect transmission such as toilets, bedding, and clothing. Pathogenic *qi* in both acute and chronic disorders was seen as entering the victim's body through the mouth and the nostrils. Most important, the notion of transmission by close and direct physical contact, including sexual and hereditary or congenital transmission, was also specified. This idea of transmission by breath or bodily fluids such as blood of the parents, urine, perspiration, and breast milk, already described in seventh-century texts, had clearly become a widespread concept. Transmission of disease by sexual intercourse was the main point developed in this late imperial period— transmission both to the sexual partner, and to the fetus in the form of fetal toxin,[73] if the intercourse resulted in a pregnancy.

Conclusion

It is quite clear to me that the sick body has been scrutinized more and more closely by medical writers, including in a social context, since the third century. By the seventh century, the basic modes of the spread of disease had been established and expressed in a language of contamination, epitomized in the word *ran*. But the term *chuanran* emerged only in the tenth century to refer more specifically to the transmission of the same disorder by contact with the sick, especially for chronic disorders like consumption. The term gained popularity in written texts, probably due to the ethical controversy launched by Neo-Confucian moralists in the twelfth century over the necessity to stay with one's sick parents and relatives despite the danger of contagion during epidemics. In that context, however, there were different perceptions of *chuanran* by doctors, nonmedical elites, and the general populace. The full complexity of the notion of *chuanran* was not reached until the late imperial period, when both the content of noxious epidemic *qi* and the types of transmission for chronic disorders were given more concrete descriptions in medical texts. *Chuanran* as a term for disease transmission also came to eclipse the other older terms containing ran to express the general idea of the spread of disease.

The growing popularity of *chuanran* since the twelfth century had an important consequence for the conceptualization of the spread of diseases. Among its many layers of meaning, transmission by contact—in particular, direct physical contact with the sick not necessarily related by blood— probably became most significant. It conveyed the sick body as a dangerous body producing contaminating breath, bodily fluids, and excrement, and as a lascivious sexual body polluting its sexual partners and producing sick infants. The sick body was dangerous even after its death, as it would pollute the environment, provoking an epidemic *qi* and contaminating not only its progeny or relatives by the process of *zhu*, but also strangers in contact with the emanating *qi*.

The impact of the idea of *chuanran* on late imperial society remains a topic to be studied. We can at least enumerate a number of new practices that revealed an increasing concern with contagious bodies. The first institutions for the segregation of leprosy patients, for instance, appeared in the sixteenth century. Unprecedented measures of segregation against smallpox were established by the Manchu government, beginning in the early seventeenth century. Variolation against smallpox was practiced after the sixteenth century, with the conviction that by so doing the vulnerable child with an innate fetal toxin could avoid contagion during an epidemic by having the toxin released under controlled conditions. And from the seventeenth century onward, community associations were organized on a massive scale to provide proper burial for exposed bodies.[74] These late imperial practices demonstrate the currency of the idea of *chuanran*, either as direct person-to-person transmission, or as the spread of disease under the influence of a contaminating, local, epidemic *qi*.

One should indeed be mindful of the multiple layers of meaning of *chuanran* that built up throughout China's long imperial history. First, the term meant contamination not only by contact with the sick, but also by contact with a pathogenic *qi*, be it epidemic or nonepidemic, an old idea originally expressed by *xiangran*. Furthermore, from the late Ming onward, many southern doctors distinguished between the noncontagious *qi* provoking Cold Damage disorders and the contagious local impure, epidemic *qi*. Second, during an epidemic and for certain chronic disorders, members of the same household or people related by blood were believed to be more vulnerable to contamination by a patient, a notion already described in seventh-century texts. Third, *chuanran* was never the only cause of the spread of any disorder. A polluted location, the weak physical constitution of the victim, bad geomancy of a residence, or moral flaws or wrongdoing were equally valid or more important causes, an idea confirmed and emphasized in twelfth-century texts. Fourth, disorders considered to be more prone to *chuanran* tended to be particularly deadly, such as severe epidemics caused by impure *qi*; chronic disorders with conspicuous poisonous sores such as smallpox, measles, Guangdong sores, and leprosy; or diseases ending in a slow, painful death, such as consumption. Some of these disorders were closely associated with sexual transmission, and all of them provoked fear or disgust in late imperial society.

The term *chuanran* reflects how Chinese medicine easily accommodated pluralistic models of events, including outbreaks of disease, imagining them as the outcome of a dynamically interacting web of influences. This approach was different from that of the Aristotelian-trained European medical scientists, whose search for the strict understanding of a sufficient cause produced in the late nineteenth century monocausal explanations—some of which had great explanatory power, but which tended, at times, to be reductionist.

Thus when Xi Liang said that people did not believe that the 1910 pneumonic plague could be transmitted (*chuanran*), he referred to one, but not all, layers of the term's meaning. He was probably referring to specific, direct, person-to-person transmission, while the populace upheld the traditional belief that they were under the influence of an epidemic *qi*, or that it was an epidemic of the noncontagious Cold Damage type, as Wu Youxing of the late Ming might have suggested. Some Chinese probably thought that running away from the place under the influence of that *qi* would keep them safe. They did not believe in person-to-person mutual contamination under that particular epidemic breath, especially when the illness did not provoke conspicuous external symptoms, or if their family members were not affected. All these ideas were built into the term *chuanran* that, nonetheless, disregarded the acuteness of epidemic diseases. Xi's perception of *chuanran* might already have incorporated modern biomedical ideas of germs, justifying Wu Lien-teh's (the head of the mission to fight the 1911 Manchurian pneumonic plague, see Sean Hsiang-lin Lei's chapter in this volume) drastic measures of quarantine, while the understanding of the populace was still loaded with traditional meanings.

This leads to a final point that I would like to stress here: the choice of *chuanran* as the Chinese term to translate contagion and infection when Western medicine was introduced into China, especially after germ theory became dominant around the beginning of the twentieth century. The complexity of the modern idea of *chuanran* at its early stage is revealed in an interesting text for a popular audience that was published in the newspaper *Dagong Bao* in the summer of 1902, ten years before the pneumonic plague epidemic and Xi Liang's comment: "These diseases are caused by minute living poisonous *chong* [*weisheng du chong*] introduced into the blood and channels, causing various disorders. These *chong* multiply very quickly, so that transmission is fast. I think that *chong* is a transformative living substance [*huasheng zhi wu*], and that there must be a *chong*-transforming poisonous *qi* [*huachong zhi duqi*] that provokes the proliferation of *chong*."[75] This passage shows the persistent importance of the traditional notions of *chong* as a polluting element, and of poisonous *qi* as constituting a pathogenic ecology. Germs (eventually translated as *weisheng wu*, or "minute living things") are here perceived as a variation of *chong* pullulating under toxic *qi*. Hence we clearly see the emergence of a biomedical perception of contagion or infection by germs, still heavily loaded with traditional ideas. The term *chuanran* facilitated and at the same time distorted the new biomedical idea it was incorporating at the early stage of the idea's introduction, partially explaining the tremendous efforts Wu Lien-teh had to make to convince people of the necessity to set up a quarantine.

NOTES

All translations are by the author, unless otherwise indicated.

1. See chapter 3. For the original source of the quote, see Xi, "Xuyan," 4.

2. A public notice in the vernacular language, published by the Bureau for Epidemic Prevention in Baoding District in *Dagong Bao* on February 25, 1911, stressed: "Plague was unheard of in China in the past. Therefore nobody knew how terrible this disease could be." The same notice also refuted the common Chinese belief of that time that the disease "was no different from some unseasonal epidemics that we have always had in the past," stating that this "new disease" was introduced from foreign countries after "the great global communication." Hence, this text clearly emphasized the newness of the plague.

3. *Oxford American Dictionary and Thesaurus*, s.v. "Contagion."

4. See Pelling, "Contagion/Germ Theory/Specificity."

5. Touati, "Contagion and Leprosy," and Conrad, "A 9th-Century Muslim Scholar's Discussion of Contagion."

6. Nutton, *From Democedes to Harvey*, 22.

7. Pelling, "The Meaning of Contagion," 16.

8. Pelling, *Cholera, Fever and English Medicine 1825–1865*, 276–85, on William Budd.

9. Ibid., 284, and Worboys, *Spreading Germs*, 126.

10. Delaporte, *Disease and Civilization*.

11. Quoted in Worboys, *Spreading Germs*, 125. The author of this article proposed three contending hypotheses on the nature of contagion: a chemical or physical theory; bioplasm, or germs; and ideas based on Pasteur's notion of living organic ferments producing zymosis.

12. The quotes are from Pelling, "The Meaning of Contagion," 20.

13. Barbara Volkmar, "The Concept of Contagion in Chinese Medical Thought," 151. This fine article is about the concept of contagion in China up to the twelfth century. Volkmar stresses the difference between the demonological view of folk medicine and the rationalistic view that assigns the cause of epidemics to cosmological and meteorological conditions.

14. *Zhou li*, 12.

15. *Shang shu*, 7:8a (in this work page numbers restart at the beginning of every chapter, so I give the chapter number after the book title to help identify the cited pages). The full phrase is *jiu ran wu su* (to have been tainted by the corrupt customs for a long time).

16. For an example of the positive meaning of *ran*, see Chen Shou, "Wu shu," 58:1350. In this story from the *San guo zhi* (History of the three kingdoms), a "barbaric group" is described as having caused upheaval in China, since it "had not been tainted with the culture of the Emperor" (*wei ran wang hua*).

17. Mozi (ca. 476–390 BCE), one of the leading philosophers of the early Warring States period, specifically compared the dyeing of silk to positive and negative moral influences on individuals. He used *ran* to express the action of one individual who was influenced by another—e.g., "King Wu was influenced by the Prince of Zhou" (*Wu wang ran yu Zhou gong*; *Mozi*, 1:11).

18. Chen Shou, "Wu shu," 60:1383.

19. Ge, *Zhouhou beiji fang*, 2:43.

20. Chia-feng Chang has published a long and interesting paper ("Yiji yu xiang-ran") on the modes of contagion in Chao Yuanfang's classic. Chang's paper discusses ideas related to contagion as found in this and other contemporary texts. By contrast, my present approach is based on an analysis of the different uses and evolution of terms containing the character *ran*. I believe that a study of the terms themselves can reveal subtle changes that often escape our modern mindset.

21. This and the preceding two examples are found in Chao Y., *Zhubing yuanhou lun*, 19:578, 48:1368, and 45:1287, respectively.

22. Apparently the same idea of contagion within the body, applicable to "the internal and pathological process in which the body slowly becomes impregnated with venomous humour, leading to the destruction of the whole edifice," was still prevalent in the West until the twelfth century (Touati, "Contagion and Leprosy," 188).

23. Chao Y., *Zhubing yuanhou lun*, 8:277; 9:302.

24. Ibid., 10:333–34.

25. Zhang Ji, *Shanghan lun*.

26. Chao Y., *Zhubing yuanhou lun*, 8:277.

27. See, for example, Sun S., *Beiji qianjin yaofang*, 9:174, for similar notions of perverse *qi*: "At times there is the qi of epidemics [*yiqi*] and vicious wind [*zeifeng*], resulting in contamination from one to another, or hot wind and *zhangqi* [miasmatic breath] that causes contamination from one to another and again results in the destruction of the entire household."

28. Li J., "Contagion and Its Consequences," 203.

29. Chao Y., *Zhubing yuanhou lun*, 24:708.

30. Wang T., *Waitai miyao*, 13:351. Chao Yuanfang provided a different explanation for the term *wugu*: "There is a bird called Innocence that hides in the daytime and flies at night. If it sees children's clothing or bedding being dried outside, it flies over it. The child who wears the clothes or sleeps on the bed with the bedding will catch

the disease" (*Zhubing yuanhou lun*, 48:1378). Chao's explanation was repeated and developed by most late imperial doctors explaining pediatric consumption. Some, for instance, considered that feathers or bugs dropped by the Innocence bird caused the disorder, as stated in the 1742 imperial compendium edited by Wu Qian (*Yizong jinjian*, 52:78).

31. Chao Y., *Zhubing yuanhou lun*, 24:702–3.

32. That the human body contained a great number of bugs was an idea present both in Buddhist and Daoist views of the body. See Strickmann, *Chinese Magical Medicine.*

33. *Chuan* refers to the classic process whereby a pathogen introduced into the body through the skin would enter the flesh and flow into the vessels and from there into the bowels (*fu*). The curability of the case depended on the path taken by the pathogen within the visceral system. See *Huangdi neijing suwen*, 19:121–123, and 56:290.

34. Li J., "Contagion and Its Consequences," 204.

35. L. Yang, "The Concept of 'Pao' as a Basis for Social Relations in China," 298–99; Li J., "Xian Qin liang Han bingyin guan ji qi bianqian" and "Contagion and Its Consequences," 203. I thank Li Jianmin for sharing his thoughts on this point with me.

36. Chapter 24 of the *Zhubing yuanhou lun* is dedicated to *zhu* disorders. For *zhu* related to *gu*, see Chao Y., *Zhubing yuanhou lun*, 24:702–3; for *sheng zhu*, see ibid., 699.

37. Chao Y., *Zhubing yuanhou lun*, 50:1401.

38. Sun S., *Beiji qianjin yaofang*, 24:439.

39. Childhood consumption (*wugu gan*) was also attributed to the milk of sick wet nurses in the eighteenth century (Wu Q., *Yizong jinjian*, 52:78).

40. The term in fact first appeared in chapter 22 of the *Huangdi neijing suwen*, in an apparently philosophical discussion of *yin*, *yang*, and *mai* (vessels), with no clear indication that sexual intercourse was involved. Zhang Ji's discussion of the "*yin-yang* exchange," even though also unclear as to its true meaning, was followed by a recipe using burned underwear close to the private parts of the man or the woman, suggesting a ritual remedy for a disorder of sexual nature (*Shanghan lun*, 7:7b–8a). This recipe is recorded in almost all later medical texts mentioning this disorder.

41. Chao Y., *Zhubing yuanhou lun*, 8:275. While discussing another closely related disorder called *laofu* (recurrence), meaning recurrent Cold Damage disease in a patient who had sex before total recovery, Chao stated that this would not happen if the man's sexual partner was a young boy (ibid., 8:277).

Wang Tao in the eighth century faithfully repeated the mechanism that Chao had described, and added a further detail: a woman who obtained an illness through this exchange could be cured if treated early enough, whereas it was much more dangerous and even fatal for a man who fell ill after such sexual intercourse (*Waitai miyao*, 2:98 and 3:124).

42. Sun S., *Beiji qianjin yaofang*, 10:191–93.

43. Xu X., *Ji shen lu*, 3:16a. The story goes on to tell us that people believed that putting a living patient inside a nailed coffin and abandoning him or her in the river would end the spread of the disease. The fisherman's daughter was treated this way but was saved by another fisherman who lived downstream. After being cured by eating eels, she married her savior.

44. Hong M., *Yijian zhi*, 7:4a–b. This collection has different editions, some of which do not specify the disorder of the woman, but all editions mention the fear that the disorder would spread by *chuanran*.

45. Chen F., *Nong shu*, 2:5a.

46. Lu S., *Wushang xuanyuan santian yutang dafa*, 470. For a description of the text, see Schipper and Verellen, *The Taoist Canon*, 1070–73. Strickmann (*Chinese Magical Medicine*, 37) reminded his readers that Liu Cunyan was the first to bring this text to the attention of the learned world in 1971, on the question of the Daoist concept of tuberculosis in the twelfth century.

47. Strickmann, *Chinese Magical Medicine*, 35–38. See his note 85 for a detailed description of the Daoist text.

48. Zhang G., *Yishuo*, 2:19b and 4:7b.

49. Chen Y., *Chen Wuze san yin fang*, 15:11b.

50. Ibid., 12b–13a.

51. Zhang Ji, *Shanghan lun*, 4b–5a.

52. *Shengji zonglu*, 29:631.

53. Volkmar, "The Concept of Contagion in Chinese Medical Thought," 159–62. See also Cheng, *Yijing zhengben shu*, 3–5; and Zhu X., *Huian xiansheng Zhu Wengong wenji*, 71:10b–11a. Volkmar points out that "all arguments against the notion of contagion were developed on practical, political, cosmological or moral, rather than strictly medical grounds" (161).

54. Chen F., *Nong shu*, 5a.

55. Gong, *Jishi quanshu*, 8:1066.

56. Ibid.

57. Many Chinese historians argue that the disease called Guangdong sores was first brought to China by European traders in the sixteenth century. Contemporary Chinese doctors, however, never considered it a disorder with a foreign origin, unlike smallpox. Judging by the first mention of the disorder by Yu Bin, an early-sixteenth-century doctor who recorded that the disorder was first noticed in the south during the Hongzhi reign (1488–1505), the disorder seems to have arisen before the massive arrival of Europeans in China in the later sixteenth century. I do not try to explain the origin of this disease here.

58. Li Shizhen, *Bencao gangmu*, 18:36. See also A. Leung, "Jibing yu fangtu zhi guanxi," 181.

59. Chen Sicheng, *Meichuang milu*, 10–11.

60. The author of the first book on leprosy, Shen Zhiwen, wrote that the disease he described was called "Guangdong sores" in the south. See his *Jiewei yuansou*, 1:3a.

61. Chen Sicheng, *Meichuang milu*, 6.

62. Wu Q., *Yizong jinjian*, 73:376.

63. Liu Chun, *Liu Chun yixue quanshu*, 40:389.

64. Xiao Xiaoting, *Fengmen quanshu*, 1:9a.

65. See A. Leung, "Jibing yu fangtu zhi guanxi." See also Marta Hanson's dissertation, "Inventing a Tradition in Chinese Medicine," in which she analyzes some Qing views on diseases caused by the warmth factor in southern China.

66. Wu Youxing, *Wenyi lun*, 42–43.

67. For some experts, epidemic *qi* emerging from the soil was characterized by dampness. The mid-Qing doctor Tang Dalie (late eighteenth century) suggested that epidemics emerging from the soil were actually caused by the dampness of the earth (*Wuyi huijiang*, 9:17b). The noxious nature of dampness was stressed first by the Yuan master Zhu Zhenheng and further elaborated by Ming and Qing doctors. See A. Leung, "Jibing yu fangtu zhi guanxi," 183–84.

68. Zhang Lu, *Zhangshi yitong*, 2:32.

69. Medical writers and scholar-officials of the Song dynasty since the twelfth century had already written abundantly on the polluting effects of filth accumulated in waterways in crowded urban areas. See Liang G., "Nan Song chengshi di gonggong weisheng wenti."

70. Zhou Yangjun, *Wenre shuyi quanshu*, 469.

71. Wu Youxing, *Wenyi lun*, 11 and 9, respectively.

72. See Marta Hanson's chapter in this volume.

73. See C. Chang, "Dispersing the Foetal Toxin of the Body."

74. A preliminary count of charitable associations in the Ming and Qing dynasties suggests at least 589 burial associations in the late part of the period. See A. Leung, *Shishan yu jiaohua*, 291–306.

75. "Shiyi yuanqi zhifa shuo [On the origins and curing methods of seasonal epidemics]," *Dagong Bao*, July 13, 1902, 2.

The Treatment of Night Soil and Waste in Modern China

Yu Xinzhong

In the history of public health in the West, the treatment of garbage and human excrement was a crucial matter in the construction of modern sanitary systems.[1] Western observers in China during the late Qing dynasty were particularly sensitive to Chinese indifference to such matters and concluded that Chinese suffered from a complete "lack of awareness of hygiene."[2] Some Japanese even considered filthiness as a national trait of the Chinese.[3] In the eyes of the foreigners, hygiene was often associated with cleanliness in the urban environment. The ubiquitous presence of human excrement and trash in late imperial cities was one of the most visible and thus most criticized aspects of Chinese life.

To the Chinese population, however, excrement was less a public health matter than an integral element of agricultural production and a precious commodity, as it was widely used as fertilizer. It became a sanitary concern only after the introduction of Western concepts of public health. Despite their rich descriptions, recent studies on modern Chinese public health have not sufficiently dealt with the question of excrement collection and use as night soil (so called to indicate that it is collected at night and used as fertilizer).[4] The latest work by Yong Xue on the treatment of night soil is a rare study of the subject.[5] Nevertheless, Xue mainly describes the complicated interaction between rural and urban areas triggered by the collection of night soil in cities and the need for it in farming villages, and does not cover issues of public health in the late Qing period. The present study aims precisely to look at the transition in the treatment of human excrement from an essentially agricultural issue to a concern of urban public health, a development that intensified in the last decades of the imperial period.

The Treatment of Night Soil and Waste in Premodern China

In late imperial China, as well as in Edo Japan, human excrement was a valuable source of fertilizer and therefore highly treasured.[6] By contrast, though it was not completely rejected, human excrement was never turned into a large-scale commodity in the West, owing to numerous reasons—including religious beliefs and the steady supply of animal manure from a relatively prosperous animal husbandry industry. In East Asia, agricultural produce traveled from villages to urban areas, whereas feces were brought from cities into rural districts to maintain soil fertility. This arrangement helped to maintain a balanced cycle in the rural and urban ecosystems.[7] While the modern sewer systems in the West were created as a response to the degenerating urban environment, due to defecation in public areas and in water sources, the practice of recycling night soil in Edo Japan contributed to a more sanitary state in the cities there. Recent Japanese studies point out that this difference is the reason for the relatively late development of sewer systems in Japan.[8] China, like Japan, must have had basic and adequate waste treatment systems in place that generally worked well with the environment.

At the central level, the Chinese government hardly enforced any general regulation of these systems. The only exception was the Jiedao Ting (Street Bureau) that managed road conditions, including cleaning in the capital and prohibiting the vandalization of roads.[9] However, in reality this organization performed only "perfunctory and routine" tasks,[10] as it often encountered difficulties at all levels, and its efforts usually petered out in the end.[11] The major task of this institution apparently was merely to make the emperor's and his officials' business tours as convenient as possible, rather than operating for the sake of urban sanitation. At the local level, the only rule regarding the management of urban environments stipulated that an official authority (*yousi*) should be in place, but no regulations were found about the personnel or the function of such an institution.[12]

The lack of toilets and efficient garbage disposal services made the urban environment in late imperial cities problematic. On the central question of toilets, it appears that while they were rare for individual households, public lavatories did exist during this time. Xie Zhaozhe (1567–1624), a scholar of the late Ming dynasty, mentioned, probably with some exaggeration, that "nowadays throughout the country, toilets are no longer necessary for households."[13] By the late nineteenth century, Miyauchi Isaburō, a Japanese visitor to China, made the following observation: "Large toilets are found everywhere in urban areas. In the daytime, local residents and passers-by would come and use these facilities."[14] Discrepancies in such observations can be explained not only by the difference in time, but also in region. Our historical accounts seem to indicate significant differences in the sanitary conditions between northern and southern Chinese cities in the late imperial period, and northern cities seem to have been worse off.

A recent study on Beijing during the Ming dynasty suggests that there were very few toilets in the capital, and the streets were often found fouled by excrement.[15] This situation continued in the following Qing dynasty. During Emperor Kangxi's reign (1662–1722), the famous literatus Fang Bao (1668–1749) wrote: "Humans live side by side with livestock, crowding this place. People feed on raw and stale food. No toilets are found in households, leaving excrement polluting and fouling ditches and roads."[16] This situation remained unchanged in the late Qing period, as recorded in a Japanese history of Beijing: "Households of the lower social classes always lack lavatories. People feel no shame at all about defecating wherever and whenever they wish." The book continued: "Even in high society, toilets remain a rarity in family houses. People are accustomed to answering the call of nature on the road at night."[17] These comments naturally refer to the habits of men. As for women in northern China, chamber pots (*mazi*) were available for ladies. A special profession of *dao mazi* (chamber pot cleaner) even existed as part of the night soil farm industry in Beijing.[18] Though public lavatories were rare in the capital in the late Qing period, they did exist, albeit in rudimentary form, and we can find records of the design and shape of these toilets in a local gazetteer: "On three sides of old-style toilets there are walls made of clay. Inside the walls is a manure pit dug out from the ground. The establishment has no shelter, no door, and no partition—indeed a very primitive installation that merely prevents passers-by from peeping at the person in this toilet."[19]

Garbage disposal also seemed to be a serious problem in Beijing during the Qing period. As an account from the mid-nineteenth century indicates, "residents dump their household wastes outside their doors. Ashes and dirt, debris and litter all pile up on the roadsides, elevating some streets and roads more than one *zhang* [3.33 meters] above street houses. To enter the houses, a ladder has to be built to go down from the road as if going down into a valley."[20]

Excrement and garbage were nonetheless treated in the capital. In the

Ming dynasty, there were dung gatherers who cruised the streets and alleys to pick up human and animal excrement as well as recyclable rubbish. They then sold the wastes to night soil plants outside the city for their living.[21] Starting no later than the Qianlong period (1736–95), a systematic structure of night soil plants (*fenchang*) handled the collection, transport, treatment, and commodification of night soil. Within areas designated by the local government, night soil plants received from workers the night soil they had collected. After proper handling, the night soil was then sold to peasants as fertilizer in the city's outskirts.[22] By the late Qing period, there were apparently many of these plants operating inside the city. During the final years of the Chinese empire (1909–11), "for the sake of sanitation, the police ordered all night soil plants in the five sections of the capital to move to the outskirts, and levied tax on the plants," triggering protests from workers in this industry.[23] Peasants dwelling on the outskirts of cities apparently went into towns to collect or purchase night soil for fertilizing purposes.

The agricultural application of night soil in northern China was recorded by the above-mentioned Ming scholar Xie Zhaozhe: "Wait until the night soil has dried on the ground, then mix it with soil to irrigate the fields."[24] Even today, northern Chinese peasants continue the same practice: Each household has an outdoor manure pit dug in the backyard. After use, the pit is covered with soil. When the contents of the pit reach a certain height, the night soil is scooped out and deposited on the side for natural decomposition. We can imagine that in the late imperial period, those peasants who cultivated large amounts of land had to collect and purchase extra night soil in towns.

Southern cities seem to have enjoyed a more sanitary environment than northern ones. In the south, the climate was milder and damper. Paddy fields also made it easy for farmers to apply night soil directly as fertilizer. The establishment of toilets and the application of night soil were naturally different from the way this was done in the north. First of all, unlike in the north, most households had their own toilets.[25] Their design was also different, with a roof to shelter users from rain and sunshine. For instance, in Fuzhou in Jiangxi Province, "peasants in this place treasure night soil as if it were gold. Beside the village dwellings, there is bound to be a toilet. The eaves of these toilets are usually lower than those of the country houses. These eaves protect people from rain and storms."[26] Due to the more intensive style of irrigated agriculture in the south, especially in the Jiangnan region, night soil for fertilization was in bigger demand. The value of night soil can be illustrated by the expression, "night soil is money."[27] Thus the level of night soil commodification was naturally higher than that in northern China. Historical documents suggest that up until the late Ming dynasty, "all toilets in Jiangnan were built in order to strike deals with local peasants."[28]

Night soil business could be carried out by individuals or by business enterprises. As already mentioned above, during the Ming period, dung pickers in cities could make a living by collecting human and animal excrement as well as recyclable rubbish on the streets and selling these to peasants or night soil industries. In Nanjing during the Wanli period (1573–1620), a man named Shao Rong "collected waste and dung and sold them for small change to survive."[29] An example of a night soil enterprise during the Ming dynasty can be found in Xuancheng in southern Zhili province, an agricultural region. A hundred *li* (one *li* equals half a kilometer) away is the town of Wuhu, a commercial city that is conveniently linked to Xuancheng by rivers and other watercourses. Owing to these favorable geographical conditions, peasants from Xuancheng "who obtain fertilizer from the town of Wuhu usually exchange firewood harvested from their land for night soil. As a result of this transaction, a certain riverside night soil dock where boats from Xuancheng usually anchor has taken on the name of 'lotus pond.'"[30] In other words, night soil markets were functioning fairly well already in medium-sized towns like Wuhu. Major southern cities such as Hangzhou and Suzhou must have been night soil marketplaces on an even larger scale. According to the agricultural text *Shenshi nongshu*, written around 1640, the night soil market in Hangzhou covered an extensive area. People from the village of Shuanglin in Huzhou, about 70 kilometers from Hangzhou, "go to the market in Hangzhou whenever they need to buy night soil." Moreover, Hangzhou was a city with more than one riverside night soil market.[31]

From at least the early Qing period on, well-organized commercial bodies that collected and sold night soil were a common institution in many large cities such as Suzhou. This profession was called the *yong* (soil) or *feiyong* (fertilizer) industry. Businessmen in these walks of life all had their specific area for night soil collection, and their ventures were mostly family enterprises that had lasted for generations.[32] Taxes they paid granted them the privilege of collecting and selling night soil in specific areas. Unauthorized collection and sale in another person's sector were prohibited as "night soil stealing."[33] The difference between this business and the "night soil plants" in the north lay in the handling of night soil. In the *yong* industry, traders did not process the night soil. They simply loaded it onto boats or carts and sold

the whole bundle to peasants. As a result of the increase in the urban population as well as the level of night soil commodification, this industry gradually expanded in the cities. In the late nineteenth century, the night soil
industry thrived even in county towns like Changshu, south of the Yangzi
River.[34]

There were apparently variations in the night soil business culture in
these southern cities. During the 1820s, Bao Shichen (1775–1855), an official in Nanjing, advised that "residents in rural areas [should] prepare a
large number of containers so that they are able to obtain night soil from
cities. In each city household, there should be barrels in place to collect
urine for the purpose of fertilization."[35] This record suggests that night soil
traders were not necessarily monopolizing the collection of night soil in
every area. The German scholar Wilhelm Wagner indicated in his 1926 book
Die Chinesische Landwirtschaft (Chinese agriculture) that night soil delivery businesses were ubiquitous in Chinese cities, operating in the form of
cooperative societies.[36] Such modes of business, however, might not have
worked in more remote regions, where peasants most likely obtained much-
needed human fertilizer by their own means. Before the establishment of
an urban sewer system in the mid-1980s, the source for obtaining night soil
for farmers in Changhua, a small town south of the Yangzi River, seemed to
be mostly the public toilets in town. At daybreak or early in the morning,
farmers pushing wheelbarrows filled with night soil that they had just collected in town were a common sight on the roads between villages.[37] Night
soil in urban areas was thus able to travel to rural places and villages, either
through business transactions or by individual peasants, keeping the cities
relatively clean. The movement of night soil was mainly a matter of agricultural development and a means of livelihood, rather than a public health
issue.

Garbage disposal in southern cities, on the other hand, was basically
done by three different parties: individuals, local authorities, and business
associations in cities. As garbage could not be recycled and commodified
completely, its disposal was generally not as profitable.[38] A portion of the
ordinary garbage, however, could still be retrieved as fertilizer, as shown in
the *Shanghai Public Health Record* edited by Japan in 1915: the annual quantity of trash collected in the International Settlement of Shanghai, which
was the combined English and American concessions, was about 130,000
tons in the six years from 1908 to 1914; about half of this was traded and
sold as fertilizer.[39] The hidden value of urban trash found in southern cities

attracted dung pickers and nearby peasants to collect garbage regularly. For example, peasants in the area around Fuzhou (in Jiangxi province) collected human and animal waste, with "the old and the young traveling in all directions . . . Dirt and mud in ditches, waste piles on roads, ashes and embers of firewood, along with feathers and bones of animals, all are [collected and] used in certain ways."[40]

Rubbish found in urban waterways was more difficult to clear away, and local authorities often had to intervene. As a government announcement of the Yongzheng period (1723–35) stated, "Along both river banks live local residents. Waste and refuse, whatever kind, was discarded into the rivers out of convenience."[41] This was particularly true in southern China where cities were found in the dense webs of rivers, canals, and lakes. Some of the rubbish that was dumped into rivers would be washed away by water, but some piled up at the bottom of rivers, making rivers silt up. The government or local gentry had to launch occasional dredging operations to clean watercourses, though such actions did not always happen in time. Sporadic records show that there were temporary cleaning activities organized by local governments. For example, in the city of Hangzhou, in the Jiangnan region, the government sent cleaning boats in the late seventeenth century to carry out a major dredging operation in the city moat, and a stele was set up afterward to prohibit further dumping.[42]

Urban business associations were responsible for the cleaning of main avenues in many southern cities. A late-nineteenth-century newspaper notes that "in large cities there are major streets and artery roads. The shops along them run good businesses and the owners hire specific people for cleaning. These shop owners, in order to save time and energy, collect money together to hire cleaners. Therefore the government need not organize cleaning operations; it is the people that take up this responsibility."[43] While major roads were cleaned by such associations, smaller alleys with no commercial enterprises remained piled with garbage. Japanese visitors to Shanghai in the 1870s found that "alleys and lanes in particular are filled with garbage and night soil, making it impossible to set foot upon them. Apparently residents in the neighborhood never find it necessary to clean up."[44] Obviously, only major streets with a good number of shops were cleaned by hired cleaners.

To conclude, cities in traditional Chinese society did organize cleaning activities that effectively removed waste and night soil from the streets. Such mechanisms were determined largely by social and commercial factors. Cleaning tasks depended on the demand for night soil for agricultural use, the density of the urban population, the efficacy of the social organization, and occasional governmental action. Southern China enjoyed better sanitary conditions owing to a larger need for night soil as fertilizer. The night soil therefore got cleared away by individual peasants and dung pickers, or specialized businesses. Moreover, towns and cities of medium and small size were more sanitary than major cities, as they were less densely populated and more accessible to peasants needing night soil.[45]

Nevertheless, there was still some association between the disposal of night soil and garbage and the question of urban sanitation in premodern southern China, as shown in Bao Shichen's comment on Nanjing in 1815: "Hardly any ditch in the city is not blocked. Night soil and waste find no way out and pollute wells, making well water bitter and salty. During summer and autumn, waves wash into inner city waterways. Along these river banks are many brothels, which clean bins and stools in the river. The polluted water flows down and is used by residents living downstream. As a result, residents in this city, old and young, drink filthy water of this kind day after day, poisoning their bodies and minds. The people in this city are known to have low taste and disposition. Knowing these poor living conditions, it becomes a self-explanatory fact."[46]

Despite such awareness, there were no deliberate and systematic efforts to improve the situation in late imperial cities. Urban filth was considered bad for health, but was not explicitly associated with contagious epidemics and never provoked integrated state actions. The great demand for human fertilizer in agricultural China seems to have preserved an equilibrium in regard to urban sanitation. Western ideas and institutions of sanitation were introduced in treaty ports only from the late nineteenth century on, but even these had to accommodate the existing traditional Chinese practices and social organizations that we have just looked at.

British Shanghai: Tradition and Novelty in Night Soil Policies

After the First Opium War (1840–42), Western concepts and practices of public health were brought into China, and the clearing of human excrement from cities became an important issue. The most significant impact was felt in the foreign concessions of treaty ports such as Shanghai, Guangzhou, and Tianjin. The International Settlement in Shanghai provides probably the best illustration of westernized policies on urban sanitation.[47] The recent publication of *The Minutes of Shanghai Municipal Council*, providing extensive information on public health in Shanghai during the late nineteenth century and the early twentieth, allows us to analyze British night soil policy in this southern city.[48]

In 1854, the Shanghai Municipal Council (SMC) was established to govern daily matters and infrastructure in the leased territory known as the International Settlement (subsequently, in the French concession, La Municipalité Française de Changhai was established). The Board of Roads and Wharfs and the Board of Police, Taxation, and Finance were set up under the SMC, and public health matters were assigned to the Board of Police. In September 1861, a veteran artilleryman named Carlyle was appointed auditor of public health, marking the beginning of integrated public health policy.[49] In 1870, the SMC appointed Henderson as the first officer of public health. In 1898, the Public Health Department was established, with Dr. Arthur Stanley being the first director.[50] From the council's minutes, we know that a Nuisance Department was in operation at least from 1867 on, with the following record offering evidence: on November 12, 1867, the Board of Directors reached an agreement that the Board of Police should manage and monitor the operations of the Nuisance Department, whose main business was to clean up night soil and waste.[51] It is clear that public health institutions such as the Nuisance Department were established in Shanghai in the 1860s, and that the clearing of human excrement in the International Settlement was immediately considered an important public health issue.

The system of clearing the city of all kinds of dirt was gradually constructed during the 1860s. In the early 1860s, temporary workers were hired by the SMC to clean up garbage and human excrement. During the council's board meeting on July 16, 1862, a public health auditor opposed the building of public toilets on the grounds that Chinese residents in the territory would use this as an opportunity to stop paying workers to clear excrement.[52] In the meeting on November 25 of the same year, the auditor reported the additional expense of contractors of rubbish boats. It was suggested that each boat be hired for an additional two dollars.[53] The minutes from October 10 of the same year suggested that the engineers in the council's employment use their trucks to carry out street cleaning tasks in order to save more than forty dollars per month compared with hiring temporary workers.[54]

These early reports show that the system was composed of both public and private financing for waste disposal. In the public sector, the Nuisance Department hired cleaners and temporary workers to clean streets, residences, and toilets. Waste, including garbage and excrement, was placed in a fixed location, and contractors from traditional networks of night soil businesses chosen by the SMC were hired to transport the waste to the countryside at a certain time of day. At the same time, some businesses and inhabitants continued to pay private contractors to clear excrement, even though this was discouraged by the SMC.[55] In other words, while night soil clearing could be done by public or private contractors, depending on individual businesses, the cleaning of streets, the clearing of garbage, and the undertaking of sanitary measures to prevent diseases remained a public responsibility of the SMC. This arrangement was in practice from the late Qing dynasty to the Republican period.

At first, the colonial government did not seem to distinguish between rubbish from excrement. Yet it did not take too long to realize the value of night soil for Chinese peasants. In the meeting of June 7, 1865, the board members asked: "Sewage and night soil are sought after by Chinese, used by them in all their cultivation. They are seen coming miles to fetch it. Might it not therefore be assumed to have a considerable yearly value?"[56] The importance of the market value of night soil was revealed in a clause added in a new contract for night soil treatment, signed in September of that year with contractor Deng Kunhe, that stated that he had to pay 505 silver dollars to the council every month, apparently for obtaining night soil. With this money, the Nuisance Department was able to pay street cleaners who had formerly been paid by contractors.[57] By June 8 of 1868, the Nuisance Department was expected to be self-supporting through the sale of night soil, and to save the SMC more than 1,600 taels (one tael equals 30 grams) of silver.[58] Yet this expectation was never realized, as the fee for night soil paid by the contractor could not cover the general cost for city cleaning, undertaken by the same contractor. Hence the council still had to pay a monthly cleaning charge to the contractor who transported the garbage and night soil to the countryside.[59]

In order to cover cleaning costs, the SMC decided in May 1869 to charge all residents and businesses in the International Settlement a fixed fee for excrement cleaning. This proposal encountered strong objections, as many people and companies paid their own private contractors to do the job. In the end, the dispute was referred to the Supreme Court for China and Japan, which had jurisdiction over English territories in those countries. The court ruled against the SMC, stating that only those whose night soil was handled by the council's contractor were subject to this fee.[60]

It is worth noting that the flush toilets were introduced to the foreign concessions in the early twentieth century, though the toilets were not very popular initially. After 1904, some shop owners intended to install this new public health equipment, but their requests were rejected by the SMC on the ground that flush toilets might pollute water sources.[61] Nevertheless, their decision could well have been influenced by the great demand for night soil as fertilizer, since the traditional commercial network of night soil treatment was closely linked to the SMC's sanitary institutions.

While it is notable that the council's sanitary efforts were still closely related to the traditional livelihood of peasants and agricultural needs, new public health ideas on aesthetics were introduced simultaneously. The notions of cleaning schedules, orderliness, and minimizing foul smells now became important in the cleaning work. At its meeting of July 6, 1869, the board came to a decision that all clearing of excrement had to be done between 8:00 p.m. and 7:00 a.m. (thus fully justifying the English term "night soil"). In addition, buckets from the settlement on night soil cleaning boats were to be securely covered.[62] In the meeting of March 19, 1886, the board instructed the police thus: "All coolies carrying night soil along the streets of the settlement in buckets that are not provided with proper cover are to be arrested and taken to the Court. If the magistrate will not punish them, the police is then instructed to take their buckets from them."[63] Later, another rule was made regarding the shape and form of night soil buckets. At its meeting on November 27, 1894, the board ruled: "After the next January first, all the coolies employed in removing night soil from the houses in the settlement must make use of airtight galvanized iron buckets for this purpose."[64]

Among these new measures, the respect for routine and regularity, and schedule and punctuality, was particularly stressed. A rule stated that in the settlement, all streets and roads, both major and minor, must be cleaned daily except on Sundays. If required, water should be sprinkled to facilitate cleaning jobs.[65] A rule regarding trash disposal stated that after 9:00 a.m., no dumping of any sort of waste on the roads was allowed: "If found, the violator will be arrested and prosecuted with no exception or excuse."[66] In addition, another mechanism was in place to monitor workers in the cleaning industry to make sure that hired cleaners, temporary workers, and contractors finished their daily duties on time. At its meeting on October 10, 1887, the board approved the following suggestion by an entrepreneur: "It is decided to instruct him to inflict the fine of five dollars if the garbage is not removed daily."[67]

Reinforcement of law and order was yet another new element stressed in the new public health policies. There are regulations for the prevention of offenses such as random discarding of litter and relieving oneself in public places. Generally, the task of enforcing these rules was performed by policemen together with public health auditors. Offenders were either fined or arrested. In the early budgeting records of the SMC, penalties and fines were listed in the annual budget. These records suggest that offenses of public health rules were frequent.[68] To improve the situation, at its meeting on December 17, 1869, the board issued the following order: "The secretary is directed to instruct the Superintendent of Police to order the force to use all vigilance in arresting Chinese found guilty of committing nuisances in the settlements." Similar rules were repeated later on.[69] Generally, though, the habits and practices of the Chinese population in the International Settlement changed only gradually. By the end of the nineteenth century, the British seemed to notice some improvement. The minutes from June 12, 1894, report "marked improvement in the cleanliness of the streets with very few arrests for sanitary offenses."[70]

Lastly, sanitary measures related to night soil gradually became public issues to be negotiated between individuals and the authorities, often represented by public health auditors. For instance, complaints about certain outdoor toilets led to their being shut down by the authorities.[71] In the meantime, new public toilets or other sewage facilities were installed.[72] Moreover, if cases were brought before the board regarding certain existing public health issues (such as garbage piles), the board would assign a specific institution or staff member to implement proper measures. For example, in the winter of 1877, a case was put forth that the mud from cleaning sewer pits was not being handled properly. The Office of Public Health conducted a survey and confirmed this undesirable situation. In its meeting of December 17 of that year, the board ordered that any sludge from sewer pits had to be transported out of the settlement like night soil and wastes.[73]

To conclude, basic night soil treatment in the concessions was not too different from traditional Chinese practices elsewhere. The public health authorities in the concessions depended on the old commercial night soil network for the employment of cleaners and temporary coolies. Although this institution might not have been available in all Chinese cities, the treatment of night soil and waste was not a novel problem in this old country. The new element introduced by the Western governments in the concessions was that night soil and waste treatment also became an issue of public health, to be regulated by new rules and aesthetics. This changing situation, with its emphasis on new aesthetics, drew attention from elites in the late Qing period, as shown in an article published in 1872 in the Shanghai newspaper *Shen Bao*: "In all Settlements in Shanghai, streets and roads are in good order, with stores and houses perfectly cleaned. Neither filth nor waste is allowed in sight. Refuse and dirt aren't allowed to pile up in public places. Some sporadic cases of rubbish on the street are cleaned by hired cleaners. Officers and patrolmen maintain and monitor the sanitary conditions. Therefore it is not necessary to speed up and cover one's nose when passing by waste. One can always take one's time and maintain one's composure . . . In our cities, on the other hand, the foul smell and filthy environment make such a drastic contrast. It is hard to measure the degree of difference between these two cases."[74]

This sharp contrast naturally drew increasing attention from the elites, especially those who had closer contact with the foreign concessions and the Western world. At the same time, modern public health concepts were gradually introduced to China by way of translations.[75] Among these were writings that urged the central government to improve urban public health conditions. For instance, Ernst Faber's *Civilization, Chinese and Christian*, which was translated and published in 1884,[76] contained a chapter dedicated to road maintenance. In this chapter, the author proposed that Chinese people should imitate the West in terms of the maintenance of public health and infrastructure. Renovation of roads and the cleaning of public areas were presented as a must.[77]

The idea of urban cleanliness increasingly came to be associated with China's much-needed modernization. Persistent bad smells, night soil, and garbage in urban public spaces became increasingly visible and less tolerable to the elites who now considered these matters as representative of the negative side of the national character, as shown in the following account in the newspaper *Shen Bao* from 1873:

It is recognized that when a place is clean, its people enjoy a good life and live happily. On the contrary, when a neighborhood is dirty, the people are subject to all kinds of diseases . . . Take Shanghai and its adjacent areas for instance. The public areas fail to maintain cleanliness. When summer comes, soaring temperatures result in a foul smell that is almost impossible to bear . . . To reflect closely on the issue, it is found that the Chinese patrol system [*baojia*] is unable to function like its counterparts in the settlements. The latter cruise the streets and maintain order every day. They dutifully perform their monitoring tasks, ensuring great cleanliness in the public areas, roads, streets, and alleys alike. Although the regulation states that public health authorities hire cleaners to clean streets at all times, the [Chinese] authority fails to implement this rule with similar efforts seen in the settlements.[78]

Sanitary Issues and Politics at the End of Imperial Rule

From the 1860s on, officials and scholars visiting Western countries and Japan were increasingly impressed by the cleanliness and orderliness of cities and wrote admiringly about them. In 1867, for instance, Zhang Deyi (1847–1918), an envoy to the United States and Europe, commented on the "exceptionally clean" streets in Japan, and on May 23, 1868, he had the following to say about New York: "Streets and roads are very broad. Houses are clean and tidy like those in Paris. This is a densely populated city where houses and shops are lined up together like those in London . . . The streets are cleaned by uniformed cleaners in the early mornings and at dusk. A special street cleaner truck is available. It cruises all the alleys in the city every day. There is a round-shaped brush in the back of the truck . . . The truck goes about the streets, turning on the brush to clean the ground."[79]

But it was the series of national crises facing China in the second half of the century, culminating in the country's devastating defeat in the first Sino-Japanese War, that transformed such admiration into a strong urge for reforms. A direct link between public health and the nation's strength was explicitly made at the turn of the century, as shown in a 1905 article in *Dongfang Zazhi*: "For thousands of years, the government and its people never recognized the crucial relationship between public health and the prosperity of a country. Road conditions and environment deteriorated gradually . . . Alas! Lack of awareness of public health will lead to disaster. The powerful countries at present all prioritize education. To fortify the power of a nation, it is necessary to improve its people's health. This makes public health the crux of education."[80] Scholars and envoys now did not merely comment on the aesthetics of clean streets in industrial countries, but looked more closely at the institutions behind such appearances.[81] The success of the Meiji reforms in Japan beginning in the 1860s additionally made Japan a model for reforms.[82] Many Chinese believed that the primary reason for Japan's success and prosperity was its modernized institutions, not the least those associated with public health. By describing such institutions and criticizing the lack of modern hygienic notions of their own people, these elites aimed at urging their government to undertake drastic reforms on the Japanese model to strengthen China as a nation.

In 1907, the author Liu Tingchun, who studied in Japan, wrote: "In its reform movement, the Japanese government considers public health a primary task and puts much effort into its operation . . . All these [public health] institutions lead to the well-being and health of the Japanese people, making society vibrant and the people energetic. This is the reason why this country is becoming one of the strongest nations in the world."[83] However, it was often the aesthetics of public health that attracted the most attention. Duan Xianzeng, a magistrate in Shandong province, visited Japan in 1905 and subsequently introduced the Japanese public health system in his travel writings as follows: "The rule of thumb for public health is cleanliness. Chinese urban areas are usually filled with rubbish, filth, and night soil, making the poor sanitation conditions a breeding ground for vermin and pests. People in this dirty environment are likely to contract diseases. It is necessary to remove these nuisances and clean up the environment."[84] For such writers, nothing reflected a declining nation better than a filthy urban environment.[85]

Recommendations for improving sanitary conditions were put into practice more generally from the last decade of the Qing rule onward. Japan remained the favorite model. In 1898, with the support of the governor general of Hunan Province, the scholar-official Huang Zunxian (1848–1905) reformed traditional night soil treatment policies on the basis of the Japanese experience. Huang established the Hunan Bureau of Public Security and Health (*baowei*) to take charge of public health matters such as the cleaning of the urban environment and food hygiene.[86] In 1897, the Bureau of Street Cleaning (*qingdao*) was established in Hangzhou, in Zhejiang Province. In this institution, the local government hired cleaners to clean the streets to maintain urban sanitation. In the summer of 1903, this organization was transferred to the supervision of the Police Department. At that time it was stipulated that all street cleaning tasks should be completed by 8:00 a.m. No night soil truck or load was allowed on major streets. Wooden garbage cans were set up on the roads.[87]

In 1905, the Qing government established a Division of Public Health under the Bureau of *jingbao* (an institution responsible for public order, disease prevention and control, and maintenance of public facilities) in the Department of Patrol Police. In the following year, the Department of Patrol Police was upgraded to a ministry, while the Division of Public Health was upgraded to a bureau and became "responsible for the control and prevention of diseases and hygiene, for medical and pharmaceutical inspections, and for the establishment of hospitals."[88] In the meantime, many public health police institutions were set up in various regions to manage urban sanitation and hygiene. From this point on, official or semi-official institutions were established in major cities throughout the country. For instance, dating back to at least early 1907, there were already cleaners working in Suzhou, with wooden trash bins installed in the streets.[89] It was the patrolmen who monitored the cleaning task. In Beijing, it was the traffic police who oversaw the street cleaning business: "When the Bureau of Work and Patrol was established, it imitated practices in the Shanghai Settlements for administration and operations . . . Patrolmen, along with policemen, oversee cleaners on their jobs . . . The patrol staff takes shifts to supervise cleaning tasks every day. There are also cleaning regulations to govern the practice."[90] In Tianjin, after the Chinese government took over local authority from the allied forces after the Boxer Uprising in 1900, it hired twenty Indian patrolmen and fifty Indian patrol police to watch over street cleaning tasks and sanitation.[91]

For night soil treatment, many Chinese municipal governments copied the model of the Shanghai concessions. In nearby Suzhou, for instance, from 1906 onward, patrol police ordered night soil traders to use wooden covers for night soil containers. Night soil coolies were required to cover buckets after making collections. Schedules of cleaning were publicly established: "In spring and summer, all night soil collection should be completed by eight o'clock in the morning. By nine in the morning, all night soil boats should leave the city. In autumn and winter, the hour for collection is nine o'clock and the deadline for boats is ten o'clock. Moreover, the night soil boats should be covered with straw mats." In addition, all night soil coolies were required to carry a tag at their waist that contained their personal information and the assigned area for their work. This tag was meant to facilitate the management of night soil workers.[92] In Beijing, after the establishment of the police administration, all night soil plants were ordered to leave the city and move to its outskirts. Some better-equipped public toilets were set up in the city.[93]

These changes were more obvious in major cities along the east and southeastern coast. A 1906 text on Suzhou noted that "in the case of streets in and around the cities, they have become much cleaner than in the old days thanks to the patrolmen's efforts and supervision."[94] Some recognized this as the most important achievement of public health in China.[95] However, these improvements were not necessarily a blessing for all the people in the country. The establishment of a central public health organization and local public health police definitely brought about extra taxation pressure on the peasants. For them in particular, these added costs never produced any substantial benefits in their lives. Moreover, additional requirements for the process of night soil treatment enforced by the public health administration, such as specific shapes and structures for night soil buckets and their covers, and hatch covers for night soil boats, as well as the tags for night soil collectors and so on naturally meant extra costs.[96] Thus it is not hard to imagine that the additional cost would be transferred to the buyer—that is, the peasant. In other words, in addition to paying extra taxes that never benefited them, peasants were threatened by rising production costs.

The traditional livelihood of the urban and rural working classes was also affected in other ways. Modern mechanized street cleaning machines, for instance, inevitably resulted in loss of employment for traditional dung pickers, while peasants living on the outskirts of cities were no longer allowed to collect night soil for fertilizer from the cities as they used to do. Last but not least, there were additional emotional costs, with the involvement of patrolmen and traders, as illustrated by an incident in Suzhou on a winter night of 1907: On February 20 of that year, a working night soil coolie passed the western Supervisory Office at the city center, where he was arrested and tortured illegally by patrolmen in that area.[97] In other words, despite the respect for tradition in the formulation of modern sanitary measures in major cities, many aspects of traditional lifestyles and livelihoods, especially for the working classes, were irreversibly changed or even sacrificed.

Conclusion

Policies for clearing the city of human excrement and garbage became part of an urban sanitation program in foreign concessions in the second half of the nineteenth century. These policies were essentially hybrid measures to satisfy both traditional agricultural needs and Western urban environmental norms, including especially the elimination of bad smells and disorder

from the streets. Such policies became a central part of the Chinese political agenda only during the last decade of imperial rule. Until then, it was
unclear despite the popular rhetoric how such policies were linked to the
prevention of contagious chronic or acute diseases and epidemics, a matter
of life and death for the population (see the analysis of this issue in Sean
Hsiang-lin Lei's chapter in this volume). Sanitary measures were more a
question of cleanliness, orderliness, and punctuality, constitutive of modern
discipline both for the individual body and for the body politic. These matters were then seen as indicative of national character and strength.

Unlike the situation in the 1950s, described in Li Yushang's chapter in
this volume, where the proper treatment of night soil in southern agricultural regions was recognized as a key factor in the control of schistosomiasis, affecting the health of millions of peasants, night soil treatment in the
nineteenth-century urban setting was more a question of hygienic aesthetics for urban-based reformers. Nevertheless, this chapter has shown that the
rhetoric on such aesthetics was an issue of overwhelming centrality in the
nationalist discourse at the turn of the century.

NOTES

I would like to express my thanks to Angela K. C. Leung for her criticisms of and
suggestions for earlier versions of this paper. It goes without saying that all mistakes
are my own. All translations are mine, unless otherwise indicated. Research for this
article was subsidized by the Foundation for the Author of National Excellent Doc-
toral Dissertation of PR China (200212).

1. Rosen, *A History of Public Health*, 107–269; Castiglioni, *A History of Medicine*,
637–47 and 746–51.

2. Yu X., *Qingdai Jiangnan de wenyi yu shehui*, 215.

3. For instance, a Japanese book on Shandong Province during the early Republican era states: "Generally, it is fair to say that the Chinese people lack public health
concepts. This makes people feel that the term 'people of filth' describes this nation
very well" (Tanaka, *Santō gaikan*, 99).

4. See the following monographs: MacPherson, *A Wilderness of Marshes*; Yip,
Health and National Reconstruction in Nationalist China; Iijima, *Pesuto to kindai Chūgoku*; and Rogaski, *Hygienic Modernity*.

5. Xue, "Treasure Nightsoil as if It Were Gold."

6. For studies on the commodification of night soil in both China and Japan, see
Li B., "Ming-Qing Jiangnan feiyao xuqiu de shuliang fenxi"; Xue, "Treasure Nightsoil
as if It Were Gold"; and Kobayashi S., *Nihon shinyō mondai genryū kō*.

7. See Takigawa, "Higashi Azia nōgyō ni okeru chiryoku saiseisan wo kangaeru"; Tokuhashi, *Kankyō to keikan no shikaishi*, 13–48; Xue, "Treasure Nightsoil as if It Were Gold," 62. In 1899, Dr. Arthur Stanley, a public health official in Shanghai, stated his opinion that this public health mechanism, which linked up urban and rural areas, was better than that of medieval England (cited in F. King, *Farmers of Forty Centuries*, 154).

8. Gesuidō Tokyo hyakunenshi hensan iinkai, *Gesuidō Tokyo hyakunenshi*, 109.

9. Regarding the situation in the Ming and Qing dynasties, see Qiu Z., "Mingdai Beijing de wenyi yu diguo yiliao tixi de yingbian," 346; and Yu X., *Qingdai Jiangnan de wenyi yu shehui*, 382–84.

10. Shen D., *Wanli yehuo bian*, 19:487.

11. Ibid., 487–88. See also Xia, *Jiu jing suoji*, 8:94.

12. Yu X., "Public Health in Qing Dynasty Jiangnan," 382–84.

13. Xie Z., *Wu za zu*, 86.

14. Miyauchi, "Shinkoku jijō tankenroku," 549.

15. Qiu Z., "Mingdai Beijing de wenyi yu diguo yiliao tixi de yingbian," 349–51.

16. Fang B., "Chen Yuxu muzhiming," 295.

17. Shikoku chūtongun shileibu (Headquarters of the [Japanese] Army in Qing China). *Qingmo Beijing zhi ziliao*, 461 and 21, respectively.

18. Wu B., "Tao dafen de," 280.

19. Shikoku chūtongun shileibu, *Qingmo Beijing zhi ziliao*, 461.

20. *Yanjing zaji*, 115.

21. Wu B., "Tao dafen de," 281.

22. Ibid., 279–82.

23. Jiang, "Dumen shi xiaolu," 258.

24. Xie Z., *Wu za zu*, 86.

25. Ibid. See also *Shoushi tongkao*, 35:262.

26. He G. et al., "Fujun nongchan kaolüe," 1:593.

27. Li B., "Ming-Qing Jiangnan feiliao xuqiu de shuliang fenxi."

28. Xie Z., *Wu za zu*, 86.

29. Wang Q., *Fang Lu ji*, vol. 1, 1285:110.

30. Shi R., *Shi Yushan ji*, 8:277–78.

31. Quoted in Zhang Lüxiang, *Bu Nongshu jiaoshi*, 56. See also Xue, "Treasure Nightsoil as if It Were Gold," 44–46.

32. Huazhong shifan daxue lishi yanjiusuo, Suzhoushi dang'an'guan, *Suzhou shanghui dang'an congbian*, 691.

33. Ibid., 691–92. Also see the stele inscription regarding the "prohibition, restraining night soil traders from occupying harbors and bullying farmers in Changzhou and Zhaowen" in Suzhou bowuguan, *Ming Qing Suzhou gongshangye beike ji*, 298–99.

34. Suzhou bowuguan, *Ming Qing Suzhou gongshangye beike ji*, 298.

35. Bao, *Qimin sishu*, 1:14.

36. Wagner, *Chūgoku Nōsho*, 48–49.

37. Author's personal experience.

38. Documents published by the Shanghai Municipal Council in the late Qing dynasty clearly echo this point. At that time, the Nuisance Department of the Shanghai Municipal Council contracted night soil and waste cleaning out to private contractors through annual public biddings. The contractors had to pay a fee for the right to clean night soil. Yet the council also had to pay the contractors a fee for waste cleaning. See Shanghai City Archive, *The Minutes of Shanghai Municipal Council*, 1890, 9:404.

39. Naimushō eiseikyoku, *Shanhai eisei jōkyō*, 296–297.

40. He G. et al., "Fujun nongchan kaolüe," 1:593.

41. Zhang Jinsheng et al., *Yongzheng Sichuan tongzhi*, chapter 13, page 561.

42. Shao, *Jieshan shiwen cun*, 10a.

43. "Chenghao jian ce shuo" (On the city moat and the erection of privys), *Shen Bao*, January 12, 1882.

44. Notomi, "Shanghai zaji," 310.

45. There are records of the contrast between villages and average-sized towns. During the Jiaqing and Daoguang periods (1796–1821 and 1821–51, respectively), literati who visited Beijing were overwhelmed by the dirt in the capital (*Yanjing zaji*, 114). See also Xue, "Treasure Nightsoil as if It Were Gold," 62.

46. Bao, *Qimin sishu*, 2:83–84.

47. MacPherson, *A Wilderness of Marshes*, 1–14; Noguchi and Watanabe, *Shanhai kyōdōsokai to kōbukyoku*, 61–62.

48. Shanghai City Archive, *The Minutes of Shanghai Municipal Council*.

49. Qiu J. and Xu, "Shanghai gonggong zujie zhidu," 117; Shi M., *Shanghai zujie zhi*, 218.

50. Shi M., *Shanghai zujie zhi*, 218; Noguchi and Watanabe, *Shanhai kyōdōsokai to kōbukyoku*, 62.

51. Shanghai City Archive, *The Minutes of Shanghai Municipal Council*, 1:181.

52. Ibid., 1:249.

53. Ibid., 1:395.

54. Ibid., 2:194.

55. Ibid., 15:670.

56. Ibid., 2:148–49.

57. Ibid., 2:184.

58. Ibid., 3:249.

59. There are frequent records of this annual contract in the council's *Minutes*. Most of these records are found in the month of August in the earlier years of occupation, and in the month of March in later years. For example, in the contract of 1900, the monthly cost for trash cleaning was 1,004 dollars. Taking out the cost of 340 dollars for night soil treatment, the SMC paid a monthly fee of 664 dollars (Shanghai City Archive, *The Minutes of Shanghai Municipal Council*, 9:404).

60. Ibid., 3:436 and 463–64.

61. Ibid., 16:4, 9–10, and 263; 17:24, 261, and 283.

62. Ibid., 3:421.

63. Ibid., 8:359.

64. Ibid., 11:500.

65. Ibid., 4:189.

66. Ibid., 8:358. See also "Does Municipal Council Fulfill Its Duty?" in *Shen Bao*, May 15, 1894.

67. Shanghai City Archive, *The Minutes of Shanghai Municipal Council*, 9:131.

68. Ibid., 3:505.

69. Ibid., 3:88, 10:144.

70. Ibid., 11:369.

71. Ibid., 3:310, 5:180–181.

72. Ibid., 4:4 and 368.

73. Ibid., 7:120.

74. "Talking Clealiness of Streets in Concession," *Shen Bao*, July 20, 1872.

75. Yu X., "Shinmatsu ni okeru 'eisei' kainen no tenkai."

76. Faber, *Zixi cudong*.

77. Ibid., 51–53.

78. "Lun Hucheng jiedao wuzhuo guan yi xiujie shi" (On the filthiness of Shanghai streets and the need for the government to clean them), *Shen Bao*, April 19, 1873.

79. Zhang D., *Xingmu qingxin lu*, 1:155–56.

80. "Weisheng lun," *Dongfang Zazhi* 2, no. 8 (1905): 156–57.

81. Many of the travel writings in *Riben zhengfa kaocha ji* are evidence of this fact. See Liu Xuemei and Liu Y., *Riben zhengfa kaocha ji*.

82. In Japan, scholars such as Nagayo Sensai and the Meiji government introduced and established institutions of public health. See Nagayo, "Shōkō shishi," 133–9; and Ono, *Seiketsu no kindai*, 98–105. Night soil treatment was also involved in Japan's national hygiene administration (Kobayashi T., *Kindai nihon to kōshū eisei*, 28–35).

83. Liu Tingchun, *Riben ge zhengzhi jigou canguan xiangji*, in Liu Xuemei and Liu Yuzhen, eds., *Riben zhengfa kaocha ji*, 328.

84. Liu Xuemei and Liu Yuzhen, *Riben zhengfa kaocha ji*, 86.

85. Zheng Guanying (1842–1922) was among the first Chinese to pay attention to public health issues. He notes in the chapter on road maintenance: "It is true that road conditions are an indication of a country's power. They also suggest whether or not the authorities perform their duty . . . Nowadays Western countries have established municipal councils to govern the maintenance of roads and other infrastructure . . . It is common in the foreign settlements to see clean streets. Chinese authorities, central and local alike, ignore the condition of roads, making streets subject to damage and vandalism. Although officials clearly recognize this situation, they take it for granted and make no effort to improve it . . . This is evidence of how local authorities fail to fulfill their duties. The government is not able to deliver any positive results; no wonder foreign powers came and had their own way" ("Sheng shi wei yan," 1:662–63).

86. Zhang Weixiong and Zheng Hailin, *Huang Zunxian wen ji*, 298–99.

87. *Hangzhoushi zhi*, 118–19.

88. Liu Jinzao, *Qingchao xu wenxian tongkao*, 119:8790–91.

89. Huazhong shifan daxue lishi yanjiusuo, Suzhou shi dang'an'guan, *Suzhou shanghui dang'an congbian*, 686–88, 691–94.

90. Shikoku chūtongun shileibu, *Qingmo Beijing zhi ziliao*, 243.

91. Ibid., 525.

92. Ibid., 243.

93. Ibid.

94. Lu Yunchang, *Suzhou yangguan shiliao*, 197–98.

95. Tanaka, *Santō gaikan*, 100.

96. For instance, in Suzhou it was required that "all tags should be renewed. The cost for tags ranges from six to seven foreign cents" (Shikoku chūtongun shileibu, *Qingmo Beijing zhi ziliao*, 243).

97. Ibid.

Sovereignty and the Microscope

Constituting Notifiable Infectious Disease
and Containing the Manchurian Plague (1910–11)

Sean Hsiang-lin Lei

In terms of accelerating China's acceptance of modern medicine, no event has been celebrated more than the containment of the Manchurian plague at the end of the Qing dynasty. Medical historians have described this achievement in various ways: as a "watershed event in the history of modern medicine [in China]," "a lesson in the importance of epidemic control and preventive medicine," an "acknowledgment of the superiority of modern medicine [over Chinese medicine]," and a benchmark that "establish[ed] the importance of public health as a national responsibility."[1] With such accolades from medical historians, one thing becomes puzzling. Why did the four relatively independent trends of development suggested in these quotes—increasing exposure to Western medicine, greater control of epidemic diseases, the state's growing responsibility for public health, and the gradual acknowledgment of Chinese medicine's inferiority—have to wait for this plague to take off all at once?

At first the answer appears to be very straightforward: modern Western medicine achieved monumental success in containing this devastating plague, whereas Chinese medicine failed miserably. This explanation, however, unavoidably raises the question of why similar results did not take place earlier in other parts of China, a country at that time infamously known as the "fountainhead" of epidemics throughout the world.[2] To put the puzzle in the form of a more specific and useful question: what was so special about the history of the Manchurian plague that it could bring about the concurrence of multiple breakthroughs in these four aspects of medical history?

In the Beginning, We Did Not Believe That This Plague Could Infect

To those who took charge of this tragic event, the Manchurian plague was indeed a very special kind of epidemic. In the preface of the two-volume official report submitted to the Qing court after the event, Xi Liang (1853–1917)—as the viceroy, the highest-ranking official in Manchuria—reflected on the major difficulties encountered in controlling the plague. Calling the foremost obstacle "the difficulty due to lack of learning among the officials and physicians," Xi elaborated:

> In the beginning, [we] did not believe that this plague could *chuanran* [spread by contagion or infection]; all the protective and therapeutic measures were based on the conventional ways that China used to cope with *wenyi* [warm epidemics]. Because practitioners of traditional Chinese medicine did not take advantage of the microscope, they had no way of sorting out the real cases of plague from those that merely resembled the plague in terms of their symptoms. As a result, whenever Chinese doctors succeeded in curing a patient who actually suffered from common cold and fever, the stubborn and conservative society would immediately grab onto this cure and claim that the *yi* could be treated easily.[3]

If one suspends the baffling assertion about not knowing that "this plague could infect"—a cryptic but crucial statement that I will decode below—this recollection clearly suggests that the Manchurian plague fundamentally challenged the traditional definition of *wenyi*: from the conceptualization of *chuanran*, to antiplague measures and the clinical procedures for identifying genuine plague cases. In their efforts to contain the plague, Xi and his colleagues had to construct the character of the disease while simultaneously trying to bring it under control. With this in mind, the historic containment of the Manchurian plague ought to be studied as the beginning of the process of constructing, instituting, and thereby coping with a new category of disease—*chuanranbing* (infectious disease). In short, the story of the Manchurian plague is about the historic shift from *wenyi* to modern *chuanranbing*, particularly the rise of the category of "notifiable infectious diseases" recognized by the state.

This radical paradigm shift took place, in the opinion of many of the participants, because the handling of the Manchurian plague was a successful, closely watched public experiment that validated the new conception of *chuanranbing* in practice. In sharp contrast, Chinese medicine was shown to be ineffective in controlling the plague, while the identity of the plague was reconstructed—conceptually, socially, and materially—to such an extent by medical scientists that its historic defeat was almost assured. The question is this: What was the historical context that allowed the Chinese practitioners of modern medicine to redefine the problem of the plague in their own terms, gain control over the social and experimental conditions, and thereby succeed in containing the plague?

The success of this public experiment was by no means simply a result of the skillful construction of *chuanranbing* by human actors. As the medical historian Charles Rosenberg points out in his introduction to *Framing Disease*, disease "serves as a structuring factor in social situations, as a social actor and mediator." Therefore, "each disease is invested with a unique configuration of social characteristics, and thus triggers disease-specific responses."[4] In light of this understanding, scholars have to ask how the special characteristics of the Manchurian plague, a pneumonic plague that was "the deadliest of all diseases" according to the historian Fabian Hirst,[5] contributed to the historic defeat of Chinese medicine. To help articulate the specific features of this plague, both social and scientific, I will maintain throughout this chapter a comparative perspective between the Hong Kong plague (1894) and the Manchurian plague (1910). Since the practical success of this public experiment was inseparable from the conceptual breakthrough, the second objective of this chapter is to capture the mutually reinforcing processes between containing and constructing the pneumonic plague in Manchuria.

The scientific construction of the pneumonic plague, a very rare and little known disease at that time, brings our attention to the final, and perhaps most revealing, point about Xi Liang's statement—his emphasis on the role of the microscope. It is surprising how little emphasis scholars have placed on the role of germ theory in containing the Manchurian plague. This dearth of information is unfortunate because that aspect of the story is actually part of a history whose significance went beyond medicine in China and into the heart of what Andrew Cunningham and Perry Williams call "the laboratory revolution in medicine."[6] Between the outbreaks of the Hong Kong plague and the Manchurian plague, the scientific community transformed the identity of plague with the aid of bacteriological research, discovering *Pasteurella pestis*,[7] the bacillus that was "the causative micro-organism of plague."[8] Dr. Wu Lien-teh (1879–1960)—a Cambridge-trained physician,

Malaysian Chinese, and hero of the Manchurian plague—was one of the key
figures in the history of the creation of new knowledge. Without taking into
account the bacteriological reconstruction of the plague, any sociopolitical
analysis would invariably give the false impression that Dr. Wu's discovery
of the pneumonic plague and the related debates over the pneumonic nature
of this epidemic had little bearing on this landmark success. Drawing on
the scholarship of science and technology studies, I will strive to provide an
analysis that integrates the sociopolitical context, the scientific controversy
over new medical knowledge, and the implementation of laboratory-based
antiplague measures.

To give a better sense of the complexity of the interrelated factors, I have
divided the rest of this chapter into six sections. The first answers the question of why the Qing state involved itself in the unconventional task of containing the plague with modern public health measures. As suggested by
this chapter's title, "Sovereignty and the Microscope," the second section
argues that the Manchurian plague was an extraordinary event partially
because it brought about an unusual alliance between the Qing state and
germ theory. By way of elaborating Xi Liang's three interrelated points concerning the shift from *wenyi* to *chuanranbing*, the third through fifth sections make visible the unusual control over social and experimental conditions. This includes the unconventional antiplague measures, perceived as
"the most brutal policies seen in four thousand years"[9] (third section), and
the blockage of the Chinese people's resistance and the challenge of Chinese medicine in response to these measures (fourth section). The fifth section decodes Xi's intriguing assertion about not knowing that "this plague
could infect"—meaning that Chinese people were surprised to realize that
the pneumonic plague of Manchuria was transmitted through a network
of infected individuals. In combination, these three sections explain how a
radically new nosology of *chuanranbing* was constructed during the historic
containment of the Manchurian plague, in opposition to the traditional conception of *wenyi*. The sixth section, the conclusion of this chapter, traces the
history of how the state turned this new conception of *chuanranbing* into
the legal category of "notifiable infectious diseases," both during and after
the Manchurian plague. Ultimately, the newly constructed *chuanranbing*,
especially the eight notifiable infectious diseases, emerged as a key aspect
of the twentieth-century history of medicine in China and thereby transformed the relationship between the state, modern medicine, and Chinese
medicine.

Sovereignty and the Microscope

In October 1910, a mysterious plague broke out in Manchuria, causing un-precedented terror due to its exceptional communicability. As migrant coolies returned home by train for Chinese New Year, this epidemic spread with a speed never seen in premodern China. Originating in Manchuli on the border between China and Russia, within two months the plague trav-eled more than two thousand miles to the province of Fengtian, threatening both Beijing and China's heartland. The unintended consequences of ad-vancements in industrial technology soon made the three railway centers of Harbin, Changchun, and Shenyang (also known as Mukden) epicenters of the plague. By any standard, the plague was a calamity.

Unfortunately—at least in the beginning—neither the Qing government nor the Chinese people expressed any interest in containing the plague by medical means. Facing such a devastating epidemic, Qing officials before the twentieth century generally would have responded with "charitable re-lief, cleanup campaigns, appeals to the plague gods, and participation in community ceremonies and processionals."[10] In 1910, if the Qing state had been considering only the horrible loss in human lives and property, the plague would never have been perceived as a national emergency that de-manded immediate medical intervention.

From its very beginning, however, the Manchurian plague was a threat to the Qing government's already shaky sovereignty. The government did not take this plague seriously until the diplomatic corps, frightened by the plague's steady progress toward Beijing, began to exert pressure on the cen-tral government.[11] According to Carl Nathan's groundbreaking research,[12] what had really provoked the Qing state to take unusual action was the concern that Japan and Russia would use plague containment as an excuse to expand their influence in Manchuria. As a result of the Russo-Japanese War (1904–5), which had ended just five years previously in Manchuria, Russia controlled the Chinese Eastern Railway stretching through the north of Manchuria, while Japan dominated the South Manchuria Railway Com-pany.[13] Both countries were claiming that since China was proving incapable of containing the epidemic, the Qing government should be relieved of its responsibilities in Manchuria, a vast land equal in size to Germany, France, and Switzerland combined. The only way to resolve this sovereignty crisis was, as Nathan put it, to organize a Chinese plague service which would "preserve, as far as possible, formal Chinese control of its administration" and simultaneously "be as 'Westernized' as possible in medical practice."[14] In fact, this was not the first time that the Qing government was forced to adopt Western public health measures for the sake of protecting its sovereignty. In order to regain sovereignty over Tianjin, the government established China's first municipal department of health in 1902, analogous to the one created by the foreign occupiers after the Boxer Uprising.[15] Perhaps having such an uneasy precedent in mind, China's vice minister of foreign affairs, Shi Zhaoji (Alfred Sao-ke Sze, 1877–1958), urgently called upon Dr. Wu Lien-teh, his old friend, to rush to Manchuria.

In the first paragraph of Dr. Wu's autobiography, *The Plague Fighter*, the young physician recalled the chilly afternoon of December 24, when he arrived in Harbin—the center of the then-rampant plague. Even before introducing himself to the reader, the author zoomed in on his own hand, which carried "a compact, medium-sized British-made Beck microscope fitted with all necessaries for bacteriological work."[16] Opening the chapter on "black death" in this way, Dr. Wu skillfully hinted that more than anything else, these materials were to play a pivotal role in containing this horrific plague.

Dr. Wu's microscope was left untouched for three days, until he finally got an opportunity to perform a postmortem upon a Japanese woman in guarded secrecy. At once he detected some organisms on this corpse that appeared to be the same *Bacillus pestis* that the Japanese scientist Kitasato Shibasaburo (1853–1931) had isolated and identified during the Hong Kong plague in 1894. Under his microscope, Dr. Wu further observed the novel fact that these bacilli were found exclusively in the victim's lungs. This important discovery suggested that the Manchurian plague was very different in nature from the Hong Kong plague: it was an airborne disease, which meant that its bacilli were transmitted directly through person-to-person contact instead of through rat fleas, as in Hong Kong's bubonic plague.[17] As a result, the pneumonic plague was considered more virulent and infectious than the insect-borne bubonic plague. Moreover, different strategies were required to control the spread of these two distinct epidemics. In order to block the transmission of pneumonic plague through human contact, public health authorities had to exercise rigorous control over human movement, while bubonic plague containment focused on controlling rats, which bore the fleas that were the primary plague carriers.

Dr. Wu immediately informed both the local officials and the officials in Beijing about his discovery. The local magistrate and the chief of police were invited to look in the microscope and convince themselves of the true cause of the plague. Their collective skepticism, however, made Dr. Wu conclude that "it was not always easy to convince persons who lack the foundations of modern knowledge and the science."[18] By itself, a microscope had no problem making visible both the plague organisms and their channel of transmission, but it exercised very limited power over people's belief and prior knowledge, not to mention changing their entrenched ways of coping with epidemic disease.

The problem of learning new information was not restricted to the Chinese people; modern-trained foreign doctors also learned the hard way about the pneumonic nature of the plague. Most of the Western-trained physicians felt confident that they were equipped with the most advanced knowledge developed since the Hong Kong plague. Four years after Kitasato had identified the plague bacillus in 1894, the French scientist Paul-Louis Simond further discovered that the plague was transmitted by way of rat fleas. The pneumonic plague was considered to be merely a derivative phenomenon, and Dr. Wu was not the first to distinguish it from the bubonic form or to describe its clinical characteristics. Pneumonic plague was initially thought to arise when a victim was infected by a bite; instead of a bubo developing, the disease spread through the bloodstream to the lungs, causing pneumonia. In previous centuries, however, pneumonic plague had been very rare, and outbreaks had remained remarkably circumscribed. According to Hirst, "it was the great pneumonic epidemic of 1910–1911 in north Manchuria which first aroused universal interests in this unfamiliar type of plague."[19]

Nothing better symbolized foreign doctors' resistance to the idea of a distinct form of pneumonic plague than the controversy over gauze masks. To protect people from direct infection through the respiratory passage, Dr. Wu designed gauze masks and demanded that both sanitary staff members and the general public wear them properly. Confident of their updated knowledge about bubonic plague, many foreign doctors—including those on the Japanese, Russian, and French staffs—doubted Dr. Wu's analysis and therefore refused to wear masks, even when they were in close contact with terminally ill plague patients. According to Dr. Wu's recollection, when the French doctor Gérald Mesny, his senior colleague on the Chinese antiplague team and the head professor of Beiyang Medical College, expressed strong resistance to his discovery, Dr. Wu felt so humiliated that he submitted his resignation to the Qing court. A few days later, however, the news arrived that Dr. Mesny had become infected with the plague when he visited the

Russian epidemic hospital without wearing a mask. Six days later, this leading figure of the antiplague team passed away, and panic erupted in Manchuria. From this point on, people started accepting the dreadful nature of
the plague, and "almost everyone in the street was seen to wear one form
of mask or another."[20] The death of Dr. Mesny was only the first in a series
of incidents by which the plague unintentionally aided Dr. Wu by stealing
away the lives of those who disagreed with him.

In contrast to the local officials, the officials in Beijing, especially Dr. Wu's
old friends in the Ministry of Foreign Affairs who had sought his assistance
in the first place, did not need the microscope to be convinced that it was a
pneumonic plague. As the tragic death of Dr. Mesny further confirmed their
trust in Dr. Wu, they were eager to turn Dr. Wu's discovery into effective
antiplague measures in order to resolve the sovereignty crisis. In a telegram
to Shi Zhaoji, the Vice Minister, Dr. Wu summarized his plan for containing
the plague: "It spread almost entirely from man to man, and the question of
rat infection may, for the time being, be left out, so that all efforts at suppres-
sion of the present epidemic may be concentrated upon the movements and
habits of man."[21] It was very daring for a young, inexperienced physician
such as Dr. Wu to suggest a suspension of all the recently established measures against rat infection.[22] Just a few weeks after Dr. Wu sent his telegram,
a Japanese-owned newspaper in Manchuria published an editorial titled
"Anti-Plague Administration Should Absolutely Pay Attention to Catching
Rats." The editorial emphasized that Taiwan, where plague had once been
endemic, had become virtually plague-free as a result of the Japanese colonial government's rigorous implementation of regulations against rats.[23]

Even after it became clear that almost all the plague victims were infected with the pneumonic form of plague, and no plague bacilli were found
in dissected rats, Dr. Kitasato, the eminent plague authority, still insisted
that the most urgent need was rodent extermination. He reasoned that once
the weather got warmer and the rats awoke from hibernation, they would
become infected by contact with plague victims, and a whole new wave of
bubonic plague would join together with the pneumonic strain and wreak
havoc across the country.[24] More importantly, when Dr. Kitasato gave a lec-
ture to the assembled staff of the Japanese consulate in Fengtian, he emphasized that pneumonic plague, relatively easy to keep from spreading overseas, might soon turn into bubonic plague, which might be carried all over
the world by shipboard rats.[25] In short, the nature of the plague—which was
contested at that time—would influence the Qing court's struggle to protect
its sovereignty in Manchuria

Knowing no cure for the present plague, however, Dr. Wu focused his energies on identifying plague cases, separating the patients from noncoughing suspects, devising plans for the proper detention of contacts, and teaching people to wear gauze masks properly.[26] In order to "police the sick,"[27] Wu recruited six hundred policemen to be trained in antiplague work, to replace the previously established untrained police.[28] As the plague spread south along the railroad, Wu also suggested that "all railway traffic between Manchuli on the Siberian border and Harbin be strictly controlled."[29] As a result, the Chinese government mobilized its troops to restrict traffic on trains and to deter foot travelers from crossing the Great Wall.

Once the antiplague campaign began to focus on controlling the movement of microbe-carrying patients, the microscope became an indispensable tool for implementing this task because it provided the ultimate criterion for the diagnosis of the plague. First of all, when conducting house-to-house visits in search of plague patients, inspectors were not allowed to fill in "diagnosis of illness" on the registration form unless they had first secured a report of *jingyan*—that is, a microscopic test—from a medical doctor.[30] This form had lines for the result and date of the test. In this sense, the identity of the infectious disease was inseparable from the use of both microscopes and germ theory. For a brief period, the Fengtian Anti-Plague Administration daily published two lists of victims in the local newspaper, one containing the names of documented victims of the plague and the other containing the names of victims suffering from "ordinary diseases." The administration showed a strong concern to differentiate the two kinds of deaths.[31] However, it is hard to believe that the microscope was involved in most of the diagnostic procedures. There were not enough instruments or trained personnel for such a comprehensive effort, and, more importantly, a microscopic test was far from the most cost-effective method for identifying plague patients.

Even ten years after the North Manchurian Plague Prevention Service was established in the wake of the initial outbreak, when another pneumonic plague broke out in Manchuria in 1921, the diagnosis procedure did not require microscopes in every suspected case. The standard procedure for the diagnosis of suspected plague patients admitted by the Harbin Plague Hospital was as follows:

As soon as the patient entered the gate of the compound and after his history had been taken in the open air, he was asked to spit into an earthenware basin. If there was blood in the sputum, if he had fever, if his facies resembled that of patients with plague, and especially if

he staggered in his gait, he was presumed to have plague and was sent
to the plague ward. In case of doubt, the sputum was collected in a
Petri dish . . . and taken to the laboratory for microscopic diagnosis.[32]

Clearly, instead of offering a universal test for every diagnosis of plague,
microscopes actually provided the certainty needed "in case[s] of doubt."[33]
The end result was that doctors did in fact find many patients who were
misdiagnosed, including those with diseases such as pneumonia, influenza,
and tuberculosis, which mimicked several of the symptoms of pneumonic
plague.[34] For the thousands of borderline cases in both 1910 and 1921, only
a microscopic test could unequivocally decide whether they were genuine
cases of the plague.

During the 1910 outbreak, confirmed plague patients were placed in
the plague hospital, while their contacts were sent to emergency detention camps that had been constructed from 120 railway wagons lent by the
Russian-controlled Chinese Eastern Railway. These plague contacts had
their pulses and temperatures taken every morning and evening, and anyone showing fever was at once isolated in a separate wagon. Once bacteriological tests had determined that someone had been infected with the
plague, the person was transferred immediately to the actual plague hospital, where he or she usually died within a couple of days after admission.[35]
Since the mortality rate in plague hospitals was 100 percent, the microscope's function of determining one's disease status gave the instrument the
power to judge matters of life and death.

"The Most Brutal Policies Seen in Four Thousand Years"

The Qing state had empowered the microscope by basing its entire antiplague infrastructure around the capabilities of this tool; in return, the
microscope legitimated the antiplague measures, which, even in the eyes
of Xi Liang, were "the most extreme and brutal policies seen in four thousand years."[36] It quickly becomes apparent why the containment policies of
the Qing government were viewed as brutal. As the historian Carol Benedict has pointed out, in many ways the Chinese response to *wenyi* (warm
epidemics) was very similar to the European response to the plague: both
peoples sought spiritual assistance, found fault with the larger environment,
and tried to shelter themselves from the poisonous atmosphere. In contrast
to the situation in Europe, however, "where government-imposed quaran-

tines directly affected people's lives, the imperial Chinese state did not impose forceful public health measures."[37] In other words, what differentiated the Chinese and Western responses to the plague was exactly the strategy Dr. Wu suggested: rigorous control over people's movements and habits.

The Chinese people strongly resisted the measures implemented during both the Hong Kong and Manchurian plagues. When the British public health authority imposed house-to-house inspections in Hong Kong and removed patients for quarantine to the ship *Hygeia*, several riots broke out among the enraged and fearful local Chinese. There was so much tension that Western doctors felt the need to carry revolvers as they reached the excited neighborhood around Donghua (Tung Wah) Hospital.[38] Furthermore, to escape from the dreadful measures imposed on them, one-third to one-half of the Chinese population fled from Hong Kong to Guangzhou, where the plague was known to be no less rampant.[39] The Chinese residents of Hong Kong apparently feared the antiplague measures more than the plague itself. Most revealingly, after the plague was under control, the Shanghai newspaper *Shen Bao* published two lead editorials urging the municipal government to prepare for a future outbreak of plague. The eight procedures suggested by the editorials all focused on cleaning, including households, streets, food stuffs, and utensils.[40] The editorials never mentioned the need to prepare for isolation stations, which, in contrast, were much emphasized after the Manchurian plague.

In Manchuria, Wu Lien-teh implemented antiplague measures that were much more rigorous and intrusive than those carried out during the earlier Hong Kong plague. With nearly twelve hundred soldiers outside and six hundred policemen on duty inside Harbin, no citizen was allowed to enter or leave his or her designated section, let alone the city limits. In addition to controlling the population, Wu had to contend with the more difficult problem of two thousand unburied corpses already piled on the ground. Stretching over one mile, the corpses could not be buried because the soil had frozen in temperatures of negative thirty degrees Celsius. Given the Chinese reverence for ancestors, Wu did not dare to carry out a mass cremation with anything less than an imperial edict. Throughout the process of plague containment, Wu's greatest concern appeared to be whether the emperor would sanction a mass cremation. Afterward, he often cited the imperial edict granting this as a milestone in the introduction of Western medicine into China.[41]

The majority of the Chinese population—who had no knowledge of the existence of *Pasteurella pestis* and no concern for sovereignty—were horrified to learn that no one taken into detention ever came back alive. In their eyes, Wu's medically directed police action and sanitary measures seemed arbitrary, despotic, and destructive. To fight the plague, Wu allowed the police force to restrict people's movements, interfere with their normal business, burn down their residences and properties, and take away their relatives—all without saving anyone who was infected. Heartbreaking stories testified to the perceived cruelty: to avoid involving family members with despotic police protocols, many plague patients crawled outside their own houses in the middle of the night, to die in the street.[42] In addition, rumors circulated widely throughout the whole ordeal. Some Chinese believed the plague had in fact been created by the poisoning of the wells by Japanese;[43] others claimed that plague patients were being buried alive by the administration. Often it was claimed that traditional Chinese medicine did succeed in curing certain patients.[44] The authority and legitimacy of the plague prevention service was challenged from many directions.

Since Western medicine offered no cure for the plague, Wu and his colleagues had no immediate means to win the trust of the Chinese people. Instead, they had to justify their apparently brutal measures on the basis of absolute necessity. From their point of view, as long as confirmed plague patients were doomed to die, the only option people had was to segregate the sick from the healthy and put the former group in a plague hospital to await their final destiny. The measures undertaken could not cure a single patient, but that was not their intended goal. Rather, by isolating diagnosed carriers of pneumonic plague from the general public, Wu and his colleagues could save many lives by limiting the further spread of the disease. While no one can say with certainty what finally stopped the plague, the total number of plague deaths per month in Harbin dropped from 3,413 to zero in just thirty days after the enforcement of antiplague measures had begun.[45] The somewhat brutal measures were thus the best available solution, even if no one was able to cure those patients infected with plague.

Challenges from Chinese Medicine: Hong Kong versus Manchuria

Practitioners of traditional Chinese medicine took offense at the conclusion, both in Hong Kong and Manchuria, that the plague could not be cured, but they encountered very different forms of the diseases than Western doctors did, and therefore experienced very different results. By claiming success in treating victims of both plagues, some Chinese doctors stood up to challenge the necessity of antiplague measures they perceived as brutal and cruel. On the basis of Chinese medicine, the Chinese-run Donghua Hospital competed with the colonial government in solving the crisis of the Hong Kong plague. The hospital's interference so irritated the colonial governor that he once ordered the gunboat *Tweed* to be anchored opposite Donghua.[46] The challenge was more daunting in Manchuria, where even the local officials at first agreed with lay people that native medicine could be effective in treating plague patients.[47] If that had indeed been the case, by forcing patients to enter plague hospitals, these antiplague measures would have deprived the patients of their only chance of being cured. In this sense, Chinese medicine constituted a serious challenge to the legitimacy of antiplague measures.

Two interesting cases reveal how the microscope played a crucial role in meeting the Chinese doctors' challenge. Told by a Western-style doctor, the first story is about a famous Chinese doctor who was hired by Donghua Hospital because he claimed to possess the ability to treat the plague during the Hong Kong epidemic. After this doctor failed to cure even a single plague patient over the course of a month, he resigned from the post with the explanation that the "plague in Hong Kong was very different from that of other places in China." The Chinese doctor was actually correct in saying so; the plague cases he treated were indeed different. The Western-style doctor went on to remind the reader that "before sending patients to Donghua Hospital, the British health authority always used a microscopic test to make sure they were genuine cases of plague. As a result, this time the Chinese doctor had to deal with the genuine cases and he surely failed in curing anyone."[48] If the famous Chinese doctor had ever enjoyed success in treating "plague" patients in the past, it was because they were not actually plague cases. As the Western-style doctor emphasized, it was crucial for the public health authorities to control the definition of plague with microscopic examinations; otherwise, it would face serious challenges from Chinese doctors and their self-serving and misguided claims of success.

The second case was documented in the official plague report to the Qing court. Early on, when the plague was rampant in Harbin but had not yet reached Fengtian, the antiplague authority rushed to send all the microscopes in Fengtian north to Harbin. As the plague spread south, the resulting microscope shortage required public health officers to identify plague patients by means of manifested symptoms, even when there were "cases of doubt." Since this method unavoidably misdiagnosed some plague patients, lay people got the wrong message that native treatments could cure plague patients. Very soon, local officials started boasting about successful cures and dismissed the modern measures of disinfection and isolation as ineffective.[49] The situation got so out of control that the viceroy had to personally order local officials to restrain from circulating these groundless success stories. In short, only when public health officers had microscopes to help identify the true plague patients—or, to put it more bluntly, only when they made the microscopic test the effective criterion for identifying borderline plague cases—could they convince local officials and the general public of the truth, that pneumonic plague was universally fatal.

It cannot be overemphasized that the two plagues were very different in terms of communicability, virulence, and transmission. Over 2,500 people died during the Hong Kong plague; 60,000 suffered the same fate in Manchuria. Being an airborne disease, the Manchurian plague was transmitted through person-to-person interaction; the bubonic plague in Hong Kong was transmitted indirectly through rat fleas. When Western doctors first learned about the germ theory of the plague in Hong Kong, they did not know that the plague was an insect-borne disease. Nevertheless, they had already recognized that the plague was not a very contagious disease, and direct body-to-body contagion seemed to be an unlikely way for it to spread.[50] Having such different characteristics, the two plagues posed very different challenges to the struggle between modern biomedicine and traditional Chinese medicine.

Perhaps due to the differences between the bubonic and pneumonic strains of plague, Chinese doctors were spared a fatal lesson in Hong Kong but were forced to observe firsthand their ineffectiveness in Manchuria. Throughout the Hong Kong plague, the Donghua Hospital continued to demand that the British government send Chinese patients to a glassworks factory, where Chinese doctors had set up a temporary plague hospital. Until the very end of the outbreak, some local Chinese still preferred medical assistance from traditional Chinese doctors.[51] Neither historical actors nor historians of the Hong Kong plague claim that higher mortality rates occurred as a result of traditional Chinese medical practices. In fact, because the citizens repeatedly debated the efficacy of Chinese medicine in the decade-long plague outbreaks, Henry Blake (1840–1918), the governor of Hong Kong from 1898 to 1904, decided in 1903 to conduct a controlled experiment between patients treated by Western medicine and those treated

by Chinese medicine. To his surprise, the difference between the two medicines in mortality rate was only 1.83 percent. The governor also mentioned a
successful treatment of a plague patient by Chinese medicine, a case which
the principal medical officer approved.[52] The governor concluded that "the
prescriptions given by the Chinese doctors are good, so far as they go."[53]
By contrast, during the Manchurian plague it was suggested that "the fatal
venture of the merchants [with Chinese medicine] was the turning point"
at which the public resistance toward the antiplague measures eased.[54]

This statement was asserted by Dr. Dugald Christie, a Scottish medical
missionary who spent three decades in Manchuria and personally witnessed
those fatal ventures. According to him, the most serious resistance to modern intervention came from local merchants in Fengtian, who found that the
public health measures severely interfered with commerce. To alleviate the
impact on their business, the local Chamber of Commerce decided to establish its own plague hospital and invited Dr. Christie to take charge of its
operation. After he turned down their invitation, the merchants invited two
famous practitioners of Chinese medicine to run their hospital. Clearly these
merchants did not prefer Chinese medicine per se; their concern was mainly
for business. Although the two native doctors treated plague patients with
acupuncture and herbs, their plague hospital did try to observe the modern principle of isolation by separating its compounds into two sections, for
plague patients and for their contacts. Nevertheless, the native doctors did
not bother to wear masks and therefore became infected and carried the
disease to the nonplague ward. Within twelve days, the two native doctors
and their 250 patients and contacts had all succumbed to the plague. Over
all, there was a 50 percent mortality rate among doctors of Chinese medicine in contrast to a 2 percent rate for practitioners of Western medicine.[55]
"It was a costly experiment, but it taught [Fengtian] a lesson," Dr. Christie
concluded.[56]

The tragic sacrifice of human lives was more than the "cost" of the
so-called public experiment; it was perhaps the necessary condition for delivering a valuable lesson.[57] This point becomes evident when we compare
the two plagues. Until recently, for instance, historians and practitioners
of Chinese medicine still suggested that "Chinese medicine was the savior
during the Hong Kong plague" and celebrated the names of the three famous Chinese doctors who courageously served native citizens during the
plague.[58] By contrast, the pneumonic and virulent nature of the Manchurian
plague made similar conclusions impossible in Manchuria. In the final

analysis, the pneumonic plague—"the deadliest of all diseases," in Hirst's words—played a crucial role in the historic defeat of Chinese medicine. Precisely because neither type of medicine could offer any effective cure to individual patients, Western medicine could demonstrate its relative, non-therapeutic strength in diagnosing and containing the plague and defending China's sovereignty.[59]

Chuanran: *Extending a Network of Infected Individuals*

From the evidence presented thus far, it may seem tempting to dismiss traditional Chinese medicine as irredeemably foolhardy. After all, Xi Liang's assertion seemingly displayed a stunning ignorance of facts that we now take for granted: "In the beginning, [we] did not believe that this plague could *chuanran*." This assertion is intriguing because, in light of Angela Leung's chapter in this volume, we know that the Chinese term *chuanran* was regularly used to describe, as she puts it, "the transmission of the same disorder by contact with the sick" from the twelfth century on. By the seventeenth century, it was further used by Wu Youxing (ca. 1580–1669) in the specific context of *wenyi*, which contaminated people "through the mouth and the nostrils."[60] Since Wu dedicated an entire book (*Wenyi lun* [On epidemics due to the warm weather]) to investigating the widespread outbreak of epidemic disease, it is particularly difficult to comprehend Xi's assertion regarding the Chinese reluctance to accept the fact that "this plague could *chuanran*." Fortunately, a plausible answer to this puzzle can be found in Xi's historic speech at the International Plague Conference after the outbreak of the Manchurian plague.

This remarkable speech was much cited as evidence that China finally "acknowledged the superiority of modern medicine over Chinese medicine" because of the Manchurian plague.[61] Right before the paragraph quoted most often, Xi actually suggested that the Manchurian plague was not an ordinary *wenyi*: the disease was something that had been completely novel to the Chinese until three or four months before the epidemic began.[62] By no means did Xi refer to bubonic plague in his statement quoted above. Because the Hong Kong plague had also spread over other areas of China and other countries—including India, Japan, the United States, and Taiwan—there were numerous recent Chinese medical books focusing on the disease of *shuyi* (bubonic plague).[63] In light of this understanding, what Xi's ambivalent assertion really referred to was the pneumonic plague, which was little known at that time even in the West.[64]

In addition to being a disease previously nonexistent in China, there was another sense in which the Manchurian plague transcended the cognitive horizon of the late Qing Chinese—namely, the fact that the specific way in which this new disease spread was almost unthinkable in traditional terms. In her chapter on contagion in this book, Angela Leung meticulously teases out layers of meanings for the term *chuanran*. According to my reading of her chapter, there existed a dichotomy between two meanings of *chuanran*: an acute and widespread outbreak of epidemic or an infection spread through direct and intimate, person-to-person contact. In the first kind of *chuanran*, epidemic diseases were transmitted by way of environmental *qi*—particularly earthy *qi*, as Wu suggested, which could enter people's bodies through the nostrils or mouth. By contrast, the second kind of *chuanran* was most often associated with nonepidemic, even chronic, diseases such as tuberculosis, leprosy, and venereal disease; it was rarely used to describe the spread of epidemic diseases. Hence we see two distinct kinds of meanings of the term *chuanran*, which were associated with two kinds of diseases—differentiable in both degree of communicability and perceived mode of communication. This internal dichotomy of meanings within the term *chuanran* might help to explain the reason why people knew that many diseases tended to *chuanran* but had never grouped these diseases together into a category of infectious diseases.

To summarize, in two separate senses, the Manchurian plague was beyond the horizon of the late Qing Chinese. First, pneumonic plague was a disease totally unheard of; second, the specific way by which the new plague spread was almost unthinkable in traditional terms. Combining two dichotomized meanings of *chuanran* in an unprecedented fashion, the pneumonic plague embodied a new conception of disease: an acute and widespread epidemic that was transmitted by direct and intimate human interaction.[65]

Nothing illustrates this novel connection more clearly than a handful of documentary illustrations called *chuanran xitong tu* (diagrams on the system of *chuanran*). Inserted within the official report on the epidemic, these diagrams were meant to display the systematic ways that plague spread out in various locations in Manchuria.[66] Take, for example, the tragic incident in Mr. Sung's shop in Liaoyang. It began when Sung found two plague corpses left in his courtyard. To avoid interference with his business, Sung and his daughter-in-law hid the corpses under piles of snow and through contact with the bodies, became infected. In less than two weeks, the plague had spread to the neighboring Yang family and took more than fifty lives among the two households. Starting with two anonymous corpses, the diagram on the system of *chuanran* for this case effectively linked fifty plague victims into a network of family members, relatives, neighbors, co-workers, and other residents of the area. As every victim was identified and linked with another, it appeared obvious that every one of them had become infected by contacting another person on the diagram. What went beyond the comprehension of Chinese people was the existence of this type of disease, a virulent epidemic that spread by way of an extended network of infected individuals. No wonder that "in the beginning, [we—i.e., the late Qing Chinese] did not believe that this plague could *chuanran*," because an epidemic that spread like the pneumonic plague had never been witnessed before and was so far beyond the traditional concepts of disease communication.

It is worth pointing out that in this chapter I have intentionally left the term *chuanran* in Xi Liang's statement untranslated, instead of rendering it as either "infection" or "contagion." While the relationship between the conceptions of contagion and infection is complicated and overlapping, "it would generally be assumed that contagion is direct, by contact, and infection indirect, through the medium of water, air, or contaminated articles," as suggested by the historian Margaret Pelling.[67] Drawing on this distinction, the most precise translation of what Xi intended to express is most likely that the Chinese people did not believe that "this plague could spread by contagion." While his intended meaning can be decoded with interpretative efforts, historians should not lose sight of the fact that his statement must have been very puzzling to his contemporaries. It was puzzling because in the Chinese language, one term—*chuanran*—was used to translate both infection and contagion. As a result, although Xi was trying to describe a novel phenomenon whose precise description demanded a distinction between infection and contagion, he was forced to use the term *chuanran*, whose meanings included both contagion and infection. Thus his language neither allowed the existence of the novel phenomenon nor was prepared to describe it. In order to capture the puzzling nature of Xi's assertion and to foreground the related issues of language and translation, I chose to leave *chuanran* untranslated.

No one took to this new knowledge more quickly than those who were physically involved with handling the sick. Having witnessed the horrific ways in which the plague had afflicted their colleagues who had dealt with patients and corpses, these people became deeply convinced of the infectious nature of the Manchurian plague. With this change of belief, according to Xi, resistance to cooperation in the medical management of the plague became a much thornier problem than previously, when people had not believed that the plague was transmitted through human contact.[68] Although the government tried to employ both carrots and sticks, many medical personnel, guards, and workers (for burying corpses) abandoned their posts until they were forced to return by the military or the police. These parallel changes in both belief and behavior reflected the fact that, at least to people involved in containing the plague, a systematic understanding of epidemic infection started taking hold among the Chinese people.

Fundamental differences in the recommendations of Western and Chinese medicine made it impossible to reconcile the two. The former recommended quarantine and isolation, whereas the latter recommended mobility. The systematic view of plague infection no doubt justified Dr. Wu Lien-teh's unconventional measures: if doctors could isolate an individual patient before he or she contacted other people, they could prevent a string of infections and save potential patients from becoming part of the system. In contrast to confining the movement of people, an important traditional Chinese practice for coping with epidemics depended on individual mobility. Since Chinese people during the late Qing period considered plague to be caused by the "earth qi" (*diqi*) of a certain place, they encouraged patients to avoid or even move out of the disease-causing location in the name of *biyi* (avoiding epidemics).[69]

In his 1910 study of the bubonic plague (*Shuyi juewei*), Yu Botao, a famous Chinese doctor and the founder of an important national association of Chinese medicine, documented two styles of *biyi* in a special section devoted to the practice. The first style focused on avoiding the hot and damp spots in one's residence, since Chinese medicine visualized the plague as originating from "hot air arising from the earth like smoke pouring out of the chimney."[70] Even when a patient was found sick with plague, Yu suggested "moving him or her outside of the house to a windy place under a big tree."[71] More important, the patient who was moved outside had to sit in an elevated chair or bed to keep a distance from the "earth qi."[72] Otherwise, moving outdoors would only worsen the situation. Rather than being concerned with the contagiousness of the patient, the author was preoccupied with the dangerous infection coming from the "earth qi."[73] The second style of *biyi* derived from the writings of the famous late-Qing intellectual Yu Yue (1821–1907). Witnessing the practice of *biyi* during plague outbreaks in the 1860s, Yu Yue described the following situation: "Once a patient was found in one household, the nearby dozen families all moved out of the neighborhood. Many were on the road but none could avoid [being infected]."[74] Instead of isolating the patient, dozens of people fled the dangerous place where that dying patient represented the first manifestation of a local epidemic.

While these two ways of *biyi* differ substantially in terms of the scale of movement, they share the concern of escaping from the hot, disease-causing *qi* of the earth. *Biyi* was a strategy designed to avoid a disease based on locality; it did not seek to avoid plague victims. As individuals abandoned their residences and joined an exodus of death, the practice of *biyi* ran the serious risk of putting more people in danger.

In light of the systematic view of plague infection, modern quarantine (*jianyi*) and Chinese *biyi* were two practices in direct confrontation. As a result, forceful implementation of quarantine and isolation meant much more than adopting a new antiplague method; in the case of the Hong Kong plague, the state could be perceived as depriving people of their very last resort. As noted above, after the colonial authorities gave in to Chinese demands for the freedom to leave the colony, eighty thousand people—one-third to one-half of the Chinese population—fled Hong Kong for Guangzhou during the plague. By contrast, during the height of the Manchurian plague, a group of more than ten thousand coolies could not force their way past the Great Wall at Shan Hai Guan because armed troops were on guard.[75] However, when a head-on confrontation seemed unavoidable, the medical officer there, a doctor named Xiao, sought approval from the central government, "if these coolies disobey the rules [against forcing their way through Shan Hai Guan], to be allowed to treat them as bandits and execute them without being charged."[76] Although in the end this horrific policy was not approved by the Ministry of Foreign Affairs, Dr. Xiao's request made clear his determination to control the movement of people coming from the plague-inflicted area.

Unlike the individualist strategy of *biyi*, blocking the network of infection is in the collective interest of the public and demands governmental intervention. As the case of Sung's shop illustrated, just one infected patient could contribute to the spread of disease by failing to cooperate fully with the antiplague authority. To highlight the lessons of this tragedy, the author concluded: "To those who hide corpses from the government and refuse to send contacted relatives to the detention camp, this [tragic incident] is their most serious warning."[77] From the systematic view of plague infection, the task of containing infectious disease went beyond any individual's immediate self-interest but demanded full cooperation from everyone. Once the government realized that "the plague could *chuanran*" by way of extending a network of infected individuals, the government had to take on the task of surveying, classifying, and controlling people, a task never called for in the traditional ways of coping with *wenyi*.

Constituting Notifiable Infectious Disease

To signal the novelty of the Manchurian plague, in many places the official report referred to the plague not with traditional Chinese terms such as *yi* (epidemic), *dayi* (great epidemic), *wenyi* (warm epidemic), or even *shuyi* (bubonic epidemic), but as *baisituo*, which is the Chinese rendition of the Japanese *pesuto*, which itself came from the French *peste*. Both the Chinese and the Japanese terms are transliterations (translations based on sound); the Chinese ideographs involved make no sense at all. In fact, Japan also used the same Chinese character *yi* (pronounced *eki* in Japanese) to call plague until Kitasato isolated *Pasteurella pestis* in Hong Kong. No one would have translated these terms in this way unless their intention was to highlight the complete foreignness of the translated concept.[78] Most importantly, *baisituo* was more than just a new disease to the Chinese; it introduced to the Qing state a new category of disease—*chuanranbing*, or infectious disease.

The category of infectious disease did not exist in traditional Chinese medicine. According to Leung, the traditional disorders often associated with *chuanran*—smallpox, leprosy (*mafeng* or *lai*), syphilis, and consumption—were never grouped together as a distinct category of disease. In premodern Chinese medicine, these diseases were prone to *chuanran*, but they did not constitute *chuanranbing*. The categorical concept of *chuanranbing* may have been introduced into China through the translation of a Japanese medical text. In his *Zhong xi yifang huitong*, published in 1909, Ding Fubao devoted a special chapter to *chuanranbing*, which, quite interestingly, still included almost all of the above-mentioned disorders but none of the major modern infectious diseases such as cholera, typhus, and plague.[79] The situation became very different when Ding made a plea to members of the provincial assembly about the relevance of the antiplague measures to local self-government (*difang zizhi*). At the height of the Manchurian plague, Ding's list of *chuanranbing* consisted of modern epidemics, most of them transliterated from the Japanese. As late as the end of the Qing dynasty, when the reform-minded Ding advocated the concept of *chuanranbing*, he still had different lists for different audiences.

The Chinese government enacted no law concerning the notification of infectious disease. Since the Hong Kong plague had been transmitted from Guangzhou, the British colonial government afterward felt it crucial to be informed of future outbreaks of plague in China. The British decided to seek this information from medical customs at Chinese seaports since the Chinese government did not concern itself with this task.[80] Within the foreign concessions, the Shanghai Office of Hygiene promulgated a regulation requiring notification of infectious disease, but it admitted it had no authority to demand notification from the citizens of Shanghai. As an alternative, it provided a financial reward to Western-style doctors who volunteered to provide the notification, and it subsequently received reports of around three hundred cases per year from 1906 to 1908. Lacking authority to impose quarantine, the sanitary authority tried to convince Chinese citizens that it was in their interest to send infected family members to the hospital; other members would then not have to bear the risk of living with a contagious patient.[81] When plague cases appeared in Shanghai's foreign concessions around the time of the Manchurian plague, the public health authority decided to seriously implement this regulation, and their efforts caused horror and strong resistance among Chinese residents.[82]

To ease the tension caused by antiplague measures, the board of directors of the foreign and Chinese sections of Shanghai held a joint meeting on the regulation of infectious disease. The Western board of directors gave in to almost all of the demands from the Chinese, including "suspending public health measures of quarantine and investigation of all the ordinary infectious diseases."[83] The directors also agreed to relax measures on cholera, smallpox, typhus and all the other notifiable infectious diseases, but they insisted on having one exception: the plague. Instead of allowing suspected plague patients to be sent to Chinese-run hospitals, as their Chinese colleagues demanded, the Western directors insisted on conducting quarantine and investigations on plague with modern medical personnel. As this case indicates, at that time plague was not an ordinary infectious disease for foreigners in China. If only one disease could be legalized as a notifiable infectious disease, it would have to be the plague.[84] It is no wonder that the Manchurian plague turned out to be the pivotal medical event that led the Chinese government to finally promulgate regulations for the prevention of notifiable infectious diseases.

It was not until the end of the Manchurian plague that Xi Liang retro-spectively issued tentative sanitary regulations. Since the regulations were specifically designed for the plague, they did not mention any other infec-tious diseases.[85] Nevertheless, notification of infectious disease lay at the heart of the interim report that the International Plague Conference sub-mitted to the Qing court. Having suppressed the plague epidemic in March 1911, the Ministry of Foreign Affairs decided to capitalize on this success with an International Plague Conference—the first international medical conference held in China, and consisting of delegates from eleven nations, including Kitasato Shibasaburo, the world-renowned Japanese scientist mentioned above. For the purpose of preventing future plague outbreaks in China, the conference passed forty-five resolutions concerning measures that the Qing government should adopt.

The conference participants discussed at length whether to recommend the official formation of a government organization to handle public health issues. They were fully aware that many suggestions would not be put into effect if there were no official with the designated responsibility of carry-ing them out. Some participants found it too idealistic to suggest that China should undertake an institutional reform and establish a central public health service. As one delegate put it, this recommendation impractically "proposes something better than we have in England."[86] Many participants also felt that, as medical scientists, it was beyond their expertise to pass a resolution concerning the reorganization of the Chinese government. On the other hand, the participants were very much concerned about making China an integral part of the global surveillance system over infectious dis-eases, especially the plague.

Starting from the first International Sanitary Conference in 1851, the fun-damental objectives of these international meetings were "to protect Europe from disease importations and to lessen the burden quarantine placed on international trade."[87] While the majority of these conferences focused on protecting Europeans from "Asiatic cholera," the emergence of plague in India "encouraged States to conclude the International Sanitary Convention (ISC) of 1897 dealing with plague"[88] and thereby gave birth to the modern international surveillance system over infectious diseases. Echoing these efforts in monitoring the outbreaks of plague, Dr. Reginald Farrar pointed out during the International Plague Conference of 1911: "Means of notifi-cation can only be had with a government department. Unless you have means of notification, you can not prevent plague."[89] After vigorous debate, representatives reached the following resolution: "With the view of giving effect to these recommendations, every endeavor should be made to organize a central public health department, more specifically with regard to the management and notification of future outbreaks of infectious disease."[90] Instead of recommending an all-embracing project for constructing public health in China, as was often claimed by Dr. Wu Lien-teh and some other scholars, the plague conference recommended that the Qing government institutionalize the notification and management of infectious disease. Partially accepting this suggestion, the newly established Republican government created the North Manchurian Plague Prevention Service in the following year, with Dr. Wu as its director. It is worth pointing out that this service was placed under the direct supervision of the Ministry of Foreign Affairs and was financially supported by the foreign-controlled Maritime Custom Service until 1929.

In 1916, six years after the Manchurian plague, the Republican government promulgated the first "regulation concerning the prevention of infectious disease." The first item stated that only the following diseases were considered *chuanranbing* and therefore subject to this regulation: *huleila* (cholera), *chili* (dysentery), *changzhi fusi* (typhoid fever), *tianran dou* (smallpox), *fazhen zhifusi* (typhus exanthemata), *xinghongre* (scarlet fever), *shifu dili* (diphtheria), and *baisituo* (plague).[91] These eight diseases were exactly the same as the set of diseases regulated by the Japanese colonial government in Taiwan in 1896, and by the government in Japan in 1897.[92] When the Meiji government started to legally recognize and regulate infectious diseases in 1879, its list included only six diseases. Although Japan did not take part in the 1897 International Sanitary Conference that focused on the plague, in that same year the Japanese government added plague and scarlet fever to its official list, thus bringing its total of notifiable infectious diseases to eight.[93] However, not all of these eight diseases were internationally notifiable during that time. As late as the thirteenth International Sanitary Conference in 1926, Japan's proposal that smallpox should be made internationally notifiable was under serious debate. In the event, the convention "provided for notification of *first confirmed cases* of cholera, plague, or yellow fever and of *epidemics* of smallpox and typhus."[94] Instead of following the international convention, the Republican government's list of eight notifiable infectious diseases promulgated in 1916 was clearly a strict copy of the Japanese list.

It is remarkable that just like *baisituo*, all of these eight names were borrowed from Japaneses translation, and at least five of them were simply transliterated. Clearly, when the term *chuanran* was used to translate "infectious disease" into Chinese, its own meaning was substantially transformed by being associated with a new set of diseases. To say the least, this definition of *chuanranbing* excluded almost all of the disorders traditionally associated with *chuanran*, with smallpox being the only exception. The Chinese and Japanese agreed on a crucial point: both individual infectious diseases and their collective category should be marked as a radical novelty in the East Asian medical universe.

Given that this regulation was the first Chinese legal document concerning infectious disease (with the exception of items from the seaport Customs Service), it effectively defined what counted as *chuanranbing* for the government. Instead of presenting a formal definition, the first article of this regulation offered an exclusive list of eight infectious diseases. Following the first article, the regulation made notification of cases of these diseases compulsory for all registered medical practitioners. It also detailed the government's responsibility in coping with these diseases, including many forceful measures that had been implemented during the Manchurian plague. This list was by no means exhaustive; both tuberculosis and syphilis were missing, for example. The main concern of this regulation was to legalize responsibilities, both of the state and of medical practitioners, regarding acute epidemics that might cause social upheaval. Given that the concept of *chuanranbing* was introduced into China mainly through official regulation and public health measures, *chuanranbing* thus became a legal and medical category of the state, a new species of disease against which the state was bound by law to take intrusive measures.

Conclusion

Robert Koch, the father of the germ theory of disease, pointed out that cholera was "our best ally" in the fight for better hygiene,[95] but it apparently took a much more virulent epidemic to serve as the catalyst for public health in China. While previous studies have rightly emphasized the role of geopolitics in transforming the Manchurian plague into a sovereignty crisis for the Qing court, little is known about the factors that turned the Manchurian plague into such a powerful ally. To repeat a quote from the medical historian Charles Rosenberg, we should search for the "unique configuration of social characteristics" of this particular plague that helped to bring about multiple breakthroughs in China's medical history.

First of all, it was very important that the Manchurian plague was a pneumonic plague. Starting with its remarkable 100 percent mortality rate, the pneumonic plague effectively denied Chinese medicine any therapeutic value and demonstrated its powerlessness in containing infectious epidemics. Second, to the late Qing Chinese the pneumonic plague exhibited the most puzzling combination of characteristics: the specific way it spread was very much like chronic or nonepidemic diseases, but in terms of the speed and scope, its transmission was way beyond the most virulent epidemics they had ever experienced. The third, and the most neglected, feature was that the existence of a purely pneumonic plague was also a new phenomenon to the international scientific community. It was during this outbreak that related knowledge was contested and then partially established.

The pneumonic plague, while known to plague experts, was greatly underestimated by the scientific community before the event. As mentioned previously, even after recognizing the pneumonic nature of the Manchurian plague, Dr. Kitasato Shibasaburo repeatedly warned that a bubonic plague might join forces with it when rats woke up from hibernation. It was only after Japanese scientists dissected more than 35,000 rats but found none infected with plague[96] that Dr. Kitasato was forced to admit, during the International Plague Conference, that "the Manchurian plague was a *pure* pneumonic plague—something that had not occurred in recent centuries" (emphasis added).[97] The plague conference opened with twelve scientific questions raised by a Chinese imperial commissioner, the majority of which were related to, if not directly concerned with, the following question: "Why should a bacillus that, as far as we know, has the same microscopic appearance and answers to the same bacteriological tests cause a pneumonic and septicemic epidemic here and only give rise to bubonic plague in India and other places where pneumonic cases occur only incidentally?"[98] Apparently, if Dr. Wu Lien-teh had not been right about the existence of pure pneumonic plague and thus played a pioneering role in advancing scientific knowledge about its nature, it is hard to imagine that the Ministry of Foreign Affairs would have been interested in holding the first international scientific conference in China, let alone having the young Dr. Wu (then only thirty-two years old) serve as its chairman, in the presence of international plague authorities. Later on, in his preface to Dr. Wu's report on the plague, Liang Qichao, arguably the most prominent intellectual in late Qing China, did not hesitate to state: "Science has been imported to China for more than fifty years. The only [Chinese] person who can face the world as a scholar is Dr. Wu."[99] In short, the last reason for the fact that the pneumonic plague served as an ally for promoting public health was because it brought a scientific victory to the Qing court. Dr. Wu's pioneering research on this rare epidemic allowed China for the first time to face the world as a country performing cutting-edge scientific research. In this sense, to go back to the title of this chapter, the new knowledge that was discovered with microscopes — not just those used by Dr. Wu, but also those used by the Japanese scientists searching for the plague bacillus in rat corpses — was crucial in resolving the sovereignty struggle over Manchuria.

The pneumonic plague was indeed a remarkable ally with multiple facets. Given the fact that it had taken such a conjunction of geopolitics and a unique epidemic to make the Qing state realize its ignorance and mistakes, advocates of public health made sure that the state implemented the painful lessons by promulgating regulations and establishing national services for preventing notifiable infectious diseases from spreading in the future.

Practically unknown in China before the event, *chuanranbing* were elevated by the official regulations concerning notifiable infectious diseases from obscurity into the state's official body of knowledge, and its moral as well as legal responsibility.[100] I use the word "constituting" in the subtitle of this chapter because the creation of notifiable infectious disease involved the construction of a new disease category as well as the transformation of *chuanranbing* into a legal institution. As *chuanranbing* emerged as a key issue in the history of medicine in China, it came to be understood as an official definition by the state, used interchangeably with *ba da chuanranbing* (eight main infectious diseases), which was the Chinese term for "notifiable infectious diseases." For Chinese people during the Republican period, *chuanranbing* was very often used in a more restricted sense, identified with these eight notifiable infectious diseases.

In addition to elevating *chuanranbing* to the status of an official governmental category, the state effectively redefined the concept of *chuanranbing* by making the microscopic test and germ theory central to its official identification. The grouping of the eight infectious diseases identified by germ theory — as revealed by their awkward-sounding names, which were improved when the Republican government reissued the regulation concerning infectious diseases in 1928 — signaled a break with the history of traditional Chinese medicine. In fact, the newly constructed official category of *chuanranbing* effectively excluded most of the traditional disorders associated with the term *chuanran*. As the result of this radical reconstruction, when control of *chuanranbing* emerged as the key project for state building, it also became the most salient weakness of traditional Chinese medicine. In the 1930s, when Chinese doctors struggled against Western-style doctors for state support, the state-sanctioned, germ-based *chuanranbing* would pose the most serious challenges for Chinese doctors as they strove to assimilate Chinese medicine into the state medical administration, and to unify the terminologies of Chinese and modern diseases in the name of scientizing Chinese medicine.

I would like to conclude this chapter with a telling example. When He Lianchen (1861–1929), a famous practitioner of Chinese medicine and the founding editor of the most long-lived journal of Chinese medicine, published a monumental compilation of medical case histories in 1929, he divided fourteen volumes into two independent series. The first series consisted of disease cases related to the traditional causes of four seasons and six excesses (*sishi liuyin*); the second was a series of cases of the eight infectious diseases (*bada chuanranbing*). To justify the organization of his compilation, He explained in the preface: "These eight diseases have *chuanran xing* [an infectious nature] and hence are very different from diseases of the Six Excesses. Besides, countries around the world have identified them as *bada chuanranbing*. Therefore, I collected cases of these eight infectious diseases and made a [separate] second series."[101] Because the concept of notifiable infectious disease was increasingly adopted by national governments, as He's remark made clear, Chinese doctors not only had to accept this official category but also employed it as an organizing principle of disease classification.

Three years later, when He was elaborating on the neglected "relationship between [Chinese] medicine and the state," he recalled his personal experience of practicing medicine in San Francisco during the plague outbreak in 1900. Since Chinatown was blamed as the source of this rampant plague, the police besieged it and harshly mistreated its Chinese residents. On the basis of his personal involvement in dealing with epidemic diseases, He emphasized that the most important relationship was indeed the one between medicine and sovereignty (*guoquan*).[102] For the sake of assisting the Chinese state to protect its sovereignty, Chinese medicine had to restructure its etiology in order to be assimilated into the newly emerging global surveillance of infectious diseases, which was designed to assist international commerce. Here we see how directly the modern transnational forces penetrated into the organizing principle of indigenous medicine by way of the state. As revealed in He's innovative efforts, the crucial transformation of Chinese medicine took place not for the sake of either medicine or science per se, but for the dual purpose of integrating China into the global systems of nation-states and capitalism on the one hand,[103] and developing Chinese medicine within such an integrated Chinese state, on the other hand. In sharp contrast, for infectious diseases such as tuberculosis that were not included in the official list, the Chinese people and Chinese doctors were still at much greater liberty to treat them in the ways they saw fit.[104] As this example suggests, if we want to understand the trajectory of traditional Chinese medicine in the twentieth century, we must pay close attention to the hybrid entities jointly created by the state and biomedicine, or—to return to my chapter's title—to the alliance between sovereignty and the microscope.

NOTES

Earlier versions of this chapter were presented at the workshop Epidemics in China (Harvard University, April 2005); the international conference Chinese History from the Perspective of Medical Healing (Academia Sinica, Taipei, December 2005); the 7th East Asian STS Conference (Kobe University, January 2007); the Workshop on Laboratory, STS and Professor Ian Hacking (Tsing-hua University, Hsinchu, November 2007); the 12th International Conference on the History of Science in East Asia (Johns Hopkins University, July 2008); and the Institute of STS Workshop (Yangming University, May 2009). I would like to thank the participants in these meetings for their questions and feedback, especially Ian Hacking, Charlotte Furth, Yungfa Chen, and Angela K. C. Leung, who urged me to think through the crucial dimensions of this history. I would also like to thank two anonymous reviewers for their helpful suggestions and Joseph Boyer and Sabine Wilms for their editorial inputs and devotion to rigorous scholarship. All translations are mine, unless otherwise indicated.

1. Chen, C. C., *Medicine in Rural China*, 20; Croizier, *Traditional Medicine in Modern China*, 45–46; Nathan, *Plague Prevention and Politics in Manchuria, 1910–1931*, 6; and Bowers, "The History of Public Health in China to 1937," 32, respectively.

2. Editorial, *National Medical Journal of China* 2 (1916): 2.

3. Xi et al., "Xuyan," 4. This document is the preface to a two-volume report called *Dongsansheng yishi baogaoshu* [Report on the epidemic in the three eastern provinces], which restarts page numbers at the beginning of every chapter. In the notes to the present article, I therefore give the chapter number after the book title to help identify the cited pages.

4. Rosenberg, "Framing Disease," xviii.

5. Hirst, *The Conquest of Plague*, 220.

6. This is the title of a volume edited by Andrew Cunningham and Perry Williams.

7. Later renamed *Yersinia pestis*.

8. Cunningham, "Transforming Plague," 234.

9. Xi, "Xuyan," 8.

10. Benedict, *Bubonic Plague in Nineteenth-Century China*, 128.

11. Wu Lien-teh, *Plague Fighter*, 18.

12. Nathan, *Plague Prevention and Politics in Manchuria, 1910–1931*. See also Flohr, "The Plague Fighter."

13. Myers, "Japanese Imperialism in Manchuria."

14. Nathan, *Plague Prevention and Politics in Manchuria, 1910–1931*, 50.

15. Rogaski, *Hygienic Modernity*, 187.

16. Wu Lien-teh, *Plague Fighter*, 1.

17. Although Chinese people had long assumed that rats played a role in spreading the plague, it was after the Hong Kong outbreak that transnational scientific elites reached the consensus that rat fleas transmitted the bubonic form of plague.

18. Wu Lien-teh, *Plague Fighter*, 12.

19. Hirst, *The Conquest of Plague*, 221.

20. Wu Lien-teh, *Plague Fighter*, 22.

21. Ibid., 12.

22. In response to outbreaks of plagues in India, an International Sanitary Convention was passed in 1903 which provided for the first time "for the destruction of rats on board ship as a protective measure against plague" (Howard-Jones, *The Scientific Background of the International Sanitary Conferences 1851–1938*, 85).

23. "Lun fangyi xingzheng yiji zhuyi bushu," *Shengjing Shibao*, January 21, 1911.

24. "Beili boshi yanshuoci," *Shengjing Shibao*, February 24, 1911.

25. Nathan, *Plague Prevention and Politics in Manchuria, 1910–1931*, 32.

26. Wu Lien-teh, *Plague Fighter*, 19.

27. Benedict, *Bubonic Plague in Nineteenth-Century China*, 163–64.

28. According to both Wu Lien-teh's recollection and the governmental report, the sanitary police established before the outbreak were not very useful in containing the plague. Wu specifically pointed out the need "to ensure better control by replacing, as far as possible, the untrained police in the routine inspection and report work by the trained medical staff. The police, thus released, could return to their proper lay duties" (*Plague Fighter*, 23). After the plague, on many occasions Wu also openly criticized those sanitary police who knew nothing about modern methods of hygiene except street cleaning. For the reasons why sanitary police were preoccupied with street cleaning, see Yu Xinzhong's fascinating chapter in this volume on night soil.

29. Wu Lien-teh, *Plague Fighter*, 12.

30. Zhang Yuanqi et al., *Dongsansheng yishi baogaoshu* 2, no. 2: 112.

31. "Diyi biao: Yibing huangzhe biao" and "Dier biao: Xunchang jibing siwang biao," *Shengjing Shibao*, January 25, 1911.

32. J. W. H. Chen, "Pneumonic Plague in Harbin," 13.

33. I would like to thank Professor Chen Yongfa and an anonymous reviewer for pushing me on the issue as to what degree the lab-based model of diagnosis, as claimed in the *Dongsansheng yishi baogaoshu* was a reality rather than an expressed ideal.

34. J. W. H. Chen, "Pneumonic Plague in Harbin," 14.

35. Wu Lien-teh, *Plague Fighter*, 27.

36. Xi, "Xuyan," 8.

37. Benedict, *Bubonic Plague in Nineteenth-Century China*, 130.

38. Sinn, *Power and Charity*, 164.

39. Sutphen, "Not What, but Where," 93.

40. "Fanghuan weiran shuo," *Shen Bao*, June 4 and 8, 1894, cited in Cao S. and Li, *Shuyi: Zhangzhen yu heping*, 346–7.

41. Wu Liande, *Dongsansheng fangyi shiwu zongchu daquanshu* 3:108 and 4:116.

42. In sharp contrast, according to J. M. Atkinson, Principal Civil Medical Officer in Hong Kong during the plague there, Chinese residents dumped the bodies of the sick and deceased onto the streets in that city. It was estimated that the proportion of bodies of plague victims that was dumped increased from 25.1 percent in 1898 to 32.7 percent in 1903 as a result of a 1903 law requiring the disinfection of houses on either side of those in which plague-infected rats had been found. See Atkinson, *A Historical Survey of Plague in Hong Kong*, 23.

43. This might be the precursor of the circulation of rumors about Japanese medicine in Manchuria, as discussed in Ruth Rogaski's chapter in this volume.

44. "Sheiwei yibing guo buke zhi ye?" *Shengjing Shibao*, January 19, 1911, and "Jingyou rushi zhi zhongyi hu?" ibid., February 23, 1911.

45. Wu Lien-teh, *Plague Fighter*, 25.

46. Sinn, *Power and Charity*, 170.

47. Zhang Yuanqi et al., *Dongsansheng yishi baogaoshu*, 1: 33.

48. Liang Peiji, "Shang fangbian yiyuan lun zhiyi fangyi shu." It is in fact unlikely that this story took place during the plague outbreak of 1894. The 1894 epidemic began in May and ended in August; Dr. Kitasato discovered the plague bacillus on June 14 of the same year. If this event had taken place during 1894, the British public health officers would have had to put into practice this new scientific knowledge within just one month of the discovery. Since in the ten years following the first outbreak in 1894, bubonic plague recurred more or less regularly in Hong Kong, it is highly likely that this event took place at a later time, if it indeed took place at all.

49. Zhang Yuanqi et al., *Dongsansheng yishi baogaoshu* 2, no. 2: 11.

50. Sutphen, "Not What, but Where," 100–101.

51. Sinn, *Power and Charity*, 180.

52. Blake, *Bubonic Plague in Hong Kong*, 6.

53. Ibid., 8.

54. Christie, *Thirty Years in Moukden, 1883–1913*, 250.

55. Bowers, *Western Medicine in a Chinese Palace*, 25.

56. Christie, *Thirty Years in Moukden, 1883–1913*, 250.

57. It is worth pointing out that if the Chinese doctors had worn gauze masks and strictly obeyed the modern rules of infection and isolation, just as Chinese doctors did in treating SARS patients in Guangdong in 2003, they would not have received such a fatal lesson in Manchuria. It is very interesting to compare the two epidemics: both involved highly virulent infectious diseases, but they led to two very different evaluations of traditional Chinese medicine. See Marta Hanson's chapter in this volume on SARS and traditional Chinese medicine.

58. Xie Yongguang, *Xianggang zhongyiyao shihua*, 297.

59. Hirst, *The Conquest of Plague*, 220. See also Wu Lien-teh, *Plague Fighter*, 48.

60. Wu Youxing, *Wenyi lun*, 11.

61. See, for example, Nathan, *Plague Prevention and Politics in Manchuria, 1910–1931*, 6.

62. "We Chinese have believed in an ancient system of medical practice, which the experience of centuries had found to be serviceable for many ailments, but the lessons taught by this epidemic, which until practically three or four months ago had been unknown in China, have been great, and have compelled several of us to revise our former ideas of this valuable branch of knowledge" (Xi, quoted in Wu Lien-teh, *Plague Fighter*, 49).

63. For examples, see Li Yushang, "Jindai Zhongguo shuyi duiying jizhi."

64. Hirst, *The Conquest of Plague*, 220–53.

65. I would like to thank Angela Leung for sharing with me her thoughts about this ambivalent assertion. Professor Leung has told me that many Western scholars found it puzzling that the Chinese concept of *chuanran* often developed along with diseases such as leprosy and smallpox, but not with the plague, which was seminal in the European notion of contagion. Her insightful remark stimulated me to think through the issue here, but the responsibility for this analysis completely belongs to me. I would like to point out that both Barbara Volkmar and T. J. Hinrichs discovered a medical/moral controversy between contagionists and anti-contagionists with regard to the appropriate response to epidemics. The contagionists in the twelfth century seemed to argue that an epidemic could be transmitted by way of direct human contact. While a more detailed discussion of the differences between my argument and their important discoveries is beyond the scope of this article, I think that it is partially caused by the lack of differentiation between contagion and infection in Chinese language.

66. Zhang Yuanqi et al., *Dongsansheng yishi baogaoshu*, 1, no. 5: 1–7.

67. Pelling, "The Meaning of Contagion," 15.

68. Xi, "Xuyan," 5.

69. Fang Xingzhun, *Zhonguo yufang yixue sixiang shi*.

70. Yu Botao, *Shuyi juewei*, 422.

71. Ibid., 423.

72. Ibid.

73. Ibid., 418.

74. Quoted in Carney Fisher, "Zhongguo lishi shang de shuyi," 706.

75. See ibid., 724.

76. Telegram from the viceroy of Zhili, January, 28, 1911, quoted in Peng W., "Qingdai Xuantong nianjian Dongsansheng shuyi fangzhi yanjiu," 69.

77. Zhang Yuanqi et al., *Dongsansheng yishi baogaoshu* 1, no. 5: 4.

78. This revealing phenomenon was pointed out by Bridie Andrews in "Tuberculosis and the Assimilation of Germ Theory in China, 1895–1937," 131.

79. Ding, *Zhong xi yifang huitong*, 96–134.

80. W. Simpson, *Report on the Causes and Continuance of Plague in Hong Kong and Suggestions as to Remedial Measures*.

81. "Chuanranbing."

82. "Shanghai jianyi fengchao shimoji," *Dongfang zazhi* 11, no. 7 (1910), 348–51.

83. Ibid.

84. Later on, when John Grant and his colleague set up a health demonstration station in Beijing, they found that in comparison to all the other communicable diseases, Chinese people expressed a distinctively different attitude toward the plague, "which is feared by everyone and consequently makes it possible to take . . . strict measures of control" (First Annual Report—Health Station 1925–1926, Appendix A, p. 7, record group 5, series 3, box 218, folder 2734, Rockefeller Archive Center).

85. Zhang Yuanqi et al., *Dongsansheng yishi baogaoshu* 1, no. 1: 12–17.

86. *International Plague Conference*, 363.

87. Fidler, *International Law and Infectious Diseases*, 12. I would like to thank an anonymous reviewer and Charlotte Furth for raising the question of the international origin of notifiable infectious diseases, and Ruth Rogaski for this reference.

88. Ibid., 30.

89. *International Plague Conference*, 362.

90. Ibid., 397.

91. Zhang and Xian, 10.

92. Liu Shiyung, " 'Qingjie,' 'weisheng,' yu 'baojian,' " 57.

93. Koseishō Imukyoku, *Isei hachijūnen shi*, 377. I would like to thank Liu Shiyung for this reference. It is intriguing that the Japanese government in Taiwan declared the set of infectious diseases one year earlier than the government in Japan itself. Unfortunately, research on this issue is beyond the scope of this article.

94. Howard-Jones, *The Scientific Background of the International Sanitary Conferences 1851–1938*, 96–98.

95. Quoted in Ackerknecht, *A Short History of Medicine*, 211.

96. Iijima, *Pesuto to gendai Chūgoku*, 188.

97. Quoted in "Beili boshi gongyan ge daibiao zhi yanci," *Shenjing Shibao*, April 6, 1911.

98. Wu L., *Plague Fighter*, 51. I would like to thank the philosopher Ian Hacking for posing this factual question to me. It motivated me to think through both the new scientific knowledge created (and contested) during this event, and the role that this knowledge played in shaping the course of the event.

99. Quoted in Yu-lin Wu, *Memories of Dr. Wu Lien-teh*, 96–97.

100. Careful readers might notice that here I use *chuanranbing* to replace "notifiable infectious disease" in the chapter subtitle. Notifiable infectious disease is no doubt a much narrower and more technical category than *chuanranbing*. Nevertheless, because the term *chuanranbing* acquired social currency through the state's official regulations and antiplague measures, these two terms were often used interchangeably during the time under study. At least, when the Republican government promulgated the first "regulation concerning the prevention of infectious disease" in 1916, the phrase used was *chuanranbing* rather than *fading chuanranbing*, the Chinese counterpart for notifiable infectious disease. I use "notifiable infectious disease" in the subtitle mainly to highlight the legal and institutional nature of this disease category.

101. He L., *Quanguo mingyi yan'an leibian*, 1–2.

102. He L., "Yixue yu guojia guanxi lun," 16.

103. For a general discussion on how transnational forces shaped the formation of the Chinese nation, and how China's local tendencies reshaped global forms in the country, see Duara, *The Global and Regional in China's Nation-Formation*.

104. Sean Hsiang-lin Lei, "Why *Weisheng* Is Not about Guarding Life."

Part II

Colonial Health and Hygiene

Eating Well in China

Diet and Hygiene in Nineteenth-Century Treaty Ports

Shang-Jen Li

In *Shanghai Hygiene,* a medical manual written for Europeans in China, the medical missionary James Henderson claimed that "of all the various prolific sources of disease, irregularities of diet are the most powerful; of all the means of cure at our disposal, attention to the quality and quantity of the ingesta are most important."[1]

During the nineteenth century, most British medical practitioners[2] in China shared Henderson's emphasis on the importance of diet for the maintenance of health. They repeatedly stressed the importance for foreigners of eating in a proper manner when living in China. Many of them were also keen observers of Chinese dietary customs and discussed extensively the healthiness, or lack thereof, of Chinese food. British medical practitioners' concerns about diet were rooted in a long European medical tradition. The Galenic six "non-naturals"—food and drink, sleep and waking, air, evacuation and repletion, motion and rest, and the passions—had long been regarded by European medical practitioners as essential factors in the maintenance of health.[3] Among these, diet was often given particular emphasis.[4] British medical practitioners had also drawn on the abundant medical literature advising Europeans in respect to hygiene while living in exotic environments.

In this chapter, I examine nineteenth-century British medical views on food, drink, and personal hygiene in China—especially the relation between diets and climates—and analyze the way theories of tropical hygiene formed the framework upon which the medical discussions of food and health in China were conducted. Current scholarship of colonialism argues that food not only formed an important part of European hygienic discourse and practice but was also a crucial aspect of European physical experiences of other cultures at the time of imperial expansion. Diet was an important component in the making of national and racial identity. In an imperial context, dietary customs often served as an important marker that distinguished the European from the other. Changing attitudes toward local food often indicated broader shifts in European positions, imperial policy, and colonial rule.[5]

Chinese Climates, European Diet

Until the mid-nineteenth century, direct commercial contact between Europe and China was largely confined to Macao, a Portuguese concession, and Canton (now Guangzhou), the only Chinese port open to European trade. The Nanjing Treaty, which concluded the First Opium War (1839–42), opened another four ports in addition to Guangzhou to foreign trade, set a fixed tariff, and gave Hong Kong to Britain. The Tianjin Treaty and the Beijing Convention, which concluded the Second Opium War (1856–60), opened more ports to commerce, permitted Europeans to travel inland in China, and stipulated that the Chinese Maritime Customs should be administered by a British inspector general.[6] Sizable European settlements gradually formed at these coastal and riverine ports, serving as the bases for Western traders keen on expanding commerce in China and for missionaries endeavoring to convert the Chinese. With an increasing number of Europeans in China, their health problems also attracted the attention of the British medical practitioners. Following the Hippocratic tradition, these men paid careful attention to the influence of Chinese environments on European health.[7] As early as the First Opium War, the perceived harmful effects of Chinese climates upon the health of British soldiers and sailors had caused medical concern. The staff surgeon T. Nelson conducted a statistical study of morbidity and mortality rates of British troops in China during both Opium Wars, and the figures were alarming: "The amount of sickness which prevailed from 1840 till 1843 on the Chinese station was indeed formidable, and produced an effect on the mind of Englishmen at home which can yet be readily traced in their estimate of the Chinese climate."[8] The Chinese climate was an obstacle to the consolidation of British military supremacy over China.

After the establishment of the treaty ports brought about more stable and comfortable living conditions in the European settlements, the alarm over

European mortality rates subsided. However, concerns about the effects of the Chinese climate on European health persisted. A number of British medical practitioners, especially those who served as medical officers in the Chinese Maritime Customs, held that the climatic conditions of China were similar to the dangerous climate of the tropics, despite the fact that most Chinese territory was not within tropical zones. Indeed, one customs medical officer stated: "There is very little of the temperate climate in any part of China, and this is true of Asia generally."[9] Another physician, Robert Alexander Jamieson, stated: "At certain seasons the conditions that surround us resemble those which constantly exist in regions proverbially fatal to European life, such as the West Coast of Africa."[10]

Customs medical officers believed that Europeans in China, just like those in other exotic and "tropical" countries, were vulnerable to its climatic influences and susceptible to certain diseases. The danger of this kind of extreme climate, Dr. A. G. Reid argued, was that it "lower[s] vitality through excessive heat, cold and humidity," and the "combined action of heat, moisture, and decomposing animal or vegetable matter under certain climatic conditions" created favorable conditions for the growth of "exciting causes" of diseases.[11] Heat was not the only problem. The extreme, unstable Chinese climate could do great harm by its sudden changes. Dr. John Dudgeon reported that the "Peking climate includes the extremes of heat and cold" and that "as a Rule," moreover, "where the cold is excessive, the rise of temperature in spring and summer is sudden and intense."[12] He claimed that "sudden changes of temperature sometimes experienced at the hills, especially during the cold nights which occasionally set in after or during the rain and when it is impossible to guard against such vicissitudes have had to do with attacks of diarrhea and dysentery."[13] It was not simply heat or cold that induced diseases among Europeans in China, but rather the sudden alternations from one to the other. Indeed, what was often referred to as "seasoning" meant not merely the adaptation of the European constitution to hot climates, but also to the different cycle and rhythm of climatic changes in exotic environments.[14]

As David Arnold argues, "calling a part of the globes 'the tropics' . . . was a Western way of defining something culturally and politically alien, as well as environmentally distinct, from Europe and other parts of the temperate zone." The tropics were not only a "physical space" but also a "conceptual space."[15] Some British medical practitioners described Chinese climates as tropical in order to register their otherness. To depict the Chinese climate as tropical also indicated that the theoretical outlook, intellectual framework, and practical measures provided by British medical practitioners were significantly informed by the medical theories developed in the tropical colonies, especially India. Henderson, for example, modeled *Shanghai Hygiene* on James Ronald Martin's *The Influence of Tropical Climates on European Constitutions* and frequently quoted Martin, James Johnson, and other British medical authorities in India.[16] Anglo-Indian medical literature also provided important references when British medical practitioners discussed the relation between diet and European health in China.

Since the seventeenth century, medical advice for travelers had stated that to preserve their health, Europeans staying in exotic environments should pay particular attention to their modes of life. British medical practitioners almost unanimously accepted the view that Chinese climates made this necessary. But they tended to be less pessimistic with regard to European acclimatization in China than their colleagues in India, who after the mid-nineteenth century were convinced that it was nearly impossible for Europeans to become acclimatized to the tropics.[17] Some of the British practitioners asserted that with proper precautions, the British could enjoy their health: "If men would be careful not to walk unguarded in the sun, and to eat and drink lightly, and to avoid catching chills, there would be comparatively little for the doctor to do."[18] The medical officer of Fuzhou reported that the oldest European male resident there was also the healthiest and asserted that "if a man is rationally careful of himself in Foochow [Fuzhou], he has more chance of living long than in England, and with, perhaps, few bodily ailments."[19]

British medical practitioners in China considered that a proper dietary regimen, often different from that in Europe, was essential for Europeans to lead a healthy life in China. The consequence of immoderation was said to be "more frequently and suddenly fatal, on account of the additional hurtful conditions introduced by the malarious atmosphere and the violence of the solar influence."[20] This opinion was of course commonplace in discussions of tropical hygiene. Drs. Müller and Manson suggested that many European ailments resulted from immoderation: "The inevitable sherry and bitters, brandy and soda, and full animal diet indulged in three times a day combined with want of exercise and a rather high temperature, induce disease which is hardly climatic although the victim may call and think it so."[21] They claimed indulgence "in too high living" was a major cause of diseases such as "tropical abscess of the liver" and "aneurism of the thoracic aorta" among the Europeans in China, noting that these diseases were seldom seen among the natives.[22] Jamieson lamented that the "foreign community in Shanghai, who, while they deny themselves no luxury which money can procure, are apparently insensible to the dangers whose avoidance is a necessity." He believed that the "alarming frequency and fatality of disease of the circulatory system among foreigners in China" should make them inspect their lifestyle. "It should be ever borne in mind," Jamieson warned, "that there are many things which may with impunity be done in Europe but which no person of prudence will attempt to do here."[23]

The medical criticism of the dietary habits of Europeans in China was similar to that of their compatriots in India in an earlier period. In the early nineteenth century, it was commonly held that the British in India not only ate excessively but also habitually consumed extravagant amounts of meat and alcohol, to the detriment of their health.[24] Some explorers and naturalists with experiences in other torrid zones such as Africa, the Amazon, and the Malay Archipelago expressed similar opinions. In his article on acclimatization, Alfred Russel Wallace argued that "the English, who cannot give up animal food and spiritous liquors, are less able to sustain the heat of the tropics than the more sober Spaniards and Portuguese."[25] It is unclear whether the Chinese considered European dietary habits extravagant, though that was probably the case. The mandarin Hang-Ki (Heng Qi) told the physician David F. Rennie and his interpreter Thomas Wade of the British legation that early in the morning he always took "some tea and confectionery" for breakfast, and then had a "light lunch" at noon and enjoyed "a meal containing animal food" at sunset. "Nothing else is taken during the twenty-four hours," Hang-Ki said, "unless it should be necessary to sit up late, when all that is indulged in is a little water that rice has been boiled in." According to Rennie, Hang-Ki considered such dietary practice crucial for achieving health and longevity and also held that "the Chinese are longer lived than Europeans," though he attributed "it to the latter being of more anxious and excitable temperaments than the former."[26]

Not every European in China, of course, consumed rich food regularly. Some of the missionary societies, for example, emphasized the importance of eating moderately in China, both for economical and hygienic reasons.[27] The missionaries also avoided extravagant consumption of food because that practice would put them in an unflattering light in the eyes of both the Chinese and their supporters at home. Some missionary organizations such as Hudson Taylor's China Inland Mission preferred eating Chinese food to ingratiate themselves with the Chinese. Other missionaries, however, chose to adhere to European cuisine and instructed their Chinese servants to cook Western meals.[28]

Medical criticism of overconsumption of animal dishes was usually directed at merchants, who might well have been indulging in that way deliberately, as a result of their aspiration to become what Benedict Anderson has described as "bourgeois aristocracy." Anderson argues that the Europeans of bourgeois and petit bourgeois backgrounds in the colonies tried to elevate their status and affirm their superiority by living in a luxurious and pompous manner in imitation of the aristocracy at home.[29] The cheaper cost of living in China also allowed Europeans with modest means to enjoy rich, meaty food and other luxuries that they could hardly afford at home. In the mid-nineteenth century, an English language student once described China as "truly a marvelously cheap country" while boasting of his gentlemanly lifestyle.[30] John Fryer, an English missionary from a humble social background who later gave up preaching to work as a translator for the Chinese government, informed his parents that he had radically changed his mode of life: "China has cured me of homeopathy and teetotalism. I believe in good exercise, good food, a glass of wine and two glasses of beer a day with plenty of beefsteak and eggs. Now and then a regular clear out with aperient medicine is all that I think one requires."[31] Regular consumption of "good food," which in the English culinary culture of that period meant a diet rich in meat, was an indication of improved social status for persons like Fryer.[32]

The medical practitioners, however, considered such dietary practices to pose serious threats to European health, and they provided advice with regard to healthy diets in China. The medical officer of the maritime customs at Fuzhou in 1871, J. R. Somerville, recommended "light, sound claret" as "the best beverage for table use in the hot season." "Malt liquor" might be beneficial to some but detrimental to others, depending on their constitutions. Somerville was not sure whether smoking tobacco was good for European health or not.[33] The recommendation of claret was consistent with most manuals on tropical hygiene.[34] According to J. Lane Notter, "the vegetable acids in light wines" could "prevent scurvy" and facilitate digestion; such wine also acted as a prophylaxis against cholera.[35] Charles Heaton also considered claret as "by far the best wine for a hot climate" because it was a "cooling drink." According to Heaton, claret was also "a blood making wine" because it contained "a small quantity of iron," and this rendered it peculiarly suitable for the tropics.[36] Somerville's somewhat eclectic advice on the consumption of beer and tobacco can also be understood in the context of the diverse medical opinions and disagreements with regard to the effects of these substances on the European constitution in the tropics. Joseph Fayrer argued that smoking "often injures the nervous system, interferes with digestion, depresses the mental as well as the physical, and muddles the intellectual powers."[37] Notter suspected that beer was rather harmful to Europeans in a hot climate.[38] W. J. Moore argued that tobacco was not as harmful as some authors assumed, but that it was not very beneficial to European health either. Among the few health benefits of tobacco, according to Moore, was that it functioned, to some extent, as a "prophylactic measure" in malarial areas.[39] With regard to the consumption of alcohol, Moore argued that "some stimulant is *actually necessary* to most Europeans in hot weather, when the heart labours and the vital energy is exhausted; and also in the autumnal season, when the physical powers are at a minimum, and malaria most prevalent." He considered malt liquors the best stimulating beverage for Europeans because they were "taken with meals, and therefore not applied to an empty stomach." Apparently, moreover, malt liquors were not "absorbed directly into the portal circulation and liver, as is the case with spirits" and hence were less harmful to the liver. Malt liquors also had a certain tonic effect that was good for Europeans working in warm climates.[40] Heaton, on the other hand, had some reservations about the health benefits of beer. He argued that beer "is a fine bitter tonic when taken in moderation, but is apt to cause indigestion, unless combined with plenty of exercise."[41]

As already pointed out, when British medical practitioners called a place "tropical," the designation had racial and moral connotations. Europeans often described the natives of the tropics as sensuous beings who indulged in nature's abundance and carnal pleasures, and often attributed the perceived moral laxity of the natives to the influence of tropical climates: "The tropical world had its own moral economy which corresponded with the character of its people."[42] This moral economy, moreover, was closely related to Europeans' own sense of identity. Ann Stoler claims that the affirmation of European supremacy "was underscored by a more explicit discourse and set of policies that tied the self-disciplining of individual colonial Europeans to the survival of all Europeans in the tropics and thus to the biopolitics of racial rule."[43] Hygienic advice on food and drink for Europeans in the tropics was often dispensed in a moralizing tone. In his exhortation against intemperance, for example, Martin argued that "the inebriate has

always been justly considered as not merely culpable in destroying his individual health, but as deteriorating the European character in the eye of the
natives, whom it is on all accounts desirable to impress with a just sense of
our superiority."[44] Moderation in food and drink formed an essential part
of self-discipline in the tropics that asserted and underlined European distinction.

Diet and Chinese Racial Character

Besides repetitively advocating dietary regimens for Europeans, several
British medical practitioners in China studied Chinese dietary habits. Their
observations and discussions took place at a time when British medical
views toward oriental customs were becoming increasingly critical. Several important studies of British colonial medicine in India argued that in
the eighteenth and early nineteenth centuries, British medical practitioners
were willing to learn from native customs and indigenous medicine. By the
late nineteenth century, European attitudes toward this issue had changed,
and many of the British medical practitioners in India no longer considered
indigenous knowledge of hygiene valuable.[45]

This deterministic view was shared by a few British medical practitioners in China. Most prominent among them was Patrick Manson, who spent
his early career in China and, after returning to Britain, became medical
advisor to the Colonial Office and founded the London School of Tropical
Medicine.[46] Manson was firmly opposed to the suggestion that the British
should adopt Chinese habits in order to adapt to the climate of China. This
was useless, according to Manson, because the characteristics of a race were
the results of the process of natural selection that worked over many generations: "Appetites bred through many generations become instincts, and
an Englishman must have his beef."[47] Manson's rejection of native food was
in accord with Fayrer, who stated:

> While enjoining moderation, I do not mean that I advise you to copy
> the natives of the country entirely of their food; you cannot altogether
> change your mode of living or the character of your aliment. Your
> stomach will no more obtain from the diet of a Hindoo all that is nec-
> essary for nutrition—though it may contain it—than it could in other
> circumstances from the blubber that delights while it nourishes an Es-
> quimo. Habit, in these things, becomes hereditary, and our machinery
> is not adapted for sudden change.[48]

Among British medical practitioners in China, Manson provided the most systematic discussion of the formation of racial constitution. As David Livingstone points out, arguments about hygiene and acclimatization were often construed in terms of natural selection and evolutionary struggle.[49] Manson framed his discussion of disease, diet, and the formation of racial constitutions precisely in this way. He utilized the theory of evolution to explain the origin of different racial constitutions and to account for the natives' possession of high immunity to certain diseases:

> The principal influences directing the development of the permanent characters of any race of men are undoubtedly the climate and the physical characters of the country it inhabits, the food it is nourished by, and the diseases that destroy or impair it. These are the great agents of natural selection; the fittest to survive under these operations propagate the race and constitute its types. This is but an extension of the Darwinian hypothesis of the formation of the variety of men, and to a certain extent has been explained by Buckle in his *History of Civilization.*[50]

Among these "agents" of natural selection, Manson considered that food and disease were of the greatest importance.[51]

Manson credited Henry Thomas Buckle (1821–62) with extending Darwin's principle to explain the variety in the human race. This betrays Manson's eclectic understanding—even misreading—of Darwin, since Buckle's outlook could be better characterized as pre-Darwinian progressivist.[52] Manson accepted Buckle's emphasis on the importance of food, but Darwin explicitly denied that food played any significant role in the formation of races.[53] Following Buckle's view and giving a twist to his argument, Manson explained racial differences so as to also explain white men's vulnerability to tropical disease and to prove European superiority: "The savage races exist by adapting themselves to circumstances, the more highly civilized races by adopting circumstances to themselves."[54] Non-Europeans were dominated by nature, while Europeans dominated nature. The perception of European susceptibility to diseases in exotic environments was an essential component of the racial identity of Europeans. Their low immunity against some tropical diseases was not a sign of degeneration, but on the contrary proved the supremacy of European civilization. As Mark Harrison says, "feelings of superiority and vulnerability were two sides of the same imperial coin."[55]

Although the Chinese had acquired higher immunity to malaria, most of them suffered from anemia. Manson observed two forms of anemia in China. One was caused by antecedent disease—that is, malarial anemia—and the other resulted from poor diet. The etiology of the two forms of anemia corresponded to Manson's two great agents of natural selection, disease and food. He concluded that universal anemia had profound influences on the racial characteristics and customs of the Chinese. Manson claimed that missionaries often sent their sick Chinese students to him for consultation or treatment, and he subsequently found that these students all suffered from anemia. He described their condition as follows:

> Taken young from the country, selected on account of their superior intelligence and physique, they at first appear eminently qualified for the life of study and originality before them. Yet in a few months many of them pine, languish, "sicken of vague disease," and are obliged to relinquish their new life and studies, from sheer exhaustion of brain and energy.[56]

These young men were "exhausted by the novelty of their work, unable from their anaemia to adapt themselves to new conditions and habits of life." Manson believed that the Chinese could only follow centuries-old routines like tilling "the same field in the same manner," or carrying "the same sort of burden the same way and over the same road." They were incapable of doing anything new because the nourishment in their systems was not enough for coping with new things. Manson inferred that aspects of the Chinese national character such as "the strong conservative propensities, the superstitious reverence for the precedent, the patience under oppression, [and] the unprogressive character of their science and arts" were "expressions of incapacity for change, for adaptation, for originality." They were the consequence of anemia, rather than the "deliberate elections of philosophic experience."[57]

With this quasi-Darwinian evolutionary account, Manson was able to provide a naturalized explanation of both the racial immunity and national character of the Chinese.[58] Moreover, he was able to accommodate both the biological boundary of races and the traditional idea of environmental modification of constitutions. Diet and disease influenced racial constitution, but the resultant racial traits were the product of the long time span of evolution; hence, there was a solid biological basis for racial differences that could not be changed within a few generations. According to Manson, there was no reason that the British in China should eat a Chinese diet, the low quality of which was amply demonstrated by the inferiority of the Chinese racial constitution, which resulted from the persistence of such a diet for generations.

Dietary Habits and Diseases of Civilization

Nevertheless, there were British medical practitioners who supported the view that Europeans in China should adopt the diet of the Chinese. Among them, John Dudgeon (1837–1901), a medical missionary of the London Missionary Society who also served as medical officer to the Chinese Imperial Maritime Customs, was the most vocal in praising the health benefits of Chinese food. In his survey of the hygienic conditions of Beijing, Dudgeon stated: "We may safely assert that the Chinese, on the whole, in regard to eating and drinking, clothing and habits generally, have found out the secrets of long and healthy life in tropical regions, namely, keeping cool, being moderate in diet, and cultivating tranquil habits of body and mind."[59] Dudgeon held that many Chinese customs were much better for health than their European counterparts. He argued that although "there are failings in the Chinese system," anyone who knew China well "will admit that the Chinese, notwithstanding their ignorance of our science, have admirably suited themselves to their surroundings, and enjoy a maximum of comfort and health and immunity from disease which we should hardly have supposed possible."[60] He recommended that Europeans learn from the ancient wisdom of the Chinese, the value of which had been proven by the mere fact that China had outlived most ancient civilizations. "This ancient Oriental people," Dudgeon said, had "a good many lessons yet to teach us in respect of living and practical health." He argued that the fact that China was still flourishing proved that there was some wisdom in the Chinese "old customs" that contributed to "this persistent vitality and antagonism to decay." Dudgeon urged medical investigations of the Chinese lifestyle, which, he argued, could lead to practical knowledge "closely related to the weal of the individual and the nation."[61] Among the "old customs," he considered Chinese dietary habits to be most worthy of European emulation.

Dudgeon praised profusely the moderate consumption of alcohol among the Chinese and argued that the British should follow the Chinese example: "Were the [British] working classes supplied with some cheap and wholesome beverages . . . the public weal and the individual health, both physical and mental, would be greatly benefited." It would also bring down the "British national drink bill" and hence bring about economical benefits.[62] Such criticism was consistent with the tradition of medical advice on the vices of alcohol, represented by the work of Thomas Trotter (1760–1832), which also accorded with contemporary medical criticism of British soldiers' excessive drinking habits in India.[63] Another great dietary error among the Europeans, according to Dudgeon, was that they ate too much meat: "The European constitution, with its inflammatory nature, fed principally on animal food."[64] On the other hand, meat constituted only a minor proportion of the Chinese diet. The major dietary item for the Chinese was rice in the south and wheat and millet in the north. Because these grains were "deficient in the flesh-forming and mineral matters," they alone could not provide enough nutrition. But the Chinese ate them "with various kinds of peas and beans in the north and fish in the south, substance rich in flesh-forming material."[65] Dudgeon particularly appreciated the way the Chinese used fish in their cuisine, because it complemented their starchy diet well. He stated that the Chinese ate a lot of seeds and fruit containing "much phosphate of lime or bone-earth," which were crucial for the formation of healthy bones and teeth. As a result, he rarely found in China "the disease known on the continent as the 'English disease,' viz., the rickets."[66] He claimed that the oriental diet was far more balanced than, and superior to, the European diet:

> Excess of the nitrogenous tends to induce diseases of an inflammatory and gouty nature, and likewise leads to fatty degeneration of the tissue. This is the prevailing type of well-fed Europeans. A lack of the nitrogenous leads to weakness, want of muscular power, and general protraction. This is the type of the badly fed poor of our large cities. In the East neither type exists, for the food of the people, whether Arab, Indian, or Chinese, comprises both sorts, nitrogenous and non-nitrogenous, in the most remarkable degree.[67]

While Manson considered the conservatism of the Chinese a pathological symptom of their anemic constitutions, and a clear indicator of both the inferior position the Chinese occupied on the racial scale and the backwardness of their civilization, Dudgeon saw that very conservatism as conducive to health.[68] He argued that the Chinese way of life was far healthier than that of the Europeans because it was natural and simple. The observation "that the Chinese . . . are subject to fewer diseases, that their diseases are more amenable to treatment, and that they possess a greater freedom from acute and inflammatory affections of all kinds, if indeed these can be said at all to exist," prompted Dudgeon to suggest that the health benefits resulting from the traditional Chinese lifestyle outweighed those of European sciences and civilization. European civilization, albeit more advanced, was artificial and complicated—hence, detrimental to health. Dudgeon lamented that "in these days of an advanced and unnatural civilization, where life and all its surroundings are so complex and artificial, it may not be amiss to take a review of a bygone yet existing civilization where life is more natural and simple."[69] While Dudgeon's urge for a temperate and regular way of life was consistent with traditional theories of personal hygiene, his medical criticism of European lifestyles had many features in common with the popular hygienic advice literature in late-nineteenth-century America and, perhaps to a lesser extent, Great Britain. The publishing success of the genre owed a great deal to the anxieties fueled by the new working environments and fast-paced urban lifestyles brought about by rapid industrialization.[70] Indeed, Dudgeon can be placed in the lineage of medical theorists of "diseases of civilization" whose most prominent representatives were Samuel Auguste A. D. Tissot (1728–97), Trotter, and George Beard (1839–83). These writers argued that the luxuries and fashions of modern material culture and the strains due to competition and a fast-paced urban life inevitably resulted in diseases.[71] It was clear that Dudgeon strongly disliked the Victorian metropolitan lifestyle. He turned his medical observation of the Chinese lifestyle into a critique of European industrial civilization.

The moderate diet of the Chinese was part of this simple lifestyle, which, according to Dudgeon, was conducive to good health. Dudgeon even argued that Europeans should assimilate the Asian dietary regimen that could reduce the risks of "high fevers, acute diseases and general inflammation." "It is here," he argued, "where Europe might with great advantage assimilate herself more to Asia."[72] Moral economy and political economy were interwoven in Dudgeon's views on diet. He argued that the Chinese diet was not only healthy but also economical, and indeed these were two sides of the same coin. "The Orientals," Dudgeon claimed, "are most frugal, making use of substances which would meet with culinary contempt in any other country." Their moderate consumption of food brought about economic benefits: "A poor man in England would starve on the food which keeps the poor man in China and all his family." Having recourse to natural theology, Dudgeon claimed that the Chinese diet also made better and more efficient use of natural resources bestowed by God on human beings: "Divine providence has filled the earth, sea, and air with things which man can eat. They [the Chinese] have a very rich variety of foods drawn from land and water which are unknown to the West."[73] With regard to eating beef, Dudgeon's conclusion was diametrically opposed to Manson's: "We should not suffer in mind, body, or estate, though the status of the national roast beef should be jeopardized."[74]

Health Benefits of the Chinese Diet

Dudgeon's positive view of Chinese food may have sounded idiosyncratic at a time when scientific racism and the European sense of superiority were rising. However, there were other medical practitioners in China who held similar views with respect to Chinese dietary customs. Charles Alexander Gordon (1821–99), a medical officer in the British army and the editor of the *Medical Reports* of the Chinese Maritime Customs, claimed: "Compared to the native inhabitants of the maritime regions of Hindustan . . . the native of the south of China is quite a superior animal." He went even further: "In many respects the labouring classes at Hong Kong contrast favourably with the corresponding classes in Britain. In personal cleanliness they are certainly superior to the 'great unwashed' of our towns, and even of the agricultural districts. In quiet industry they beat the Englishman hollow."[75] Gordon attributed the good health of the southern Chinese to their diet. He observed that they consumed a lot of pork, and he explained:

> One of the powerful causes of the active and energetic character of the southern Chinaman as compared to the cold-blooded Hindoo, who inhabits a corresponding latitude, is to be found in the meat-eating propensities of the former, and the vegetarian diet of the latter. If, as is said, but a very small amount of animal food is required in the torrid zone, John Chinaman is guilty of a degree of extravagance.[76]

In Gordon's account, the influence of diet on constitution was so great that it could even undermine the racial hierarchy between the Chinese and the English.

James Watson, a medical officer in the northern treaty port of Niuzhuang, articulated a similar view, although he favored the northern Chinese rather than their southern compatriots. He praised the physique of the northern Chinese:

The men are tall, large and well built. The women away from the towns and cities have clear complexions. The skin of men and women is much whiter than that of the Chinese of the south. But for the peculiar Chinese eyes and general absence of hair on the face, the men might be mistaken for English if appropriately dressed.[77]

Watson claimed that throughout the history of China, most of the rulers had been northern Chinese, and that people from the Niuzhuang region and other parts of Manchuria could be trained to be good soldiers. He held that "they are potentially a great people . . . and it is highly probable that in the future they will exercise a healthy influence upon China." Watson also attributed the quality of these people to their diet, consisting mainly of millet plus some fish and vegetables. Moreover, "here spirits, as an article of diet, are used advantageously, and very rarely abused."[78]

According to the observations of Gordon and Watson, the quality of a race was not innate but could be modified by dietary factors. Their arguments highlight the complexity of the concept of racial constitution and the ambiguity of the idea of racial hierarchy. They also showed that British medical practitioners' outlooks on native food were more varied in China than in India. This is an interesting contrast since the opinions of British medical practitioners in China were significantly informed by the observations, concepts, and theories of Anglo-Indian medicine. Some of these differences were certainly due to different backgrounds and theoretical positions of individuals. Dudgeon's favorable views on Chinese food, for example, could be related to his Glasgow background and Scottish Presbyterian upbringing. He considered Chinese dietary and agricultural practices in general to have made very efficient use of natural resources and reduced waste to a minimum. They appealed to his vision of the moral economy of health, which was rooted in Scottish Presbyterian theology. In the 1870s, moreover, Scotland began to experience a painful economic decline after the long boom since the end of the Napoleonic Wars. Dudgeon's elevation of Chinese diet and lifestyles was also a critique of the social and economic conditions of Scotland.[79] On the other hand, it is not surprising that Manson, whose parasitological research in China had contributed enormously to the medical knowledge that tropical diseases were caused by parasites and their insect hosts rather than by direct climatic influences on European constitutions, held a more biological and deterministic view on the links between diet and racial constitutions, although he did not downplay the significance of food or hygiene either.

Another important factor in shaping such attitudes was the nature of the British presence in China and the power relations in the treaty ports. The argument that ideas and practices of personal hygiene were closely related to the rise of racism in the nineteenth century is well founded, but the hygienic, racial, and moral connotations of "the tropics" varied for Europeans in different imperial contexts. Tropical hygiene dealt with both the physical and the moral aspects of health. Dietary practice was not only a measure adopted to ward off diseases; it also often had the effect of strengthening racial boundaries and confirming European supremacy. Hygienic regimens were not only a method of maintaining health, but also a way of distinguishing and distancing the European self from the native other. Recent historiography of colonial medicine has established that European medical attitudes toward native lifestyles changed in accordance with shifts in colonial rule and imperial policy. In her examination of the colonial culture in Indochina, Stoler notices a significant shift in French attitudes toward local customs: "Adaptation to local food, language, and dress, once prescribed as positive signs of acclimatization, were now the signs of contagion and loss of (white) self. The benefits of local knowledge and sexual release gave way to more pressing demands of respectability, the community's solidarity, and its mental health."[80] In the East Indies, the fact that many Dutch children preferred local food to European dishes often caused great anxiety among their parents and was frequently cited by medical practitioners and education reformers as an indication of parental negligence and schooling failures prevalent in the colony. "Food," according to Stoler, "was remembered as a principal arena in which Dutch fears about contact and contamination were played out but also as a site where the seductive pull of Javanese ways often proved too powerful to resist."[81] E. M. Collingham claims that the Anglo-Indians' perception of their bodies underwent a significant shift in the first half of the nineteenth century. "The body of the nabob" in the eighteenth century "was envisaged as an open body, in flux with its environment," and the "practices which surrounded it allowed adjustment to the circumstances of life in India," but with the advancement of the Anglicizing "reform" in the early nineteenth century, bodily borders between the British and the Indians were consolidated.[82] Harrison argues that with the expansion of British colonial activities in India, there also appeared a hardening of the view of racial differences. The high mortality rate of the troops during the war against the Marthas, the expansion of European settlements into less salubrious areas, and the need to emphasize racial distinction in order to promote the impression of British superiority to the natives all contributed to the rise of scientific racism. The mutiny of the Indian troops in 1857 reinforced the skeptical and pessimistic views on European acclimatization in the tropics.[83]

The relationship between Britain and China was somewhat different. China was not a colony. Although the British government had repeatedly subjugated China by military force, its interests in China were mainly commercial. The "unequal treaties" signed between China and Britain and the treaty ports system were mainly designed to open the Chinese market to British commerce and to facilitate trade. The maintenance of racial distinctions and the British sense of superiority in China were never as urgent as in India. While many British in China were convinced that European constitutions and civilization were superior to those of the Chinese, it was not so exigent for them to underpin and display their sense of superiority by deprecating the food of the natives. The policing of racial boundaries and the restrictions on adaptation and assimilation of local habits in the Chinese treaty ports were not as vigorous as in British India during the same period.

British medical practitioners in the late nineteenth century were still interested in discovering useful hygienic information from Chinese customs. Watson, for example, was keen on finding out "the effect of millet on European constitutions." He was supplied with an occasion to test this when the British consul sentenced a European sailor to seven weeks of solitary confinement for "several serious offenses." Instead of putting him on bread and water, Watson fed this sailor "solely on millet and water." He found that the sailor was not only in perfect health but had even put on some weight at the time of his release.[84] Dudgeon claimed that the Chinese had "succeeded intuitively, or as the result of their long experience, in the attainment of the maximum of nourishment with the minimum of cost, which ought to be the object of every people and not alone of a Government dietary for soldiers and sailors."[85]

In the late nineteenth century, European chemists and medical scientists conducted systematic investigations into the nutritional value of different food items, analyzing and measuring their chemical contents. In an age of nationalism and imperialism—when international competition in terms of military strength, economic productivity, and colonial efforts intensified—scientists and medical practitioners tried to find healthy and economical diets for their nations, especially for soldiers and workers.[86] In Britain, many studies were conducted on the relationship among food, health, and econ-

omy. There were lively discussions on what constituted proper diets for soldiers and laborers, utilizing the results of recent chemical analyses—such as
those of Justus von Leibig and William Prout—of the principal constituents
of food.[87] Some authors voiced concern that the improper ways of cooking
in Britain reduced the quality of food and wasted a large amount of fuel,
and that poorer families were suffering from such waste.[88] There were official investigations of the diet of the laboring class, to examine the connection between their nourishment and health.[89] Medical practitioners, chemists, and politicians were debating the makeup of an appropriate diet for
a British soldier that could both provide ample nutrition for the man and
reduce the burden of military budgets.[90] While the British medical practitioners' criticism of foreign traders' eating habits at the Chinese ports can
be considered a continuation of the tradition of dispensing dietary advice
for the upper classes, represented by the eighteenth-century medical man
George Cheyne, their attention to Chinese food was part of a growing medical interest in discovering an appropriate yet economical diet for soldiers,
sailors, and the working classes, which arose in the second half of the nineteenth century.[91]

Conclusion

In a study of the changing meanings of the Chinese concept of *weisheng*,
Ruth Rogaski argues that the divergence between British medicine and Chinese medicine was not as great in the mid-nineteenth century as claimed
by many European medical practitioners, and that there "actually existed
many points of similarity between the medicine of British physicians" and
"that of Chinese healers, especially with regard to their conceptualization
of disease etiology." Rogaski also argues that although both British and Chinese medical practitioners identified miasma as a major health threat, Qing
medical thinkers planned prevention for individuals, whereas the British
countered miasma through sanitary engineering. Their "great divergence"
lay in "organization and action" rather than "underlying premise" and "was
primary political, and not medical, in nature."[92] She further points out that
British medical practitioners in China also paid great attention to "planning prevention for individuals," and that many of them considered learning from Chinese practices of personal hygiene valuable. This is particularly evident in British medical discussions on the effects of Chinese diets
on European constitutions. The outlooks of British medical practitioners

on this issue were closely related both to domestic medical discussions and to colonial medical experiences. Their discussions responded to the health concerns of Europeans in China, and they also participated in metropolitan debates on issues such as soldiers' diets, the economy of health, and the relations between races, civilizations, and evolution. When studying Chinese dietary customs, British medical practitioners relied heavily on the conceptual framework and theoretical resources provided by tropical hygiene, especially the work of their colleagues in India. In this respect, British medical practitioners in China can be regarded as part of the imperial medical network that was characterized by "polycentric communications" between different colonies and imperial outposts.[93] The different attitudes toward indigenous diets by British medical practitioners in India and China, moreover, had to do not only with the different medical outlooks of individual practitioners but also, more important, with the different nature of the British imperial presence in these two countries.

NOTES

1. Henderson, *Shanghai Hygiene*, 3–4.

2. At this time, the medical profession in Britain did not have a unified system of education nor a single qualification. Many of the medical missionaries and the medical officers of the Chinese Maritime Customs were members of the Royal College of Surgeons or licentiates of the Society of Apothecaries, instead of holding the license of the Royal College of Physicians. To call them physicians or doctors would be anachronistic. Hence I use the term "medical practitioners" throughout this article.

3. See Rather, "The 'Six Things Non-Natural'"; Jarcho, "Galen's Six Non-naturals."

4. Indeed, diet occupied a prominent place in Galen's medical theory. See Grant, *Galen on Food and Diet.*

5. Collingham, *Imperial Bodies*, 69–72, 156–59; Stoler, *Carnal Knowledge and Imperial Power*, 198–201.

6. Although the Tainjin Treaty was signed in 1858, the Qing government reneged on its pledge to allow British and French Legation to enter Beijing. As a result, hostilities resumed, which ended in the sacking of the Summer Palace and the signing of Beijing Convention in 1860. Fairbank, "The Creation of the Treaty System"; Cain and Hopkins, *British Imperialism*, 422–46. On the locations and the opening dates of the treaty ports, see A. Porter, *Atlas of British Overseas Expansion*, 92.

7. On the eighteenth-century revival of Hippocratic ideas about climates and health, see Riley, *The Eighteenth-Century Campaign to Avoid Disease.*

8. Nelson, "Medical Results of Recent Chinese Wars," 205.

9. Dudgeon, "Dr. John Dudgeon's Report on the Physical Conditions of Peking ... (First Part)," 82.

10. Jamieson, "Dr. Alexander Jamieson's Report on the Health of Shanghai for the Half Year Ended 30th September, 1873," 55.

11. Reid, "Dr. A. G. Reid's Report on the Health of Hankow," 46.

12. Dudgeon, "Dr. John Dudgeon's Report on the Physical Conditions of Peking ... (Second Part)," 36.

13. Dudgeon, "Dr. John Dudgeon's Report on the Health of Peking," 7. On diseases induced by sudden changes of climate, see also Müller and Manson, "Drs. Müller and Manson's Report on the Health of Amoy for the Half Year Ended 31th March, 1872," 22.

14. Harrison, *Climates and Constitutions*, 44–48.

15. Arnold, "Introduction," 6. See also D. Livingstone, "Tropical Climate and Moral Hygiene."

16. Henderson, *Shanghai Hygiene*, 1 and 3. See also J. Martin, *The Influence of Tropical Climates on European Constitutions*.

17. Harrison, *Climates and Constitutions*, 48–56, 80–88. On the history of tropical hygiene, see Harrison, *Public Health in British India*, 36–59.

18. Stewart, "Dr. J. A. Stewart's Report on Health Conditions in Foochow," 65.

19. Ibid.

20. Jamieson, "Dr. Alexander Jamieson's Report on the Health of Shanghai for the Half Year Ended 30th September, 1871," 41.

21. Müller and Manson, "Drs. Müller and Manson's Report on the Health of Amoy for the Half Year Ended 30th September, 1871," 11.

22. Ibid. See also Manson, "Dr. P. Manson's Report on the Health of Amoy for the Half-Year Ended 30th September 1881," 1. British medical men also observed the prevalence of hepatitis and liver abscess among Europeans in India and considered hepatitis an endemic disease of India. See Arnold, *Colonizing the Body*, 30, 36, 72, 82. Arnold conjectures that the high incidence of liver disease was probably caused by amoebic dysentery and excessive consumption of alcohol.

23. Jamieson, "Dr. Alexander Jamieson's Report on the Health of Shanghai for the Half Year Ended 30th September, 1873," 55.

24. Collingham, *Imperial Bodies*, 27–30; Harrison, *Climates and Constitutions*, 80–88. The criticism was still voiced in the late nineteenth century by medical men such as Joseph Fayrer, an authority on diseases in India. "As a general rule," according to Fayrer, "people eat too much in India—more than they can assimilate, or is needed for nutrition," and this resulted in "disordered digestion, faulty assimilation, disordered liver, bowel complaints, and the presence of effete matter in excess in the blood" (Fayrer, *Tropical Dysentery and Chronic Diarrhoea*, 362).

25. Quoted in D. Livingstone, "Tropical Climate and Moral Hygiene," 104.

26. Rennie, *Peking and the Pekingese*, 121.

27. See, for example, A. Jones, *North China English Baptist Mission*. Stoler also warns that the picture of "bourgeois aristocracy" should not be taken as character-

istic of European communities in the colonies. Many of the Europeans were in fact laborers, servants, and "poor whites" (*Race and the Education of Desire*, 101–16).

28. Roberts, *China to Chinatown*, 75–79.

29. B. Anderson, *Imagined Communities*, 136–37. See also Collingham, *Imperial Bodies*, 150–65.

30. Quoted in Spence, *To Change China*, 115.

31. Quoted in ibid., 142.

32. On the symbolic significance of meat consumption in English culture, see Fiddes, *Meat*.

33. Somerville, "Dr. J. R. Somerville's Report on the Health of Foochow," 29.

34. Fayrer, for example, advised new arrivals in India "to prefer light wine, such as claret, to beer, [and] beer to spirits" (*Tropical Dysentery and Chronic Diarrhoea*, 362).

35. Notter, "The Hygiene of the Tropics," 38.

36. Heaton, *Medical Hints for Hot Climates*, 7.

37. Fayrer, *Tropical Dysentery and Chronic Diarrhoea*, 363. See also Somerville, "Dr. J. R. Somerville's Report on the Health of Foochow," 29.

38. Notter, "The Hygiene of the Tropics," 38.

39. Moore, *Health in the Tropics*, 212.

40. Ibid., 221–22, emphasis in original.

41. Heaton, *Medical Hints for Hot Climates*, 7.

42. D. Livingstone, "Tropical Climate and Moral Hygiene," 108.

43. Stoler, *Race and the Education of Desire*, 45.

44. J. Martin, *The Influence of Tropical Climates on European Constitutions*, 130.

45. Harrison, *Public Health in British India*, 39–41, 52–54; Arnold, *Colonizing the Body*, 40–43, 52–54.

46. On Manson's career, see Haynes, *Imperial Medicine*.

47. Manson and Manson, "The Drs. Mansons' Report on the Health of Amoy," 32. Eating beef was a dietary custom that often got singled out as an indicator of the racial difference between Europeans and Chinese. The anti-Chinese propaganda of the nineteenth-century American labor union movement, for example, argued that— as Sen. James G. Blaine put it in an 1879 speech—"you cannot work a man who must live on beef and bread alongside a man who can live on rice. In all such conflicts, and in all such struggles, the result is not to bring up the man who lives on rice to the beef-and-bread standard, but it is to bring down the beef-and-bread man to the rice standard" (quoted in Shah, *Contagious Divides*, 167).

48. Fayrer, *Tropical Dysentery and Chronic Diarrhoea*, 361.

49. D. Livingstone, "Tropical Climate and Moral Hygiene."

50. Manson and Manson, "The Drs. Mansons' Report on the Health of Amoy," 30. Manson coauthored this report with his brother David, who came to Amoy in 1873 but was transferred to Takow, Formosa, in 1875. Like his elder brother Patrick, David Manson also received his medical training at Aberdeen University (see Wong and Wu, *History of Chinese Medicine*, 413, 417).

51. Manson and Manson, "The Drs. Mansons' Report on the Health of Amoy," 30.

52. Influenced by contemporary physiological writings, especially J. Franz Simon's *Animal Chemistry* (1845–46), Buckle believed that the laws of climates, which were mediated by food, determined the accumulation and distribution of wealth. See Stocking, *Victorian Anthropology*, 112–17, 137–40.

53. C. Darwin, *The Descent of Man*, 246.

54. Manson and Manson, "The Drs. Mansons' Report on the Health of Amoy," 32.

55. Harrison, "'The Tender Frame of Man,'" 70.

56. Manson and Manson, "The Drs. Mansons' Report on the Health of Amoy," 30.

57. Ibid. Other British medical men also observed malaria-induced anemia among the Chinese. For example, Underwood reported that "the chief results of malaria, seen in those long resident, are anaemia, not generally pronounced, and an infirmity of temper, and disposition to be worried by petty annoyances that would hardly be noticed in health" ("Dr. G. R. Underwood's Report on the Health of Kiukiang," 19).

58. The association between anemia and effeminacy was common in nineteenth-century medicine. Manson's description of the universal anemia among the Chinese also suggested that they were feeble and effeminate, and hence an inferior race and nation. For a study on how American physicians reflected gender norms and the "moral management of women" in their research on chlorosis in the late nineteenth century and the early twentieth, see Wailoo, *Drawing Blood*, 16–45.

59. Dudgeon, "Dr. John Dudgeon's Report on the Physical Conditions of Peking . . . (First Part)," 80.

60. Dudgeon, "Diet, Dress, and Dwellings of the Chinese in Relation to Health," 257–58. Dudgeon's paper was included in a series of publications resulting from the International Health Exhibition at South Kensington, London, in 1884.

61. Ibid., 258.

62. Ibid., 304–5.

63. Trotter, *An Essay Medical, Philosophical and Chemical on Drunkenness*. On medical criticism of British soldiers' alcoholism in India, see Arnold, *Colonizing the Body*, 80–83, and Harrison, *Public Health in British India*, 62–63. It seems that medical men with military or overseas experience were particularly concerned about the immoderate consumption of alcohol among the British. Trotter was a naval surgeon.

64. Dudgeon, "Diet, Dress, and Dwellings of the Chinese in Relation to Health," 332.

65. Ibid., 261.

66. Ibid., 292.

67. Ibid., 314–15.

68. Dudgeon, *The Diseases of China*, 63–64.

69. Dudgeon, "Diet, Dress, and Dwellings of the Chinese in Relation to Health," 258–59.

70. For an analysis of this genre of medical literature in the American context, see Fellman and Fellman, *Making Sense of Self*. For an example of British medical authors' contributions to this genre, see Evans, *How to Prolong Life*.

71. For the history of diseases of civilization, see R. Porter, "Diseases of Civilization." See also Cheyne, *The English Malady*; Tissot, *An Essay of Diseases Incidental to Literary and Sedentary Persons*; and Trotter, *A View of the Nervous Temperament*.

72. Dudgeon, *The Diseases of China*, 61.

73. Dudgeon, "Diet, Dress, and Dwellings of the Chinese in Relation to Health," 311.

74. Ibid., 322.

75. Gordon, *China from a Medical Point of View in 1860 and 1861*, 27. See also Gordon, *An Epitome of the Reports of the Medical Officers*.

76. Gordon, *China from a Medical Point of View*, 28.

77. J. Watson, "Dr. James Watson's Report on the Health of Newchwang," 12.

78. Ibid. Sturdy northern Chinese and effete southern Chinese were not merely stereotypes fabricated by Europeans in China, but also appeared in nineteenth-century Chinese medical literature. See Hanson, "Robust Northerners and Delicate Southerners." Whether there was any exchange of these medical ideas between the Europeans and the Chinese is an issue worthy of further exploration.

79. See Shang-Jen Li, "Moral Economy and Health."

80. Stoler, *Carnal Knowledge and Imperial Power*, 69.

81. Ibid., 199.

82. Collingham, *Imperial Bodies*, 79.

83. Harrison, *Climates and Constitutions*, 58–152. See also Harrison, "'The Tender Frame of Man.'"

84. J. Watson, "Dr. James Watson's Report on the Health of Newchwang," 13.

85. Dudgeon, "Diet, Dress, and Dwellings of the Chinese in Relation to Health," 261.

86. Kamminga and Cunningham, Introduction; Kamminga, "Nutrition for the People"; Finlay, "Early Marketing of the Theory of Nutrition"; Milles, "Working Capacity and Calorie Consumption."

87. Dunell, "Great Britain. Food."

88. Berdmore, "The Principles of Cooking," 205–6, 250.

89. Fiddes, *Meat*, 24.

90. Blyth, "Diet in Relation to Health and Work," 341–46; De Chaumont and Francois, "Practical Dietetics," 68–69.

91. On the relation and transition between eighteenth- and nineteenth-century medical concepts of diet in Britain, see Turner, *Regulating Bodies*, 177–95.

92. Rogaski, *Hygienic Modernity*, 82, 103.

93. Harrison, "Science and the British Empire," 63. See also Chambers and Gillespie, "Locality in the History of Science"; MacLeod, Introduction.

Vampires in Plagueland

The Multiple Meanings of Weisheng *in Manchuria*

||

Ruth Rogaski

Historians of colonial medicine take many different approaches to their subject. Some may explore the organization of the medical infrastructures established by colonial regimes. Others may analyze health statistics—disease incidence, disease mortality, numbers of vaccinations, numbers of visits to hospitals or clinics—in order to discern how well (or how poorly) the health of a colonized population was served. Others may search for indigenous resistance to biomedicine, seeking to highlight the injustice and violence that often accompanied public health interventions. But while colonial medicine generated statistics, institutions, and resistance, it also generated meaning. Colonizers and colonized alike imbued medicine and public health with sometimes profound significance. As historians of the cultures of colonialism, we need to examine how these narratives embodied painful and contentious divides of race, class, and nation. At the same time, however, we must be open to evidence that confounds our received expectations about these very same divides.

This chapter explores the multiple meanings that some Chinese and Japanese attributed to biomedicine and public health activities in Manchuria during the first half of the twentieth century. As I have argued elsewhere, a broadly defined, comprehensive biomedicine/public health/state nexus—known as *weisheng* in Chinese and *eisei* in Japanese—emerged as a central vehicle for the expression of hope and anxiety about modernity in East Asia in the late nineteenth century and the early twentieth.[1] During the period of Japanese presence on the northeast Asian mainland, "hygienic modernity" became a vehicle for the expression of power, fear, and hope in the region's complex informal and formal colonial settings.[2]

In order for the historian to explore these multiple meanings, "texts" from a variety of sources—ranging from articles published in elite scientific journals to village rumors and urban legends—must all be consulted.[3] From this broad swath of sources, from among many possible themes and meanings, two intriguing but complicated notions arise. One, voiced in elite writings, was the definition of Manchuria as a singularly diseased environment, a place whose very terrain seemed to be replete with the seeds of contagion. The work of many Japanese physicians, public health workers, and administrators reflected an almost Hippocratic obsession with the airs, waters, and places of Manchuria. In these writings, diseased land, diseased animals, and backward people intertwined in Manchuria to produce a dangerous plagueland that required the utmost vigilance and effort to control. From rumor, memory, and popular culture, a different interpretation of medical efforts to control the plague emerge: the image of Japanese doctors as embodiment of evil, white-jacketed agents of empire who gouged out organs and stole (or intentionally tainted) the blood of their victims: monsters or vampires who employed the techniques of hygienic modernity to kill and conquer.[4]

While these themes provide a rich basis for the exploration of meanings of hygiene in a colonial setting, we must not assume that these understandings were easily divided into those of the colonizer and those of the colonized. Many Japanese may have envisioned Manchuria as a plagueland, an unhealthy zone steeped in harmful microorganisms, but the concept of Manchuria as a backward source of plague also informed the work of Chinese elites. Similarly, stories and rumors that Japanese public health workers were propagating the germs of disease may have spread among many Chinese in Manchuria during the Japanese occupation, but before the occupation, ethnically Chinese doctors had been the target of similar stories. The image of Japanese *eisei* as the primary embodiment of medical evil may have been most clearly cultivated after the end of the Second World War, with the public exposé of the activities of the Japanese Imperial Army's biological warfare laboratory, Unit 731. Ultimately, an examination of the meanings attributed to public health and biomedical activities in Manchuria helps to blur the border between colonizer and colonized, a line vividly demarcated in most contemporary mainland Chinese scholarship on Japanese science in Manchuria.[5] At the same time, such an examination blurs the borders between fact and imagination, statistics and culture, rumors of vampires and the actual existence of vampires.

Manchuria as Plagueland

As it did in Taiwan and elsewhere in the empire, modern hygiene (*eisei*) figured prominently in the tool kit of Manchuria's Japanese planners. In particular, the public health network established by the South Manchuria Railway Company (Mantetsu) became a jewel in the crown of Japan's empire. Dalian (then known as Dairen), the port city at the southernmost tip of the Liaodong Peninsula, served as the starting point for Japanese medical modernity in the early twentieth century, with a state-of-the-art bacteriological laboratory and massive modern hospital.[6] By the 1930s, Xinjing—literally the "new capital" of Manchukuo, the Japanese puppet state in Manchuria, and previously and later known as Changchun—was slated to become "the first city in Asia in which all [new] residential, commercial, and industrial buildings were equipped with water closets."[7] But these utopian colonial projects, planned by an urban intelligentsia to incorporate the best things that hygienic modernity had to offer, faced a particular challenge in Manchuria. Japanese publications on the environment and health of Manchuria inevitably painted the region as an epicenter—if not the epicenter—of disease in East Asia. For all of its attention to hygienic modernity, the project of Japanese settlement in Manchuria was constantly haunted by the specter of that least modern of diseases, the plague.

Perhaps the modern world's most dramatic outbreak of plague took place in Manchuria when pneumonic plague, easily transmitted from person to person through the air, claimed as many as 60,000 lives in the winter of 1910–11.[8] This terrifying epidemic came at a pivotal time in northeast Asian history: just before the fall of the Qing dynasty, a year before the end of the Meiji reign in Japan, and the same year that Korea became a colony of Japan. As detailed by Sean Hsiang-lin Lei in this volume, the Manchurian plague epidemic was a critical event in the last year of the Qing government's existence. Through participation in epidemic-prevention work led by doctors of biomedicine, the Qing dynasty displayed its medical modernity to the world in an attempt to retain its sovereignty over its waning empire. Similarly, the great epidemic of 1910–11 was a central experience for the rising empire of Japan: coinciding with the first decade of Japan's intense investment in the Liaodong Peninsula with the South Manchuria Railway Company.

My use of the word "plagueland" to describe Manchuria harkens back to this extremely formative moment, but it was not the only moment when plague was present in Manchuria. Although the disease never returned with such terrifying virulence, the western regions of Manchuria—particularly the Kerqin grasslands, bordering the Mongolian plains (near Tongliao); and the northern Transbaikal region (near Manzhouli)—were endemic zones for plague, and frequent, though usually limited, outbreaks were a constant threat. After the 1910–11 epidemic, cases of plague arose in Manchuria with astonishing frequency: in 1920–21, 1927, 1928, 1933, 1934, 1935, 1936, 1939, 1940, 1941, 1942, 1943, and 1944. During each outbreak, deaths ranged from around one hundred to several thousand.[9] Similarly, "plagueland" might also be used to symbolize the frequency of epidemic outbreaks of other infectious diseases in Manchuria, particularly cholera—which hit major cities along the South Manchuria Railway in 1907, 1919, 1926, and 1932.[10]

In his magisterial work on plague in modern China, Iijima Wataru has shown how plague helped define the shape of modern China's state, as Chinese *weisheng* bureaucracies arose for the control of the disease under conditions where inability to control plague would mean the loss of China's sovereignty.[11] Plague was also a central event that helped shape Japan's imagining of Manchuria and, along with this imagining, shaped Japan's governance and scientific infrastructure in the region. The challenge of contagious disease control brought municipal and rail administrators, military personnel, consular officials, physicians, and research scientists into a web of cooperation. The fear of contagious disease may even be seen as a factor that directly generated a significant part of the structures of scientific study in Manchuria. Mantetsu and the Manchukuo government also maintained several agricultural experiment stations, a central laboratory, the Mainland Institute of Science, two cattle disease prevention institutes, two hygiene institutes, and a network of thirty hospitals, several of which conducted medical research. Even the famed reports of local society produced by Mantetsu's research department, while providing details on the Chinese economy and customs, also included detailed information on climate, soil composition, vegetation, and animals. In many ways, much of the professional probing of the environment was related in one way or another to the production of knowledge for controlling contagious disease, the major impediment to Japanese control of and the advent of modernity in Manchuria.

Nowhere was the perception of Manchuria as plagueland more apparent than in the writings on settler hygiene produced in the 1930s and 1940s.[12] Maintaining health in Manchuria's environment had always been a concern to the Japanese professionals and merchants who lived in cities along the rail lines since the turn of the century, but in urban settings the natural environment could be managed through urban infrastructure. For the hundreds of thousands of Japanese brought in under the Manchukuo-era Farm Colonization Program, resettlement directly on the land of the Manchurian frontier posed a hygienic conundrum of an entirely different order.[13] As the mass agricultural resettlement program was planned and executed, physicians, scientists, and public administrators published numerous studies and informative pamphlets on how to survive in Manchuria's unhealthful environment.

Taken collectively, these publications express an almost Hippocratic obsession with the potential effect of Manchurian air and land on Japanese health.[14] All of these texts begin with sections on Manchuria's climate and local environment, which include discussions of temperature, humidity, and sunlight. In these writings, composed long after the germ theory of disease had been widely accepted, the climate appears as the crucial determinate of disease. Extremes of temperature are bad for health: the burning heat of Manchurian summers gives rise to gastrointestinal diseases, while the frigid and sunless winters force people to pack themselves into stuffy rooms and ruin their lungs.[15] Not only is the climate of Manchuria different from Japan, it is different from the climates commonly encountered in European and American colonies. While the West's imperial experience was primarily with tropical diseases, the landmass of Manchuria encompasses arctic, temperate, and even tropical climates: therefore Manchuria is home to arctic, temperate, and even tropical diseases. As a result, Japan's scientists, and Japan's colonists, had to be particularly vigilant and persistent in their management of Manchuria's complex disease environment.[16]

Managing Plagueland: Japanese Epidemic Control in Manchuria

To manage this environment, an elaborate network of physicians, laboratories, health departments, and sanitary police evolved under the Japanese administration of Manchuria during the first half of the twentieth century. The focus of much of these *eisei* efforts was to protect the flourishing trade, massive investments, and burgeoning populations of the big cities along the South Manchuria Railroad. Robert Perrins, in his detailed work on the public health of Dalian, has described the extensive safety net that protected the health of that city. The South Manchuria Railway Company, the regional Kantō (Kwantung) government, and the Kantō Army all main-tained units that policed, tabulated, and provided for the health of Dalian and surrounding areas. The jewel in the crown for this network was the South Manchuria Railway hospital, opened in 1927 to great fanfare. Perched on a hill high above the city's bustling port, the massive hospital possessed "gleaming patient wards, a well-stocked pharmacy, and surgeries and labo-ratories equipped with the latest instruments from Japan and Germany."[17]

As Perrins has noted, however, the gleaming facilities of the SMRC hos-pital were not meant for the Chinese of the city, but almost exclusively for its Japanese residents. This exclusivity was a telling symbol of the nature of Japanese *eisei* infrastructure and policy in Manchuria from the beginning of the twentieth century through the end of Manchukuo: public health was not conceived as a set of services meant to maintain the well-being of the broad mass of people. Instead, *eisei* touched the Chinese population pri-marily in times of crisis, particularly during the outbreak of epidemic dis-ease. For most Chinese in the Japanese-administered territories, *weisheng* (public health) was experienced almost exclusively as *fangyi* (epidemic control).

To understand this phenomenon, one must read between the lines of existing publications from Japanese public health units. The reports and statistics generated by the SMRC include mortality statistics, statistics on contagious disease, numbers of hospital patients, numbers of vaccinations, and numbers of disinfections performed by SMRC personnel. The sick and the vaccinated are always delineated by nationality: Japanese, Chinese, and foreigners. In these extensive reports, one cannot fail to notice the remark-ably small numbers of Chinese who seemed to have come in contact with the daily functionings of the SMRC health bureau. A handful of patients here, a few dozen vaccinations there: the numbers are entirely unrepresen-tative of the overall Chinese population of the region.[18]

The numbers of Chinese touched by the Japanese *eisei* network spiked, however, during times of epidemic disease. When plague or cholera threat-ened, physicians, police, and military personnel sprang into action. In 1919, to fight cholera in the port of Dalian, officials showered ship passengers in formaldehyde, conducted door-to-door inspections in laborers' quarters, quarantined Chinese neighborhoods, burned corpses, and administered nine thousand doses of cholera vaccine to Chinese laborers. In spite of these efforts, the city experienced over six thousand deaths due to cholera in that year alone.[19]

Epidemic control extended to the more remote regions of Manchuria, especially in the towns along the western branches of the South Manchuria Railway. As the railway stretched into the eastern Mongolian grasslands, it ran up against a terrain where plague was a frequent occurrence. In towns such as Tongliao, Changling, and Nong'an (to the east of Changchun), plague cases cropped up with alarming frequency: for example, in the thirty-six years from 1916 to 1952, Nong'an township experienced plague outbreaks twenty-five times.[20] Outbreaks in the areas along the railroad mobilized the SMRC *eisei* network. Physicians and technicians from the company, backed up by military and police personnel, raced to the scene and enacted standard epidemic-control procedures: quarantine, inspections, and corpse disposal. In 1931, the Japanese Army occupied all of Manchuria. After the establishment of the puppet government of Manchukuo, epidemic-control work in Manchuria grew more complicated, more militarized, and more powerful than ever before.

One example of the astonishing scale of epidemic control in Manchuria under the Japanese occupation can be found in the 1940 outbreak of bubonic plague in Jilin Province, which centered on the city of Changchun (then Xinjing or Shinkyo, the "new capital" of Manchukuo) and the surrounding towns along the rail line, especially the mid-sized town of Nong'an. Mainland Chinese scholars—using a rich variety of sources, including Manchukuo government documents, SMRC reports, Japanese military documents, and the recorded recollections of Chinese townspeople—have painstakingly pieced together the events of this outbreak and subsequent epidemic-control activities. The picture they reveal is that of a people assaulted and terrorized not only by plague, but by the measures used to control the plague.

The first signs of plague appeared in Nong'an, a town about sixty kilometers west of Changchun. A central authority was set up in Changchun to oversee plague control efforts. It included representatives from a bewildering array of entities: the SMRC health bureau, the Kantō government, Changchun's mayor and police, Manchukuo's imperial household and Red Cross, and the Japanese military police. While the SMRC, with its long experience of plague prevention, played a major role in the work, it is very clear that the Kantō Army oversaw all operations. In Changchun, efforts focused on the area near the train station, the busiest hub of the SMRC transportation network. From October to December 1940, over 207,000 passengers were injected with antiplague vaccine, an average of three thousand injections a day. Eight physicians were on hand at the train station around the clock, inspecting the crowds and pulling aside anyone who showed signs of plague. Entire neighborhoods in the city were put under quarantine. Chinese workers' dormitories were disinfected with Chloropicrin, a potent substance that had been used in the chemical warfare arsenals of the First World War. Eventually, the poorest sections of the Chinese areas were put to the torch.[21]

Antiplague interventions were even more dramatic in Nong'an. During the summer and fall of 1940, two waves of epidemic-control attacks swept through the county seat. Over a thousand antiplague personnel descended on the town in rail cars and a convoy of trucks, accompanied by close to a thousand police and Kantō Army soldiers. They set up roadblocks, shut down businesses, and quickly erected a *cordon sanitaire* around the town. Twenty-four isolation sectors were established, each cut off from the other with fences made from reed mats and barbed wire. Watches were set up along rooftops to make sure no one escaped the quarantine. Doctors conducted daily physical examinations of the population and isolated anyone who had a fever. In the words of one witness, Nong'an resembled a battlefield, and the people were terrorized more by plague prevention than the plague itself.[22]

Residents recalled the horror of being subjected to the Japanese *eisei* regime. Several households secretly buried family members who had died, only to have the sanitary police dig up the graves and perform open-air autopsies on the bodies. Relatives looked on as their loved ones had their "torsos slit open and their hearts dug out." Stories began to circulate that the Japanese doctors had come to kill Chinese and steal their organs.[23]

Many of the residents' fears centered on the Japanese doctors' use of the hypodermic syringe to extract blood and to administer injections. People began to talk of two types of injections: the "Blood-Measuring Needle" and the "Extermination Needle." Japanese physicians had come to the town to steal organs and blood; in the worst-case scenario, they injected Chinese with unknown substances that led to death, not a cure.[24]

After weeks of inflicting extreme *eisei*, the plague-prevention teams withdrew, leaving a bewildered population to ponder the isolation, mutilation, and mysterious injections it had endured. Out of a population of approximately thirty thousand, Nong'an experienced 298 deaths from plague. But stories of diabolical Japanese physicians wielding needles and knives continued to circulate in the region.

Interpreting Stories of Vampires Where Vampires Were Real

How to interpret stories of evil associated with agents of colonial medicine has recently engrossed historians of Africa. Luise White has written a history of how Africans expressed their understanding of colonial exploitation through the genre of stories about men who stole blood, the *bazimamoto*. *Bazimamoto* were associated with a variety of professions connected to the colonial state: firemen, policemen, game wardens, and doctors, all of whom drained the blood of Africans so that whites could make medicine from the blood. In presenting these vampire stories, White does not seek to expose how Africans misunderstood biomedicine. Instead, she insists that she takes the stories "at face value," as descriptions of "the aggressive carelessness of colonial extractions."[25] She demonstrates how the repetition of formulaic elements in stories turned the stories into truth for the African speaker and listener alike. It is important to note, however, that in writing her history, White does not have to believe that agents of the colonial state actually sucked blood. What is important for the historian is that the subjects she studies think the stories are true: as White puts it, "vampires are a story, but belief in vampires is a fact."[26]

Nancy Rose Hunt, when dealing with similar stories of bloodsucking doctors in *A Colonial Lexicon*, reminds us that truly bloodcurdling things did take place under colonial rule in the Congo. Foremost among the horrors was the dismemberment inflicted on many during King Leopold II's *Heart of Darkness* reign in the Belgian Congo. Against this backdrop, Western doctors dug up human bones (to procure skeletons for research and teaching), extracted lymph through painful lumbar punctures (a test for sleeping sickness), and performed thousands of autopsies on adults and infants alike. On this last point, Hunt's interpretation is quite stark: in Africa, she suggests, "a key incentive for colonial medical research . . . was implicitly the ready availability of a dead and dissectible subject population."[27] Dismemberment and violence were part and parcel of colonial rule. It is not surprising then that the Africans in Hunt's book believed that white doctors drank the blood of Africans or chopped up their bodies to make canned meat.

Nevertheless, no matter how seriously these Africanists say they are taking the stories of their informants, in all these examples rumor is still perceived as metaphor. The researcher is quite certain that white doctors, no matter how racist they might have been, in fact did not drink African blood, nor did they make Africans into Spam. In spite of insistence on "taking stories at face value," in these works there still exist two separate worlds of belief, one mistaken or at the very least metaphorical (colonial doctors who committed inhuman atrocities), and one true, grounded in fact (colonial doctors who were part of an inhumane system, but who did not commit atrocities).

But what happens when some of the stories about vampires are true?

The Chinese accounts of their experience in Changchun and Nong'an in the 1940 plague are horrifying enough, but they might easily be interpreted as the misunderstandings of a population unversed in the scientific principles of epidemic prevention. In this perspective, during the necessary course of plague-prevention work, common people mistook doctors for monsters. However, a different understanding is generated when we discover the name of the man who directed the entire plague-prevention process in the 1940 Changchun outbreak: Ishii Shirō, the director of Unit 731, the Japanese Imperial Army's infamous biological warfare division. Under the euphemistic name of Epidemic Prevention and Water Purification Department, Unit 731 personnel participated in and coordinated the epidemic-prevention strategies. Documents even place Ishii himself in Nong'an in the fall of 1940. The people of Nong'an were quite correct in suspecting that a monster walked in their midst. In essence, their stories of vampires were real.[28]

We are thus forced to read the fears of Nong'an townspeople against the backdrop of truly terrifying atrocities: the Japanese germ-warfare program, the activities of the infamous Unit 731. Formed in 1932, Unit 731 was headquartered in Pingfang, on the outskirts of the city of Harbin. In this massive military and laboratory complex, doctors and scientists of the Japanese Imperial Army developed biological and chemical weapons, often in cooperation with scientific personnel already stationed in Japan's Manchurian *eisei* network. The state-of-the-art facilities included bacteriological laboratories, clinical wards, areas for breeding huge quantities of fleas and rodents, a military airstrip, extensive dormitories for scientists and their families, cellblocks for prisoners, and a massive crematorium. In experiments reminiscent of the atrocities perpetrated by German doctors in Nazi concentration camps, Unit 731 physicians conducted diabolical experiments on human prisoners, most of whom were Chinese captured by Japanese secret police in and around Harbin. Captives of Unit 731 experienced lingering deaths in experiments that seemed especially tailored to the Manchurian environment: exposed to frostbite in the Manchurian snows or exposed to the germs of bubonic plague, administered through shrapnel cuts, fleabites, or the hypodermic syringe. To discover the pathways of disease in living systems, doctors performed vivisections on doomed experiment victims, cutting up chest cavities and removing the organs of still-living subjects. During the war, the Japanese army used biological weapons developed at Pingfang against Chinese civilians. Outbreaks of bubonic plague caused by Unit 731 attacks in eastern and central China are well documented, and evidence of other attacks continues to emerge.[29]

Any story of evil Japanese doctors who "rip open bodies" and inflict the "Needle of Extermination" must therefore be considered within the context of the atrocities committed by Unit 731. But even before the existence of Unit 731 and well beyond the range of its activities, there existed in many parts of China a consistent narrative genre about the evil Japanese physician. The story of the martial arts figure Huo Yuanjia is one of the more famous in this genre. Huo was the renowned founder of the Jingwu Athletic Association (*Jingwu tiyu hui*), a physical-culture organization that flourished in Republican-era China. He died in Shanghai in 1913, not long after he won a well-publicized fight against a Japanese judo expert. Chinese documents from as early as 1925 claim that Huo died from injections administered to him by Japanese physicians who wished to kill him as revenge for beating the Japanese martial arts master. The story of how Huo's disciples avenged his death became the basis for the popular movies featuring Bruce Lee, Jet Li, and many other martial arts stars.

Another example is centered in Manchuria, enshrined in the museum that was the home of Puyi, the last Chinese emperor and the figurehead ruler of Manchukuo. On the second floor of the mansion, between the bathroom and the meeting room, lies the room where Puyi received his morning grooming. A barber's chair, looking more like an elaborate dentist's chair, was positioned in front of a large mirror. There Puyi would get a shave and trim each day. Next to the chair stood a table with what appears to be an open doctor's kit on top. Within this kit, various ampuls and hypodermic needles are visible. An explanatory sign for the room states that Puyi's Japanese doctors injected him with hormone treatments as part of his daily grooming ritual. The sign and the setting seem to suggest that Puyi's physicians did not have his best health in mind when they administered these injections. Downstairs in the formal reception rooms of the mansion, other exhibits describe the sad fate of one of Puyi's consorts, who was killed as a result of constant mysterious injections administered by Japanese physicians.

Visions of nefarious Japanese injections abound in northern Chinese memories from the second Sino-Japanese War. At the site of my previous research, Tianjin, I encountered the belief that Japanese military doctors had purposely caused the cholera epidemics the city experienced in 1937, 1938, and 1943. Newspapers from northeast China in the early 1950s reported the recollections of peasants who were victims of diseases that were caused by injections meted out by Japanese doctors.[30] Particularly in recollections of the war, the Japanese doctor with his syringe seemed an omnipresent symbol of the evil and duplicitous nature of the Japanese occupation of China.

Herein lies one of the difficulties in interpreting stories about evil Japanese doctors. The colonial archive tells us that Japanese physicians administered examinations, quarantines, and vaccinations on a mass scale in order to control epidemics in Manchuria. Yet the far less accessible evidence from Unit 731 demonstrates that Japanese physicians also perpetrated singular atrocities in Manchuria using the tools of biomedicine. Can we simply sidestep the questions of intent, harm, and misunderstanding in examining Chinese tales of the evil behind Japanese *eisei*? In analyzing these widespread suspicions of Japanese medicine and public health, one runs up against the problems of representation and truth, history and justice.

It is imperative that scholars establish, to the fullest degree allowed by available evidence, the exact extent of the Japanese military's experimentation with biological weapons and document atrocities committed in Japanese colonial hospitals and laboratories.[31] On the other hand, it is important that scholars be able to ponder some of the widespread and varied rumors of evil Japanese doctors as rumor—as a narrative genre that tells its own sort of truth, a truth experienced by Chinese who faced the sometimes monstrous forces of hygienic modernity both before and after the Japanese occupation.

Managing Plagueland across the Colonial Divide:
Antiplague Measures before 1931

To place these rumors in their appropriate context, we need to understand popular reactions to epidemic-control efforts made before Manchuria came under Japanese control—that is, when Japanese doctors worked with an international mix of doctors, including those who were ethnically Chinese, to control plague in Manchuria's unforgiving environment.

During the pneumonic plague epidemics of the 1910s and 1920s, Japanese were certainly not the only physicians who carried out mass inspections, autopsies, and disposal of human bodies. As Mark Gamsa points out in his research on the 1910–11 plague in Harbin, the biomedical paradigm taught in London and Paris was the shared template guiding the actions of foreign and Chinese "plague-fighters" alike.[32] Accompanied by armed soldiers, medical personnel from Russia, Europe, America, Southeast Asia, Japan, and the Qing empire conducted invasive inspections, destroyed neighborhoods, separated families, and forced individuals into hospitals from which they would never return. As Sean Hsiang-lin Lei notes in his chapter in this volume, Qing observers called the plague-prevention measures "the most brutal policies seen in four thousand years."[33] The "brutal policies" were carried out by actors from many nations and ethnicities, including Chinese.

Among the most shocking and invasive procedures were the postmortem autopsies performed on victims. These were often conducted in the open air, with little or no barrier to shield the gruesome procedure from the eyes of others. Several factors contributed to the existence of these open-air autopsies: the harsh, frigid conditions of the Manchurian winter, the sense of panic about the plague's spread, the need to confirm plague cases and generate accurate statistics, and, quite possibly, the physicians' apparent disdain for the coolie class who were most often the plague's victims. These factors caused physicians to abandon any concern for the sensitivities of the victims, their families, and any potential laypeople who may have witnessed the procedures.

Japanese photographers captured several autopsies for inclusion in official reports on antiplague measures. Some images portray doctors in makeshift morgues, standing over cadavers in the final stages of disembowelment. Other photos show medical personnel in the field, kneeling beside a freshly felled plague victim and preparing to conduct an autopsy while curious bystanders look on.[34] The inclusion of these photographs in official reports suggests that the compilers saw in them a narrative of heroic physicians who struggled to achieve scientific accuracy in the midst of a harsh, primitive environment. One can imagine that Chinese lay observers who might have witnessed the procedures would draw different conclusions.[35]

While these photographs appear in Japanese reports on the plague, perhaps the most graphic description of open-air procedures performed on Chinese corpses comes from a report by the head of the North Manchuria Plague Prevention Service, the famous (ethnic Chinese) physician Wu Lienteh. In his words:

From suspected corpses or dead found in the streets, cultures from the spleen were obtained. A simple method was employed: skin over the spleen was painted with tincture of iodine, and a short sharp knife sterilized with iodine was inserted and some contents withdrawn. Cultures on agar were made, and the knife rubbed on two glass slides for microscopic examination. The whole operation usually took two minutes. In view of the very cold weather, strong wind and frequent exposure of corpses in the streets, such quick operations were necessary. All cadavers found in the streets were sent to the common cremation pit to be burnt.[36]

Given the horrors of plague in Manchuria and the Draconian methods used to fight the disease, it is not surprising that stories of other meanings began to circulate: stories that described what it meant to be the object of these bizarre and violent interventions. Wu's writings present some of the rumors, stories, and fears he encountered as a Chinese physician of biomedicine during his plague-prevention work in Manchuria. There were rumors that the doctors themselves had brought the plague and that it would simply disappear if only the antiplague doctors would go away. It was said that medical personnel not only intentionally spread the plague, but also "poisoned wells, flour, and food."[37] Rumors spread that "something uncanny" happened within isolation hospitals; the fact that patients went in but never came out was because of the evil actions of the doctors themselves, and not the plague. Wu describes the situation that he and other medical personnel encountered during the 1921 outbreak:

> The past week has been a very anxious one for our anti-plague staff for the concentrated suspicion of and prejudice against our policy of removal of the sick to hospital, isolation of contacts, systematic inspection of inns and other sources of infection, closing of theaters, low brothels, etc., coupled with the restriction of railway traffic and our inability to cure the plague victims resulted in numerous rumours to discredit our dangerous and humane mission.[38]

In this quote and elsewhere, Wu lists the numerous traumatizing interventions that make up antiplague work but seems stunned that these radical methods would generate a set of meanings at odds with the lofty intentions of his medical staff. The objects of epidemic-prevention interventions—in Wu's accounts always coolies, miners, laborers, soldiers, gamblers, and other undesirables—seem remarkably ungrateful for the heroic efforts of science to save them. Their stories of body snatching, poisoning, and germ warfare are the irrational ravings of the uneducated and uncivilized. While Wu critiques the Manchurian underclass for its overactive gothic imagination, he seems immune to the horror lurking within his own narrative: medical technicians who sneak up to corpses on the street, dab the bodies with red paint, plunge in a dagger, and cut out pieces of spleen; family members separated from their homes at gunpoint and taken off to unknown places, never to return; and mass cremation fires which "burnt fiercely in the open" because the "fatty constituents of the cadavers helped to keep up the fire once it was lit," leaving, at the end of the day, "only white crumbled bones as residue."[39]

Medical Ecology: Probing the Link between Animal and Man

After the 1910–11 epidemic, the control of plague in Manchuria hinged upon the scientific investigation of Manchuria's small, ground-dwelling mammals, including the rat but focusing particularly on the tarbagan, a type of marmot. The tarbagan was identified as the main vector for transmitting plague to humans in the 1910–11 pneumonic plague epidemic. The pelt of these small, furry creatures once found a worldwide market, and thousands of Chinese (along with Russians) made a living trapping the animals. In the aftermath of the epidemic and the International Plague Conference, one of the plague-prevention techniques taken up by the North Manchurian Plague Prevention Service included the establishment of "tarbagan skin disinfection stations" designed to eliminate remnants of *Pasteurella pestis* from the millions of pelts collected in the region.[40]

After the 1910 outbreak, both Chinese and Japanese scientists and public health experts scoured the Manchurian plains for specimens of burrowing mammals. Several of Wu's North Manchurian Plague Prevention Service reports show that organization's obsession with the tarbagan. Chinese scientists trapped, measured, weighed, gassed, and dissected the animals. Photographs show scientists on the plains taking the temperature of live tarbagans with rectal thermometers.[41] Japanese scientists performed similar procedures, but sometimes with different goals in mind. Well into the 1920s, scientists were still uncertain exactly how plague spread from animals to humans. In 1928, both Wu's plague-prevention service and Japanese scientists from the Mantetsu Hygiene Institute conducted investigations around an outbreak of plague in the vicinity of Tongliao, in the Kerqin grasslands. Wu hypothesized that an epizootic among rats had preceded the outbreak among humans. However, the Japanese scientists came up with different results. To disprove Wu's assertion, they collected 57,216 small mammals from the Tongliao area. Assays showed no substantial plague bacteria in the animals, and none whatsoever in rats. The Japanese scientists concluded that the "rats were entirely innocent" in the epidemic, and that the spread of the epidemic was due instead to the "conditions in which the uncivilized natives live." The report concluded: "the infections seem to have been carried by the ignorant natives themselves."[42]

In the scientific imagination, the primitive and unhealthy nature of Manchuria was most dangerously manifested in the intimate proximity between its human and animal populations. The etiology of the plague, a disease born in wild animals but spread to humans, placed humans firmly within the web of biological phenomena. A central task of *weisheng* and *eisei* was to understand the medical ecology of Manchuria: to unravel the relationships between vectors and man—or, rather, to see man as part of an intertwined disease-producing environment. Testing, examining, and observing man was part and parcel of testing, examining, and observing nature.[43]

Chinese and Japanese scientists both engaged in this medical ecology pursuit. Just as the pith-helmet-wearing, jodhpur-clad scientist in the field examining tarbagans may have been Chinese or Japanese, the man in the distinctive early-twentieth-century biohazard suit, with its frightening Ku Klux Klan–like pointed hood, may have been a Chinese public health worker or a Japanese scientist. The medical ecology of plague control required an understanding of the intersections among microorganisms and two types of mammals: rodents and humans. In the eyes of those dedicated to using the tools of science to control the plague, rodents and humans alike had to be captured, categorized, probed, and autopsied in order to stop the microorganism from spreading. The political control of this Manchurian plagueland necessitated the violent control of life-forms on the macro and micro level. As the Japanese achieved political ascendancy in Manchuria after 1931, the challenge of epidemic disease shaped—and warped—the practice of the biomedical sciences.

The Ubiquitous Needle

Many of the legends about Japanese doctors revolve around the hypodermic needle. Unlike African *bazimamoto* stories, in Chinese evil-needle stories Japanese doctors do not use the syringe to extract blood. Instead they use the needle to inject pathogens into Chinese bodies without the victims' knowledge. The Chinese victims are sometimes willingly under the medical care of Japanese physicians (as in the legends of Huo Yuanjia, who sought out Japanese treatment for tuberculosis). However, for our purposes, more interesting is the suspicion that seemed to arise from Japanese mass vaccination projects, a central aspect of Japanese colonial *eisei* administration.

Frank Dikotter, in his recent work on Chinese consumer and drug cultures, has shown that the hypodermic syringe became a commonplace object in Chinese urban society in the first half of the twentieth century. According to Dikotter, the Chinese welcomed the needle as a fast and easy way to access both cure and pleasure. Laymen injected themselves with a variety of things, from vitamins to opiates, while the "popular belief in the efficacy of injecting medicine" caused patients to demand that doctors inject them with biomedicines, the most popular being the much sought-after syphilis treatment, Salvarsan.[44] While the needle may have become familiar in many circles, it still carried with it a complex assortment of meanings. As Dikotter puts it, "the syringe represented many things to many people, from an object of fear to a potent symbol of healing power, an emblem of medical authority or a marker of drug addiction."[45]

In Dikotter's work, needles are primarily objects that are embraced by Chinese consumers. The Chinese feel comfortable with them and use them with ease themselves. Such ease, however, may not have been felt by those Chinese who lived far from the urban centers of drug use and biomedical clinics, or by those who were injected by anonymous doctors in the midst of Japanese epidemic-control campaigns. Stories about the nefarious uses of injections stem from two possible sources: the ubiquitous identification of biomedicine with the hypodermic needle, and the increased use of mass vaccination campaigns by Japanese public health authorities to control numerous types of contagious disease outbreaks in northeast China. To understand the rise of rumors about the intent of Japanese *eisei* activities, it is necessary to first shed light on the material culture of biomedicine as practiced in Manchuria by Japanese physicians and public health workers, and to highlight the role of the syringe within this material culture.

Iijima Wataru and others have noted that although the Japanese government had established a large network of hospitals along the South Manchuria Railway, the vast majority of those who made use of those hospitals were Japanese. Iijima reminds us that in spite of the importation to Manchuria of various public health schemes from Taiwan, vaccination was the primary manifestation of *eisei* activity.[46] The hypodermic needle was the medium that represented *eisei* in the common experience of Chinese in Manchuria. It is not surprising that some Chinese offered interpretations of Japanese *eisei* through interpretations of the significance of the needle.

Japanese physicians carried the needle to even the most remote corners of the Manchurian plains. For some dwellers in rural Manchuria, their first encounters with a needle (and with Japanese doctors) came under fairly benign circumstances. For Japanese medical students and medical professors, field trips to offer health clinics to remote Manchurian villages became a sort of annual summer vacation event. Beginning in the summer of 1924, the Manchuria Medical School, under the sponsorship of the South Manchurian Railway Company's Public Health Office, sent small groups of physicians, medical students, and technicians to travel for one month in the Kerqin grasslands, providing medical services and investigating the *eisei* situation among the natives. The goals of the expedition were numerous and grand. By offering medical care, the mobile medical teams were to bring the light of civilization to a remote place. At the same time, their hygiene investigations in the easternmost parts of the railway network would help protect the *eisei* of southern Manchuria and its growing Japanese population. The expeditions were conceptualized within an overall framework of nurturing benevolence and mutual understanding between the peoples of Manchuria. Organizers pointed out that Christian missionaries had sacrificed their lives to bring modern medicine to the Chinese, but antiforeign feelings had led to the destruction of hospitals and religious institutions. In the contemporary situation of competition between various foreign concerns in China, it was important for Japanese medicine to demonstrate benevolence in order to win over the hearts and minds of the natives. For this reason, the Japanese would risk their lives to bring medical relief to the miserable sufferers of eastern Mongolia.[47]

Eastern Mongolia, or the western parts of what was to become Manchukuo, was a site of perpetual interest for Japanese scientists. This was the border where the fertile Manchurian plain turned into the shifting grasslands and deserts of the Mongols, in the area where today's Inner Mongolia meets the northwestern sections of Jilin province. From the perspective of *weisheng*, this area was a dangerous site, for it was home to bubonic plague. Plague outbreaks took place there in 1928, 1935, and 1936, just as the Mantetsu rail lines were expanding into the region. To a Japanese administration that had lived through the great Manchurian plague of 1910–11, the hygienically backward Kerqin grasslands loomed as a perpetual threat to the Japanese presence in Manchuria. Beginning in 1924 and then continuing every year for the next twelve years, faculty and students from the Manchuria Medical School spent their summer vacation bringing biomedicine to this dangerous area in order to bring benevolence to the natives and protect the endeavors of the Japanese empire.

The work of the mobile medical teams was quite diverse. They took photographs of local suffering, generating the usual colonial archive of horrific images: victims of tertiary yaws with noses and lips half eaten away, monstrous births, missing appendages, deformed bone structures. At the same time, they took photos of wild landscapes and had a particular fondness for photographing camels and piles of cow manure. The teams tested water, commented on local foods and customs, and made notes on the flora and fauna of the region, with particular emphasis on the relationship between humans, insects, and domesticated animals. But their primary business was to cure the bodily ills of the local inhabitants.

The extensive records of each expedition allow us a glimpse into the physical constituents of biomedicine as experienced by the region's people. Many of the objects used by the mobile medical teams were designed to pierce or probe inside the skin: needles for sewing wounds, needles for administering smallpox vaccinations, a tool for puncturing the chest cavity, speculums (for vagina and anus), blood-drawing needles, and finally a wide assortment of hypodermic needles and ampuls for giving injections.[48] The needle was frequently employed among remote populations by these Japanese visitors.

Needles were also central to the Japanese investigation of Manchuria's medical ecology. On each trip, mobile medical teams surveyed the natural environment of the grasslands and the place of native people within it. Scientists drew blood from people and animals alike to understand flora and fauna on a microscopic level. Mobile medical teams were not the only investigators to do this. Mantetsu surveys of agriculture and land use (information used by American scholars to understand village society) also frequently included information on the diseases of livestock, tested by drawing blood from cattle and sheep. These investigations overlapped with medical and anthropological investigations of the blood of different ethnic groups conducted in the name of *weisheng* or *eisei* during the Manchukuo regime.[49]

The hypodermic needle was a part of studying the nature of Manchuria, but it was also a central tool in the prevention of disease. The needle gained increasing prominence during the Manchukuo regime as Japanese epidemic-control activities penetrated even the most remote areas of Manchukuo. An example is the Japanese management of a localized outbreak of bubonic plague in the Kerqin grasslands in 1935. After the Mukden Incident and under the Manchukuo regime, Japanese administrators were able to marshal far more resources in the area than what had been represented by the mobile medical teams of the previous decade. Over one thousand police, military, and health personnel did door-to-door (or yurt-to-yurt) inspections of hundreds of thousands of people. With the plague inspections came vaccinations: in one month in 1935 alone, Japanese *eisei* personnel injected almost 200,000 people in the region with a plague vaccine.[50] From this documented example, we can see that Japanese public health and epidemic-control efforts not only touched cities, but spread to the farthest edges of the empire. Mongol nomads living in yurts, Russian pioneers in logging camps, and monks cloistered in lamaseries on the edges of the grasslands experienced the Japanese medical presence, usually in the guise of the public health worker wielding a hypodermic needle in the company of a military escort wielding a bayonet. After Japan's occupation was completed in 1932, the Japanese wielded the hypodermic needle on a mass scale in the name of the state and military. Chinese suspicions of the needle—and of *weisheng* interventions—emerged in this politically charged environment.[51]

This preliminary investigation reveals several important insights. First, hypodermic needles were an integral part not only of Japanese public health activities in Manchuria, but also of the general scientific investigation of Manchuria's natural environment by Japanese scientists. Second, Japanese medical and scientific personnel ranged far and wide across Manchuria, and the needle went with them wherever they went. Finally, the use of the hypodermic needle in Japanese *eisei* activities increased after 1932 and particularly after 1937, as war brought more soldiers, more doctors, and more disease to Manchuria.

Speaking with Vampires in Manchuria

What has not been well documented—and what can never be accurately determined—is the specific extent of the Japanese military's biological warfare attacks, specifically the geographical scope and frequency of the intentional spreading of infectious disease outside of the Pingfang laboratories. In mainland Chinese scholarship on the Japanese medical presence in Manchuria, the overwhelming emphasis is on exposing the evil intent of Japanese physicians, including those affiliated with Mantetsu public health infrastructures. The stories that trace outbreaks of epidemic disease in north and northeast China in the 1930s and 1940s to the machinations of Japanese doctors wielding hypodermic needles go unexamined or are taken at face value.

In the present research climate, it is unacceptable to suggest that the frequently encountered stories of Japanese spreading disease through vaccination may be examined as a formulaic rumor. The trope of Japanese medicine and public health as inherently evil dominates official public discourse. It forms a central element in both official and unofficial expressions of Chinese nationalism. These rumors—if they are rumors—cannot be seen as products of subaltern sensibilities or confusions, but are the very stuff of national identity, groomed and perpetuated (though also slightly contained) by national elites through official government institutions: textbooks, research institutions, and museums.[52] The story of northern China as victim of Japanese colonial medicine and public health frames almost all inquiry within China. My discussion of rumor, needles, and Japanese *eisei* violates taboos by blurring the line between truth, representation, and rumor. The scholar working on twentieth-century China, in contrast to the scholar of twentieth-century Africa, is not at liberty to profess a postmodern embrace of representation while simultaneously maintaining a modern belief in what is true and what is not. The foreign scholar who does this in China runs the risk of being accused of sympathies with right-wing Japanese challenges to the credibility of Chinese war memory.

Many Chinese suspicions about Japanese public health and medical activities revolve around specific aspects of the material culture of biomedicine: the "entangled objects" at the intersection of contact between Japanese physicians and a Chinese public.[53] But this is not a story of exchange, circulation, and colonial encounters; it is instead about the understanding of a tool that was wielded by the colonial specialists, a tool that had the power to penetrate the skin of the colonized in order to cure, or perhaps in order to kill.

How then are we to make sense of Chinese tales of Japanese physicians not bringing benevolent public health through hypodermic needles, but inflicting disease with them instead? Carlo Ginzburg, in his work on tales of witchcraft and werewolves in Europe, suggested that rumors should be read as reflections of beliefs stretching back to an ancient past. Details in stories provide glimpses into a shared mentality of a peasant world, of old traditions and tales.⁵⁴ Certainly tales of armies secretly poisoning their enemies in war — by poisoning wells or by intentionally spreading "pollution" — are frequently encountered in the Chinese historical record. Barend ter Haar, in his recent monumental work on the telling of stories in Chinese history, has identified specific genres of rumor related to the stealing of "life force," "organ theft," "fetus stealing," and other mysterious bodily injuries perpetrated on innocents, dating back as far as the Song dynasty. Often in these rumors, the scapegoats are identified as liminal figures (such as old widows or monks) or outsiders (those from other villages or provinces or, in the nineteenth century, foreigners from another country). Ter Haar finds little truth in any of these stories, even those that emerge from Qing court cases where the authorities tried and convicted perpetrators for crimes such as organ theft. While he allows that "at least a few details must be actually true for [the stories] to remain credible" and thus widely disseminated, for the most part he sees such rumors as the products of social chaos, created in times of stress such as famine or wartime; metaphors that reveal the tensions between in-groups and "the other."⁵⁵

That Japanese would be accused of wide-scale poisoning of Chinese could be seen as an expected continuum of a tradition — only in this instance, the vehicle through which the poisoning was accomplished had changed from poisonous bugs (*chong*) slipped into a well to injections, from the nefarious extraction of organs through supernatural means to the nefarious extraction of organs in the scientific laboratory.

Tales of evil physicians should also be placed in the context of popular beliefs that accompanied the evolution of biomedicine in Europe. Historians of medicine usually pay far more attention to colonial "misunderstandings" of public health interventions, forgetting that in England riots broke out in reaction to government cholera control activities in the 1830s and 1840s. British working-class city dwellers were convinced that they were being sent to hospitals so that medical students could cut up their bodies — a fear with solid foundation after the passage of the Anatomy Act of 1832, which mandated that bodies of the destitute who had died in the workhouse and other public institutions would be used as cadavers for medical instruction.⁵⁶ The belief that foreigners cut out various body parts of the Chinese and used them to make medicine resonated not only with traditional Chinese beliefs that men could actually seek human organs for use as medicines, but was also part of a worldwide reaction to an emerging biomedicine, one that cut bodies both living (surgery) and dead (autopsies).⁵⁷

However, stories that equated Japanese injections with poisoning and germ warfare emerged in a specific environment of Japanese imperialism. Liu Shiyong has noted that beginning in the 1920s, Japanese public health in Taiwan relied increasingly on vaccination to prevent epidemic disease.[58] A similar trend can be discerned in Manchuria. There, the increased reliance on vaccination to control cholera, typhoid, and plague coincided with increased violence and presence of soldiers. There may have been an overall shift in Japanese science that led to an increased reliance on needles in public health, but in Manchuria, the incidence of disease and the administration of its control were inseparable from military invasion.

Chinese stories of Japanese doctors' injecting disease reflect fears of Japan's remarkable power and ability to penetrate China seemingly at will. Luise White has interpreted stories that link biomedicine to vampires as tales of unfair victimization: "Bazimamoto stories are those in which Europeans get the upper hand. They [Europeans] were not necessarily smarter than Africans, but they had better tools, more power, and most especially, better drugs."[59] The legend of the death of Huo—the kung-fu master whom the Japanese could defeat only through the surreptitious use of hypodermic needles—closely fits this sort of interpretation. In these stories, Japanese technology helps explain Chinese defeat. The coincidence of military invasion and mass vaccination helped to generate more rumors, beyond those resulting from the occasional encounter with Japanese medicine within a Japanese hospital setting. As we have seen, Japanese public health personnel brought the syringe into the far reaches of Manchuria. Mass exposure to the needle on a wide scale helped to create a unified genre of rumor across a broad geographical area.

Japanese scientists did not use needles just to inject substances into or draw them from humans: the blood of animals was also scrutinized through the same method. Indeed, humans and animals in Manchuria existed on an ecological continuum for many Japanese researchers. That man was a natural object for Japanese experts in biology and public health is perhaps most graphically demonstrated in photographs from plague-prevention work in Manchuria. The official Japanese history of the great Manchurian plague of 1910–11 contains photographs of Japanese scientists performing autopsies on the frozen corpses of donkeys, followed immediately by photographs of Japanese scientists performing autopsies on the frozen corpses of (Chinese) humans. Bodies of both animal and human subjects are splayed in similar positions and displayed in similar settings, and the scientists are garbed in similar white coats and masks. The overall effect of this sort of continuity is to position both human and animal as objects of scientific penetrating, probing, and disemboweling. In this light, tales of evil injections can be read as resistance to the objectifying intent of science, a response to being callously examined and injected by Japanese scientists, along with the rest of nature. Medical ecology may have been an advanced approach to the study of disease, but in the colonial setting, and under conditions that saw the erosion of medical ethics, medical ecology represented an opportunity for the emergence of medical atrocities.

In spite of the prevalence and intrigue of these rumors, these were obviously not the only meanings that Chinese gave to the Japanese biomedical presence. Chinese elites analyzed Japanese public health activities in newspapers and journals, joined with Japanese in joint public health administration in cities such as Dalian, and studied medicine under Japanese mentors in institutions such as the Manchuria Medical School. As Ming-cheng Lo has shown in her work on Taiwanese physicians under Japanese colonialism, elites within the Japanese empire frequently negotiated their identities as colonial moderns through medicine and hygiene.[60] Ideally, research into rumors of evil needles should specify who may have authored such beliefs and uncover when such beliefs became widespread. Rana Mitter has demonstrated how tales of spontaneous Chinese resistance against the Japanese in Manchuria were primarily the product of nationalists organized south of the Great Wall. The actual response within Manchuria to Japanese expansion was diverse and ambiguous, and could not entirely be encompassed by a narrative of heroic resistance.[61] It appears that discussion in print of the evil intent of Japan's *eisei* activities emerged after 1949, with the establishment of the People's Republic of China and the official exposure of Unit 731 by the Chinese government. Certainly such rumors have merged with mainland Chinese constructions of war memory, and war memory forms a major basis for contemporary nationalism, including the official kind nurtured by the present government. These eliding associations remind us of the complexity of exploring tales and rumors dealing with Japan.

Ultimately, however, no consideration of needle rumors can separate itself from the legacy of Unit 731. Currently, scholars in China, and some in Japan, are making painstaking attempts to expose evidence of Japanese wartime atrocities masquerading as epidemic-prevention interventions.[62] In the interests of justice, this work must continue. Many difficulties remain, however, not the least among them being the question of how to adequately document truth in order to give it a separate existence from fiction or rumor.

Perhaps there is another way to think through this conundrum. In some ways, this blurring of benevolence and amorality in the case of Japanese *eisei* in China may be a highly indicative example of a truth about modern biomedicine and public health. Scholars writing about the subject have faced two analytical paths: either it brings the desirable benefits of health and modernity (who among us does not want clean toilets and vaccinations for her children?), or it is a mode of social control, a coercive force, which, in creating modernity, limits the range of possible expressions of humanity. It is perhaps most advantageous to see these two paths as not mutually exclusive interpretations. The history of biomedicine and public health (*weisheng*) has in fact inextricably combined the two: health and violence, cleanliness and coercion, religious benevolence and scientific objectification.

Dipesh Chakrabarty has challenged scholars to "write into the history of modernity the ambivalences, the contradictions, the use of force, and the tragedies and ironies that attend it." He has suggested that the ironies of modernity are nowhere more evident than in the history of public health, modern medicine, and personal hygiene. Chakrabarty points out that the triumph of an ultimately beneficial and benevolent modern health "has always been dependent on the mobilization, on its behalf, of effective means of physical coercion."[63] There is perhaps no clearer example of this than the Japanese exercise of *eisei* in Manchuria during the first part of the twentieth century. Tales of the Japanese physician dispensing disease through the hypodermic needle embody the frustrations and suspicions caused by occupation, inscribed upon one of the most common objects that lay at the literal point of Japanese-Chinese contact. The difficulty in the present PRC political climate of recognizing the dual nature of *weisheng*—at once brutal and modern—lies at the base of mainland Chinese constructions of national identity. It is also a paradox that lies at the base of our own understandings, as scholars, of the nature of hygienic modernity.

NOTES

All translations are mine, unless otherwise indicated.

1. Rogaski, *Hygienic Modernity*.

2. For a recent exploration of the role of hygiene in the Japanese colonization of Korea, see Henry, "Sanitizing Empire."

3. A noteworthy example of scholarship that probes voices high and low for understandings of public health work in China is Gamsa, "The Epidemic of Pneumonic Plague in Manchuria 1910–1911." This exemplary work, which focuses primarily on Russian and Chinese epidemic-prevention activities in the 1910s and 1920s, has helped inform my own thinking about the legends and metaphors that surround health and disease in Manchuria.

4. My use of the term "vampire" here is inspired by Luise White's pathbreaking work, *Speaking with Vampires*. I will discuss White's method of interpreting vampire stories in Africa later in this chapter.

5. As Gamsa has pointed out in "The Epidemic of Pneumonic Plague in Manchuria 1910–1911," this line is far too clearly demarcated in much Western scholarship on colonial medicine.

6. On Dalian's public health, see Perrins, "Doctors, Disease and Development."

7. Young, *Japan's Total Empire*, 249.

8. Classic studies on the 1910–11 outbreak include Nathan, *Plague Prevention and Politics in Manchuria, 1910–1931*, and Wu Lien-teh, *Plague Fighter*.

9. For a chart tabulating plague outbreaks during the occupation years, see Xie Xueshi, "'Xinjing' shuyi moulue," 113.

10. On Dalian's experience with cholera, see Perrins, "Doctors, Disease and Development," 116–17; also Sun Chengdai et al., *Diquo zhuyi qinlue Dalianshi congshu*, 14–64.

11. Iijima, *Pesuto to kindai Chūgoku*.

12. Young, *Japan's Total Empire*, 307–411.

13. As Prasenjit Duara has pointed out, this conception of Manchuria as a "wild, empty frontier" was an inaccurate fantasy: much of the allegedly empty frontier had been peopled and cultivated by Chinese farmers for decades (*Sovereignty and Authenticity*, 171–77).

14. Some examples include Toyoda H., *Toman to eisei*; Minami Manshū Tetsudō Kabushiki Kaisha; Eiseika, *Manshū fūdo eisei kenkyū gaiyō*; Uruno Katsuya, *Manshū no chihōbyō to densenbyo*; and Toyoda Taro, *Manshū no iji eisei kotoni densenbyō*.

15. Uruno, *Manshū no chihōbyo to densenbyo*, 26.

16. Toyoda H., *Toman to eisei*, 1–17.

17. Perrins, "Doctors, Disease and Development," 104.

18. See statistics in the SMRC annual reports, Minami Manshū Tetsudō Kabushiki Kaisha; Eiseika, *Minami Manshū Tetsudō fuzokuchi eisei gaikyō*.

19. Perrins, "Doctors, Disease and Development," 104.

20. Xie X., "'Xinjing' shuyi moulue," 117.

21. On the plague situation in Changchun, see ibid., 72–83.

22. On the Nong'an experience, see ibid., 84–94.

23. Ibid, 89.

24. On needles, see ibid.

25. White, *Speaking with Vampires*, 5.

26. Ibid., 308.

27. Hunt, *A Colonial Lexicon*, 191.

28. Xie, 110. Xie Xueshi holds that the Changchun plague was a "test run" for Unit 731's 1940 germ-warfare attack on Zhejiang.

29. The most recent monographs on Unit 731 in English include Harris, *Factories of Death*, and Barenblatt, *A Plague upon Humanity*.

30. These stories about Japanese doctors were particularly prevalent in Chinese media during the germ-warfare allegations against the United States in the Korean War. See Rogaski, "Nature, Annihilation, and Modernity."

31. An example of recent Japanese scholarship in this vein is Suenaga, *Senji igaku no jittai*.

32. Gamsa, 166–67.

33. Xi, "Xuyan," 8, quoted in chapter 3 of this volume.

34. Examples of these photos can be found in Kantō Totokufu Rinji Bōkibu, *Meiji yonjūsan-yonen Minami Manshū "pesuto" ryūkōshi*.

35. These images continue to be circulated today in surprising venues, with re-markable interpretations. One autopsy photograph from the 1911 plague, captioned "child victim," has even been used in a present-day anti-Japanese Web site with information about Unit 731. See http://www.aiipowmia.com/731/731child.html.

36. Wu Lien-teh, "The Second Pneumonic Plague Epidemic in Manchuria, 1920–21," 274.

37. Ibid.

38. Ibid., 275.

39. Ibid., 274.

40. Wu Lien-teh., *A Treatise on Pneumonic Plague*.

41. Wu Lien-teh, "Plague."

42. Ando, Kurauchi, and Nishimura, "A New Plague Endemic Area in the North-eastern Part of Inner Mongolia." On earlier debates between Chinese and Russian scientists about the tarbagan theory, see Gamsa, 172–74.

43. On ecology, medical ecology, and empire, see Anker, *Imperial Ecology*, and Mendelsohn, "From Eradication to Equilibrium."

44. Dikotter, *Narcotic Culture*, 179–80.

45. Ibid., 190.

46. Iijima, *Pesuto to kindai Chūgoku*, 178–86.

47. Manshū Ika daigaku; Minami Manshū Tetsudō Kabushiki Kaisha. Eiseika. *Manshū Ika Daigaku daiikkai Tōmōjunkai shinryōhōkoku*.

48. Ibid., 4.

49. On ethnicity in Manchukuo, see Tamanoi, "Knowledge, Power, and Racial Classifications."

50. See Minami Manshū Tetsudō Kabushiki Kaisha; Eiseika, *Kōtoku ninendo pesuto bōeki gaikyō Kōtoku ninendo pesuto bōeki gaikyō*.

51. The public health situation in other parts of China also changed radically after the outbreak of total war in 1937. The threat of contagious disease under conditions of war led Japanese authorities to administer preventive vaccinations frequently

and on a very large scale. For example, in Tianjin in 1939, the combined forces of the Japanese military, the Japanese concession health department, and the collaborationist government health department conducted 213,000 cholera vaccinations, 217,000 smallpox vaccinations, and 9,000 typhoid fever vaccinations. See Rogaski, *Hygienic Modernity*, 272–73.

52. This is demonstrated by the graphic displays of Japanese doctors conducting experiments on Chinese prisoners at the Unit 731 museum outside Harbin and the Jiu-yi-ba Museum in Shenyang.

53. The term is taken from Thomas, *Entangled Objects*.

54. Ginzburg, "Clues: Roots of an Evidential Paradigm."

55. Ter Haar, *Telling Stories*, 97. He argues that Qing officials possessed a "demonological paradigm" that made it impossible for them to understand the difference between "real" people and "fictional" characters. As a result, for ter Haar, "it is difficult, even with the benefit of hindsight, to determine when we are dealing with false accusations and when with genuine events" (191).

56. On the Anatomy Act, see Richardson, *Death, Dissection, and the Destitute.*

57. On these beliefs, see ter Haar, *Telling Stories*, and P. Cohen, *China and Christianity.*

58. Liu S., "'Qingjie,' 'weisheng,' yu 'baojian.'"

59. White, *Speaking with Vampires*, 115.

60. Lo, *Doctors within Borders.*

61. Mitter, *The Manchurian Myth.*

62. See Rogaski, "Nature, Annihilation, and Modernity."

63. Chakrabarty, "Postcoloniality and the Artifice of History," 288.

Have Someone Cut the Umbilical Cord

Women's Birthing Networks, Knowledge,
and Skills in Colonial Taiwan

Wu Chia-Ling

As part of a seminar on children's welfare that was held in Taipei's Public Hall in 1940, a group of distinguished Japanese doctors, professors, public health officials, and social welfare advocates debated why so few Taiwanese women made use of modern midwifery.[1] Magara Masanao, chair of the Obstetrics Department of Taipei Imperial University, observed that of the nine thousand women giving birth each year in Taipei City, supposedly the most developed area in this showcase colony of Japan, only two thousand sent for licensed midwives or obstetricians for childbirth. Magara inferred that it was because "Taiwanese are stingy with money" and believed they would rather have cheaper lay (unlicensed) midwives. Gotō Kioshi, a professor at Taipei Imperial University, argued that it was rather due to women's shame at exposing their naked bodies to strangers during childbirth. Tachikawa Yoshio, the vice president of the Taiwan Social Welfare Society, suggested that in addition to the factor of expense, lack of scientific knowledge was the key reason. Sota Nagamune, a researcher of vital statistics under the governor general of Taiwan, agreed that the Taiwanese population had low hygienic literacy and proposed a more active system of public midwives to approach these women. Sota's proposal was immediately supported by the participants and thus became the seminar's recommendation.

This scene provides a snapshot of how elites portrayed birthing women in the colonial period. These top Japanese policymakers saw Taiwanese women as conservative, insufficiently educated, and backward, and their unlicensed birth attendants as ignorant of basic hygiene. Although desiring to reduce maternal and neonatal mortality for the Taiwanese, these

Japanese male elites adopted a so-called deficiency model, which viewed women as needing to be educated and improved. By the 1940s, infant mortality rates and maternal death rates were higher for the Taiwanese population than for the Japanese population living in Taiwan. Browsing published governmental reports, medical journals, and social welfare monographs, I found that Taiwanese women were repeatedly blamed for these discrepancies.

The birthing system in Taiwan underwent a significant transformation in the first half of the twentieth century (see table 1). After 1895, the distinctive Japanese project of scientific colonialism included building a modern public health system, establishing institutionalized medical education, and promoting scientific ideas on personal hygiene as important components of medical modernization.[2] While battling infectious diseases like malaria in Taiwan was the first priority for the Japanese colonial state,[3] efforts to improve maternal and infant health also gradually gained attention. Cosmopolitan midwifery was introduced with the establishment of its education system, licensing regulations, and public midwifery programs. Public officials, local doctors, and even certified midwives served as agents of this new project. Birthing women were mostly viewed as the passive recipients of this new hygienic practice, or as stubborn opponents of modernization. Experts represented women in statistical reports without names or identities. In the most formalized data, the women were voiceless and faceless.

Why did women use or not use cosmopolitan midwifery? How did they view their birth attendants? How can we avoid the elites' passive and derogatory image of women and instead view them as active agents shaping midwifery in colonial Taiwan? In contrast to the pages and pages of male elites' observations and comments, how would women tell their own stories?

Feminist scholarship stresses the importance of taking such women's voices seriously as it probes how cosmopolitan science and medicine transformed the institution of motherhood and the experience of mothering. The abundant literature on scientific motherhood and the medicalization of childbirth critically evaluates the early-twentieth-century ideology that scientific principles should guide child rearing and childbearing.[4] Further, feminists politicize the growing involvement of medical and scientific experts in women's reproductive labor.[5] Beyond analyzing the intervention of the male-dominated state and professional actors, they explore women's agency during this process. Rather than viewing women as socially con-

Table 1. The development of certified midwifery services in Japan and Taiwan

Year		
1868	Japan	Regulation banning illegal midwives
1875		Registration of midwives
1876		Midwifery education at medical school
1899		Japanese Midwifery Act
1902	Taiwan	Regulation banning illegal midwives
		Midwifery education at medical school (for Japanese nurses only)
1907		Midwifery training program at medical school (open to Taiwanese)
1922		Public midwives services
1923		Taiwan Midwifery Act
1926		Short training program and licensing for traditional midwives
1927		Private midwifery school offered by Taiwanese obstetricians

trolled or passive receivers, such scholars argue that women were able to mobilize around motherhood issues and claim authority to negotiate their childbearing and child-rearing practices.[6] The stories of those who stayed within the indigenous birth system can illuminate the evolving and complex tangles connecting gender and class roles, scientific and technological development, and personal struggles.

More recently, science and technology studies (STS) has emphasized the importance of treating both users and nonusers as essential actors in the network building of new technological systems.[7] Feminist STS scholars focus on how women actively participate in the development of technology, as well as how they negotiate the meaning of technology while using it.[8] In examining the nonusers, they argue that resistance to new technology is neither irrational nor heroic, but is a common occurrence when a sociotechnical system changes.[9] Nonuse is not just about ignorance and deprivation but includes a voluntary dimension that deserves systematic investigation.[10]

These insights inform my study of birthing women's stories in the colonial period of Taiwan. I place birthing women's oral histories at the center of my analysis and explore how we can reinterpret the transformation of the birth system by incorporating their voices. For this purpose, I conducted interviews between 2003 and 2006. The twenty-one women I interviewed were born between 1910 and 1927 and had their first child between the late 1920s and the late 1940s. The oldest woman I met was ninety-five years old, and she could still bend down to tighten the shoelaces of her sneakers. For women in their early eighties at the time of my interviews, I often jokingly complained that they were too young for my research project, and they seemed very happy to hear such a comment. Although the four youngest grandmothers did not give birth until after the end of colonization, all inter-viewees recalled observations of their mothers' or other women's childbirth experiences in the colonial period, adding valuable data for my analysis.

All but one of the women could clearly specify the type of their birth attendant: eleven of them had licensed midwives as their birth attendants throughout their reproductive cycle; five had the assistance of their rela-tives or other elderly women, or they "cut the umbilical cord" themselves; and four had a combination of birth attendants. According to government statistics, by the end of the colonial period fewer than half of all women in Taiwan were using licensed midwives. My sample had a higher percentage than this, probably because the snowballing method of finding interview-ees tends to reach middle-class families first. Still, my sample is diverse across social classes and a wide range of childbirth experiences. The pur-pose of this chapter is not to represent all women's experiences but to offer counterarguments and critical explanations by revealing the underrecorded life histories of birthing women in the colonial period. I also analyzed medi-cal journals, state policy documents, and other secondary resources, mainly to compare and contrast my subjects' claims with those of the authorities.

Women's Memories of Their Lay Birth Attendants

According to the accounts of governmental health officials during the Japanese colonial period, modern midwifery is a sign of the progress of civilization. Even before formal midwifery education was available to the Taiwanese people, the Japanese government attempted in 1902 to ban un-certified Taiwanese midwives.[11] Medical records, newspaper stories, and public health reports claimed that these midwives' ignorance of antiseptic practices was responsible for the high rates of neonatal tetanus as well as puerperal fever. Carol Laderman's description of how lay midwives were portrayed in Malaysia during British colonial rule could also apply to their Taiwanese counterparts: "Childbirth customs were described at length as examples of superstition: the midwife's practical role was neglected in favor of her ritual activity."[12]

As the high rate of infant mortality became a serious problem in the eyes of public officials, almost all discussions on reducing infant mortality in colonial Taiwan emphasized the importance of replacing traditional midwives with midwives who had received a modern biomedical education.[13] Such views were shared by biomedically trained Taiwanese doctors. As both Yang Cui and Fan Yanqiu stress, the Taiwanese elite emphasized midwifery training and maternal services even more actively than the Japanese public health officers, implying that they too rejected indigenous midwifery.[14] However, accounts other than those of medical professionals and public health officials offer a divergent understanding of why women kept using unlicensed midwives.

Lay Midwives as Capable, Experienced Women

Who were these lay midwives?

> "[The lay midwife was usually] an old woman. She was capable and diligent, and people would ask such an *a-pô* to cut the umbilical cord."
> "Who was better? *Sán-pô* or *a-pô*?"
> "There was no difference. The real difference lay in your own birth; if your birth pain lasted longer, then it was more painful. That's the real difference."[15]

In the official statistics, midwives are often grouped into a single category called "lay midwives," but in my sample noncertified birth attendants were quite diverse: women's mothers, mothers-in-law, other female relatives like aunts, the birthing women themselves, and lastly certain old women in the neighborhood, referred to by women like Tumei in the interview above as *a-pô*. *A-pô* literally means "old woman" in the Taiwanese Hokkien dialect, in contrast to *sán-pô*, which refers to educated and licensed midwives. As another woman named Afang observed, "in every township, there seemed to be a woman who knew how to cut the umbilical cord,"[16] and such women were often called *a-pô*. Nevertheless, the indigenous midwifery system was not centered on *a-pô*. Some women's close family members did attend births, but not as regularly as *a-pô*. The women I interviewed who had cut the umbilical cord themselves usually did not attend other women's births. Their mothers and mothers-in-law helped only their immediate family members and did not serve the rest of the neighborhood. This shows that at least in the 1920s and 1930s, folk knowledge on assisting birth was prevalent to some degree, but was neither simply limited to a small number of old women like *a-pô*, nor widely known and practiced by every woman.

The term *a-pô*—consisting of the sound *a*, an honorific, and *po*, which means grandmother—shows the first feature of these traditional birth attendants: they were senior community members. Often they were themselves the mothers of many children.

For example, a woman named Aluan described how her mother's sister-in-law assisted her in childbirth during the war. She stressed that the aunt had herself given birth to twelve children, "winning a gold medal from the Japanese government" (which at that time stressed a pronatalistic policy). An *a-pô* or an elderly female relative was the kind of woman "who *was able to* do it" or "who *knew how to* cut the umbilical cord" (emphasis mine).[17] In this context, age meant plentiful physical experience as well as capabilities.

Since not all women who gave birth to many children became birth helpers in the neighborhood or among family members, some other features also counted. My interviewees emphasized certain unique characteristics of these women helpers. Tumei stressed that these old women were "capable and diligent."[18] Aluan observed that women who were "brave, smart, and big-hearted"[19] tended to be asked for such help. They were so skillful that some women saw no difference between the lay and the licensed midwives, as Tumei claims in the quotation at the beginning of this section. The appreciation of such capability even led Ayu, a middle-class woman living in one of the most prosperous urban areas in Taipei, to have her mother serve as her birth attendant in the late 1940s, "because she was so capable of doing the job."[20] Compared to the denunciation of lay midwives by officials, birthing women saw these midwives as respectable, experienced women from the community or the family circle. What exactly were the skills and birthing knowledge that made these lay birth attendants so trustworthy?

Lay Midwives and Their Skills

In women's birth narratives, to give birth is practically equated with cutting the umbilical cord:

> "We had hardship, and we all gave birth ourselves, and cut the umbilical cord ourselves. First you prepared the scissors, then you used

string to tie the umbilical cord, and then you cut it. You need to tie it really tightly so that it would not bleed . . . Then we used sesame oil to spread on the umbilical region."

"How did you know how to do this?"

"My mother-in-law delivered my first three children. After she died, since I had seen how she did it, I delivered the rest of my children myself."[21]

In Chaodi's words, the phrase "giving birth" also means "cutting the umbilical cord." This association implies that accompanying the birthing woman during labor pains was not the core of the indigenous birth system.[22] The families of the women I interviewed often did not fetch a midwife until they could not stand the labor pains, and they said that these helpers stayed with them only for a short time. Tumei even emphasized that sometimes it was not until after the newborn came out that an *a-pô* was called in to cut the umbilical cord: "Since she was our neighbor, she was really close by."[23] The standard tasks of the *a-pô* in my interviewees' descriptions were to cut the umbilical cord and to bathe the baby, and with that she had finished the job.

Although the *a-pô* may not have stayed with the birthing woman for a long time, several of the interviewees could describe events that had happened seventy years ago in amazing detail. Cutting the umbilical cord emerged as the best-remembered process in women's narrative of their childbirth. What Chaodi described in the interview cited above was a typical account in my sample, with only slight differences. Some women emphasized that the umbilical cord needed to be tied twice, with the second knot done after the cord had been bent down toward the child's lower abdomen. Thread made from ramie fibers was recommended for tying the cord. Some women remembered that alum powder was spread on the umbilical region after the application of sesame oil. To tie, to cut, and to apply sesame oil— the women's collective description was very similar to the so-called folk practice recorded in Japanese by the governmental investigators.

Cutting the umbilical cord served as a key point of criticism aimed at lay midwives, due to the frequency of neonatal tetanus. Both doctors and policymakers, Japanese and Taiwanese, claimed that tetanus was the major cause of death among Taiwanese newborns, although the infection was almost never seen in Japanese babies. They used the high rate of neonatal tetanus among the Taiwanese population to justify their efforts to encourage the use of aseptic instruments for cutting the umbilical cord, in order to prevent any subsequent infection of the cord. The rate of infant mortality caused by tetanus was often cited as evidence that the replacement of indigenous practices with modern techniques of midwifery was necessary.[24]

Nevertheless, the link between neonatal tetanus and the single factor of traditional birth attendants was shaky. First of all, the incidence of tetanus as a cause of neonatal death might have been overstated. Medical professionals admitted that tetanus was hard to diagnose,[25] and the first statistics reported by the pediatricians of Taipei Imperial University did not even contain any category for tetanus.[26] Great interregional variation existed. For example, tetanus was listed among the ten leading causes of infant deaths for two of the five prefectures in the 1920s but not shown at all in the other three, and the overall leading category of diagnosis was "unknown."[27] Therefore, doctors doubted the statistical accuracy of neonatal tetanus counts as well.[28] In one of the most detailed statistical studies of infant mortality, Dr. Li Tengyue (Ri Tōgaku), a researcher from Taipei Imperial University, found that according to death reports over half of all victims of neonatal tetanus died within five days of birth. This fact could imply misdiagnosis. Li noted that newborns who died of tetanus typically exhibited symptoms only from the fifth to ninth day after birth, and died one to three days after that. Therefore, it was unlikely that most of those who died within five days of birth were victims of tetanus.[29] I suspect that tetanus was overdiagnosed, for it was easily attributed to the indigenous practice of midwifery. Despite recognizing the faulty accuracy of the data and the possibility of misdiagnosis, Li still insisted on the prevalence of neonatal tetanus that was due to the ignorance of both lay midwives and parents.[30]

Besides, proper cutting of the umbilical cord was only one of the steps that would prevent the introduction of bacteria (*Clostridium tetani*) into the umbilical wound; the overall improvement of living conditions also played an important role. Instead of stressing the importance of upgrading the overall environment, it was easy for the elites to blame either ignorant lay midwives or the filthiness of the Taiwanese population in general. No colonial investigators attempted to actually correlate outcomes with the practices of midwives on the ground.

How do we reevaluate indigenous midwifery practices? Some of them can be traced back to pediatric medicine in the Chinese tradition, which has been defended as scientifically effective by a number of scholars. Ping-chen Hsiung) has detailed how the best practices of Chinese medicine included sterile procedures as early as the Sung dynasty.[31] In the eighteenth century, the Qing government's official medical encyclopedia laid out the correct procedures for safely cutting the umbilical cord: first heat the scissors in a flame, and then cut the umbilical cord, cauterizing the wound.[32] Other medical books at that time recommended that people should tie off the cord before cutting it, or apply powder to keep the wound dry. These procedures of tying before cutting, heating the scissors over a fire, and applying power have been well recorded in Chinese medical books since the eighteenth century. Xiong believes that such procedures reflect an understanding of the risk of infecting umbilical wounds and were strictly sterile by today's biomedical standards.

As Fu Daiwei argues, it is rash to assume a complete lack of sterile procedures among the lay midwives in colonial Taiwan.[33] The women I interviewed did talk about some possibly useful procedures that were also recorded in the medical books. Tying off the umbilical cord about three centimeters from the baby's navel before cutting it was an almost universal practice. Some women even remember clearly tying the second string before cutting. This act (tying the cord tightly near the naval area) does in fact lower the baby's chances of getting tetanus.[34] Applying powder to dry the wound was also mentioned in some of the interviews. Alum powder has been proven to have a sterilizing effect.[35] However, none of my informants mentioned heating the scissors used for cutting the cord.

One noteworthy practice was the use of sesame oil. It was unanimously mentioned by the women I interviewed, but it is not discussed in Xiong's study. Even today, some of the licensed midwives in Taiwan still use sesame oil routinely in their treatment of the umbilicus. Sesame oil was used to heal wounds in Chinese medicine as early as the Ming and Qing dynasties.[36] For example, the text *Complete Essentials of Materia Medica* (*Bencao beiyao*) by Wang Ang (1615–ca.1685) published in the Qing dynasty, lists "pain-relieving and tissue-building" among the therapeutic effects of sesame oil.[37] In sixty-three formulas for external application to heal sores recorded in the Chinese medical books, sesame oil appears eight times, ranked as the fourteenth most popular ingredient among 121 Chinese herbs.[38] A number of randomized controlled clinical trials have also demonstrated the healing effects of sesame oil.[39] Hence it is possible that sesame oil served as protection against infection.

Although the ethnographic gap in infant mortality between Taiwanese and Japanese residents in Taiwan began to widen in the 1910s, in 1906, before Japan's public health project was widely launched, the two populations were not far apart: the infant mortality rate in 1906 was 166.5 per 1,000 births for the Japanese population, and 154.1 for the Taiwanese population.[40] The rate of neonatal death for Taiwanese was about the same as in France and Belgium before widespread access to biomedical midwifery.[41] Such a relatively good health outcome was not attributed to the possible contribution of indigenous midwifery practices by the public health officials at that time. In the governmental and professional literature on birth, the early claim by one Japanese doctor regarding Taiwanese health that "although they do not have hygienic knowledge, they might have experimented with some methods to maintain their health" did not apply to traditional midwifery.[42]

The Transformation of the Lay Midwife

Women's birthing stories also remind us not to essentialize the so-called indigenous midwifery. While I have shown the element of traditional Chinese medicine in the lay midwives' practices, Ayu's detailed description of her mother's way of delivering her own babies in the 1940s demonstrates an accommodation of biomedicine:

> "My mom was very capable when giving birth. When she gave birth to my younger sister, I knew that she cut the umbilical cord herself . . . When she felt pain, she boiled the water first and prepared the scissors, and then after the baby had come out, she tied and cut . . . She was very brave, very healthy . . . When I gave birth, she cut the umbilical cord for me . . ."
>
> "You did not send for a *sán-pô*?"
>
> "My mom was so capable of doing the job, so it was better to have her . . . She put some sesame oil on the umbilical region and then *covered the area with gauze.*"
>
> "*Gauze? Where did the gauze come from?*"
>
> "*She bought it from the drugstore.*"[43]

By the time Ayu gave birth to her own first child in the late 1940s, the political regime had changed; Japan had ended its colonization in 1945, and the Nationalist government had come from China to rule Taiwan. Ayu, once a librarian in the colonial period, was married to a mainlander, a government official who had immigrated to Taiwan due to the Chinese civil war. Ayu and her husband chose to live with her parents after marriage. In this middle-class family, Ayu still had her mother as her birth attendant. Such birth attendants, listed under the category of "unqualified birth attendant" in the new government's official statistics, assisted at more than 30 percent of births from the late 1940s to the early 1960s.[44]

Most of the women I interviewed who did not use licensed midwives for their first childbirth persisted in this behavior after the end of the colonial period. Yuzhi had her last child in 1963. At that time, she gave birth at home with the assistance of her sister-in-law, since her former birth attendant—her mother-in-law—had died.[45] Chaodi also did not have a certified midwife for her later children in the early 1950s; her mother-in-law had died by that time, so she delivered her subsequent seven children herself.[46] The change of government, or the advancement toward modernization, seems hardly to have transformed these women's perception of birth risk or birth attendance patterns—the belief persisted that certified midwives were not needed.

Nevertheless, Afang's story demonstrates that so-called lay midwifery may have undergone some changes. The use of sesame oil was not abandoned, but with the availability of gauze in drugstores, sterile procedures were more carefully carried out than before. As Aluan vividly described to me, when a certified midwife came, the air smelled of iodine solution, but when it was a lay helper delivering babies, you could smell sesame oil.[47] Afang's story shows that sesame oil could have been combined with iodine solution, as some biomedical practices were not limited to medical professionals and became part of folk knowledge. Other interviewees mentioned using hot water or rice wine to clean the scissors when they gave birth by themselves in the 1950s or 1960s, demonstrating that sterilization had become routine practice. As shown earlier, we can trace the so-called indigenous birth system back to traditional Chinese medicine, and biomedical knowledge must have been incorporated into the lay practices to some extent. The boundary between lay or indigenous and professional or biomedical was not fixed.

I want to emphasize here that these women were not unaware of the dangers of birth. Some of them had heard about women who had died in childbed, but they still believed that birth was a normal event unless something went wrong. Mostly judging from their own bodily experiences, rather than the perception that danger could be expected, they often stated that they knew that in normal births, the woman could basically manage things on her own. Only two of my interviewees (Chaodi and Ayu) had experienced difficult births, and both had fetched licensed midwives for help. When Ayu gave birth to her second child, she bled too much, and her mother therefore suggested that for her third child it was better to send for a *sán-pô*. From these women's accounts, we can see that certified midwives were typically utilized only when the birthing women perceived a risk. However, some women sent for *sán-pô* even when expecting a normal birth.

Birthing Women Meet Modern Midwives

How did women meet their modern midwives? The public health officials in the colonial period often assumed that once women had modern hygienic knowledge, they would abandon the use of traditional birth attendants and consult formally educated midwives. Therefore, officials viewed the promotion of hygienic knowledge as a useful strategy to increase women's willingness to have modern midwives attend their births. Modern midwifery was promoted through various exhibitions. For example, an exhibition on hygiene held in Taipei in 1925 included an important section that urged people "to send for sán-pô for childbirth" and displayed some biomedical equipment for delivery.

Such exhibitions—as well as other activities for promoting health, like establishing consulting centers and disseminating health advice books— continued to increase after the 1930s in the name of child protection.[48] This was carried out under the assumption that the acceptance of modern hygienic knowledge would cause women to appreciate the new practice of midwifery.

To the frustration of doctors and public health officers, Taiwanese mothers did not embrace the project of scientific motherhood very well. Only a small number of them could read, so it was doubtful whether the popular advice books were widely circulated or read, and not all women visited exhibitions. Sakai Kiyoshi, a pediatrician, complained that the less educated and poorer mothers in the rural areas should be the real target, but the mothers who came to the 1925 exhibition were mostly middle-class women.[49] Furthermore, the consulting services were so unpopular that Sakai considered replacing them with home visits.[50]

Instead of associating the choice of birth attendants only with the mothers' scientific literacy, I would like to emphasize the importance of social networks here. Through what kind of networks did birthing women encounter modern midwives?

The *sán-pô* is my husband's elder sister. She came to our home to assist at the birth . . . She did not establish her own clinic; her husband
wouldn't let her do that. And she gave birth to five children and was
busy with her own children [she probably did not have the time to be
a full-time midwife]. She assisted at the birth of our family members.[51]

Ade's *sán-pô*, her sister-in-law, was among the first formally educated midwives in Taiwan, trained in a modern Japanese midwifery program. In
Japan, giving birth with the assistance of scientifically trained midwives
was viewed as an important step toward modernization from the 1870s on,
early in the Meiji period.[52] By the time that Japan took over Taiwan in 1895,
the formal licensing and education system for midwives had been established for twenty years in Japan, and the transfer of that system to its first
colony, Taiwan, did not take long. In the early days of colonization, dozens of
certified Japanese midwives moved to Taiwan to practice midwifery, mainly
to serve Japanese women. A formal midwifery education program started
in colonial Taiwan in 1902, and in the first few years only Japanese nurses
were allowed to be trained.[53] It was not until 1907 that the first Taiwanese
women were qualified to become certified midwives in Taipei Hospital.[54] In
that year, eleven graduates were issued certificates, including Mary Helen
Mackay, daughter of the influential missionary Dr. George Leslie Mackay.[55]

Since education credentials served as the major qualification for admission to midwifery programs and less than 10 percent of Taiwanese girls attended primary school before 1920 (the proportion reached 20 percent in
1933), daughters from middle- and upper-class families were the first to become students at the most formalized midwifery programs offered by the
government.[56] Like Ade herself, her sister-in-law was born into a rich land-
lord family; her fathers and brothers practiced medicine themselves, and
she entered the most formalized midwifery program. Only around twenty to
thirty Taiwanese women graduated from this program each year from 1911
to 1945, while more than 100,000 Taiwanese women gave birth each year.[57]
The midwifery training later included a short, three-day program for traditional birth attendants, and in the 1920s Taiwanese doctors started to offer
private midwifery education. With various types of training programs, by
the end of colonization in 1945, an estimated two thousand women had received some form of biomedical midwifery education in Taiwan.

Ade's birth attendant, her sister-in-law, had received the most formalized level of midwifery education, but she assisted only her family members. In his position as the official examiner for midwifery licensing after

the late 1930s, Magara Masanao once complained that some Taiwanese treated the midwifery license only as a class symbol, rather than taking midwifery as a professional vocation.[58] In keeping with this statement, Ade observed that reluctance from her sister-in-law's husband and the need to fulfill family obligations prevented the sister-in-law from adopting a career in midwifery. In this case, the midwife's certificate did not simply become a woman's dowry to marry up, as Magara believed often happened, but it facilitated the sister-in-law's role as the family's birth helper. In Ade's husband's family, "most women were assisted in birth by her."

While Ade's story demonstrates that the use of modern midwifery was embedded in young women's class mobilization, other women of the upper-middle class whom I interviewed took the presence of a *sán-pô* at their births for granted in the 1930s. In addition to Ade, my informants included a woman who married into a family managing a gold mine, a daughter of a theater owner and his concubine, and a woman from a gentry family. When I asked them why they had sent for *sán-pô*, their narratives often clearly distinguished their licensed birth attendants from the birth attendants of poor peasant women, emphasizing that they lived in urban areas or that they could afford *sán-pô*. Huamei, a woman who gave birth for the first time in Kaohsiung in the 1940s with licensed midwives, claimed that "having a *sán-pô* assist birth was safer. And for me it was affordable."[59]

Indeed, to some extent, having a *sán-pô* already entailed a risk perception that was not based on bodily experiences, as the previous section has shown. Aying observed:

> *Sán-pô* received an education, and we should only send for those who graduated and are licensed. We should not ask someone else to attend the birth. If the birth goes all right, it's all right, but if it goes wrong, [having someone other than a *sán-pô* attend it] will be terrible.[60]

Nevertheless, such discourse was not always stressed by another type of women who used *sán-pô*. They did not take having *sán-pô* as a must, but merely as an option. The other significant group of women among my interviewees who utilized *sán-pô* were new internal migrants who had moved to urban towns because of marriage or for work, and who had met trained midwives in their urbanized neighborhoods. Afang's story illustrates this:

"Why did you send for a *sán-pô*?"
"Because I didn't know how to do it myself! . . . I did not know any of those old aunties. If there was an experienced auntie nearby, people

usually would just utilize her . . . For every rural town, there was an old auntie who served like a midwife, knew how to cut the umbilical cord . . . I never had that; I had *sán-pô*."[61]

Afang, an energetic ninety-year-old, surprised me twice when I asked her why she had sent for a *sán-pô*. She first answered that it was because she did not know how to deliver babies. I repeatedly asked her whether she would have delivered her babies herself if she had known how to do it. She said yes and was impressed that some women just knew how to do that. Being able to deliver a baby by oneself constituted a valuable skill for Afang, and she recognized that she did not have it. And then, she surprised me again by emphasizing that she did not know any old women in her town since she had moved there only after marriage. She was a new resident there. Having a *sán-pô* was thus considered an inevitable choice for a woman lacking a family network or community resources like an *a-pô*. Similarly, another woman named Meili had moved to a new town after marriage; her birth attendant was the mother of her new friend in the neighborhood, who happened to be a certified midwife. Meili emphasized that it was not due to her license or certification, but because of her neighborhood familiarity that she had turned to this woman. Like my other upper-middle-class interviewees, she associated such a network with the difference between rural and urban environments, contrasting them this way: rural areas had bigger family networks and thus women there used older female relatives, while women in nuclear families in urban areas had lost their family connections and thus used *sán-pô*, the community healers.

Afang reflected on the gradual emergence of the nuclear family in Taiwan's first wave of industrialization during the colonial period.[62] Due to the growing sugar industry, people migrated to newly industrialized towns. Women followed their husbands to these towns, worked as full-time housewives in their nuclear families, and often lost touch with the network of their maternal families. Certified midwives were also more accessible in these more urban areas; according to Hong and Chen, the number of certified midwives per ten thousand birthing women in urban areas was three to five times higher than that in rural areas.[63] The residents of such newly industrialized towns tended to use licensed midwives as birth attendants. It is also noticeable that, like Afang, such newcomers' narratives often did not distinguish significantly between certified midwives and traditional helpers. For example, Aluan had previously used a *sán-pô* as her birth attendant, like many other workers in the sugar factory. However, when she fled to the countryside during the war, she returned to her family network and there used an *a-pô* for her birth. She did not view such a switch as bringing increased danger to her.

Therefore, a woman's network matters. It seems that upper-middle-class women met their midwives in their family circles, and new internal migrants met theirs in their industrialized towns. The urban-rural divide was more associated with the resources of birth attendants, rather than simply with the ability to appreciate newly introduced scientific ideas. The women I interviewed did not always view their use of modern midwives as more civilized or scientific. Rather, women may have seen modern midwives as an inevitable choice when lacking a familial network.

Conclusion

Childbirth is not simply a personal, one-day event isolated from historical and social context. Childbirth politics stands out as a quintessential "microcosm in which the relationships between rapid technological progress and cultural values, normative behaviors, social organization, gender relationships, and the political economy can be clearly viewed."[64] In this chapter, I have used twenty-one women's birth stories to offer a different delineation of the birthing system in colonial Taiwan. Specifically, birthing women and their lay birth attendants were often devalued by the Japanese male elite as backward, irrational, and insufficiently educated. Using written official texts as data, contemporary historians could easily reproduce this viewpoint of women as the main obstacles to the expansion of the new public health system. Fu refers to such denunciations made by the elite agents of modernization at that time as the first wave of stigmatization of traditional birth attendants.[65] The second wave of stigmatization may have come from academic writing today. By allowing women to narrate their own stories, we can offer a different angle on such historical changes.

From these women's perspective, lay birth attendants were not old, uneducated women who lacked modern scientific knowledge, but rather respected, brave women with appreciated skills, possibly originating in the traditional Chinese medical system. Some of the nonusers of the newly introduced midwifery system were excluded from the system because they did not have access to such resources, while others chose to stay with lay midwifery, either viewing it as being of high quality or assuming—based on their own experiences—that birth is a normal event that does not require medi-cal intervention. While traditional midwifery was often accused of leading to high rates of infant death, we have reason to doubt the direct causal link between traditional birth attendants and these mortality rates. For those women who started to use modern midwifery, I emphasize that they did so because trained midwives had become part of their networks, and the admi-ration of new hygienic knowledge came with their class identity, not because they specifically valued modern midwifery. Therefore, it is too simplistic to use scientific literacy as an explanation for the divide between the women who used and the women who did not use certified midwives.

Ming-cheng Lo argues forcefully that when analyzing colonial medicine, we should treat indigenous professionals as critical contributors to the pro-cesses of building modernity.[66] How can we extend such an angle to the lay public, such as these birthing women in Taiwan? One important step would be to present women's accounts and to avoid blaming women. Today, to explain Taiwan's high cesarean rates, most researchers still use the defi-cit model—the lack of scientific knowledge—to present birthing women's ideas and thoughts on birthing.[67] The often-mentioned policy implication is that women need to be corrected through education. If we do not adopt the methodology of feminist and STS studies to take the accounts of women users of technology seriously—no matter whether the issue is the nonuse of a new midwifery system in the colonial period, or the excessive use of ob-stetrics in the twenty-first century—women remain easily blamed, both by public health officials and by academic researchers.

NOTES

This chapter is sponsored by the project of the Academia Sinica called The Idea, Organization, and Practices of Hygiene in Han Society from the Traditional to the Modern Period. I thank Angela K. C. Leung and other team members for their con-tinuing comments and support. Fan Yen-chiou, Jender Lee, and Charlotte Furth com-mented on earlier versions of this essay, and their insights have inspired me to make some major changes here. I appreciate very much all the copy-editing work and stimulating encouragement from Sabine Wilms. I thank my research assistants Chiu-Chu Cho, Komiya Yukiko, Tabata Mayumi, Denzel Chen, Nien-Yun Liu, and Chun-Liang Liu for their great help and inspiration. All translations are mine, unless other-wise indicated.

1. All the comments and the quotation in this paragraph come from Taiwan sha-kai jigyōsha, "Jinteki shigen jūjitsu to jidōhogo," 77, 81, 82–83.

2. Fan Yen-chiou, "Riben diguo fazhan xia zhimin Taiwan de renzhong wei-sheng." Many scholars of Asian medicine employ the term "cosmopolitan medicine" (and hence "cosmopolitan physicians") to avoid the colonial or neocolonial bias implied by the terms "modern medicine" or "Western medicine." See Leslie, Introduction, 8; Lo, *Doctors within Borders*, 6. Nevertheless, I preserve the usage of "modern medicine" or "Western medicine" if such terms were used in the historical data.

3. See the chapter in this volume by Lin and Liu.

4. See, for example, E. Martin, *The Woman in the Body*; Apple, *Mothers and Medicine* and "Constructing Mothers."

5. Litt, *Medicalized Motherhood*, chapter 1.

6. Davis-Floyd and Sargent, "Introduction: The Anthropology of Birth," *Childbirth and Authoritative Knowledge*, 11–17; Litt, *Medicalized Motherhood*, chapter 1.

7. Bijker, *Of Bicycles, Bakelites and Bulbs*; Claude Fisher, *America Calling*; Kline and Pinch, "Users as Agents of Technological Change."

8. McGaw, "No Passive Victims, No Separate Spheres"; Wajcman, "Reflection on Gender and Technology Studies."

9. Oudshoorn and Pinch, *How Users Matter*.

10. Wyatt, "Non-Users Also Matter."

11. Hong Y, and Chen, *Xianshengma, chanpo, yu fuchanke yishi*, 29–32.

12. Laderman, *Wives and Midwives*, 103.

13. Takagi, *Taiwanjin no eisei jōtai*; Horiuchi, "Taiwan nyūyōji shibō no bōshi-saku"; Ri, "Taiwan ni okeru shōni shibōritsu oyobi nisan shōni sibōgen-in no tōkei-kansatsu"; Haebara, "Taiwan ni okeru nyūyōji shibō ni tsuite" and "Taiwan ni okeru nyūji hashōfū ni tsuite."

14. Yang C., *Riju shiqi Taiwan funü jiefang yundong*, 503–4; Fan Yen-chiou, "Riben diguo fazhan xia zhimin Taiwan de renzhong weisheng," 240–42. See also Wu Z., *Yaxiya de guer*, 112–13.

15. Author's interview with Tumei (all of the interviewees' names have been changed to protect their privacy), April 4, 2005, Yunlin. Tumei had her first child in 1935 with a certified midwife and all her other children with lay midwives.

16. Author's interview with Afang, September 16, 2005, Taipei.

17. Author's interview with Aluan, December 7, 2003, Taipei.

18. Author's interview with Tumei, April 4, 2005, Yunlin.

19. Author's interview with Aluan, December 7, 2003, Taipei.

20. Author's interview with Ayu, September 9, 2005, Taipei.

21. Author's interview with Chaodi, March 28, 2005, Taipei. Chaodi, a coal miner's wife, gave birth to her first child in 1929.

22. This finding contrasts with Leavitt, *Brought to Bed*, chapter 4. Leavitt found that the company of other women (including friends, relatives, and midwives) was significant for birthing women's psychological support, throughout the nineteenth and early twentieth century in America.

23. Author's interview with Tumei, April 4, 2005, Yunlin.

24. Haebara, "Taiwan ni okeru nyūyōji shibō ni tsuite"; Ri, "Taiwan ni okeru shōni shibōritsu oyobi nisan shōni sibōgen-in no tōkeikansatsu."

25. Hayashizawa, "Shoseiji hashōfū no jikken," 63.

26. Sakaue, "Shoseiji hashōfū ni tsuite oyobi sono nirei," 37.

27. Taiwan sōtokufu keimukyoku, *Taiwan keisatsu oyobi eisei tōkeisho*, 88.

28. Sakaue, "Shoseiji hashōfū ni tsuite oyobi sono nirei, 38; Ri, "Taiwan ni okeru shōni shibōritsu oyobi nisan shōni sibōgen-in no tōkeikansatsu," 1441–43.

29. Ri, "Taiwan ni okeru shōni shibōritsu oyobi nisan shōni sibōgen-in no tōkei-kansatsu," 1441–43.

30. Ibid., 1443.

31. Xiong, *Youyou*, 65–82.

32. Cited in ibid.

33. Fu D., *Yaxiya de xin shenti*, 94.

34. Klein, *A Book for Midwives*, 191.

35. Lusby, Coombes, and Wilkinson, "Honey," 299.

36. X. Fu, Wang, and Sheng, "Advances in Wound Healing Research in China," 3.

37. Ang, *Complete Essentials of Materia Medica*, 4:6.

38. Quoted in Xu Y. and Chen, "Pifu chuangyang zhengzhi sixiang yu shengji lei fangji de yanjiu," 183.

39. Ang et al., "Evaluating the Role of Alternative Therapy in Burn Wound Management," 15–18; Li Wei, Chen, and Guo, "Shirun shaoshanggao zhiliao ruchuang 33 li liaoxiao guancha," 31.

40. Hatori, "Taiwan oyobi nanpō shokuminchi hikaku eisei tōkei," 172–73.

41. Morel, "The Care of Children," 198.

42. Taiwan nichinichi shinpōsha, 8.

43. Author's interview with Ayu, September 9, 2005, Taipei. Emphasis mine. Ayu's mother gave birth by herself in the 1920s and attended the births of Ayu's first two children in the late 1940s.

44. The Nationalist state relied on certified midwives to "retire" lay birth attendants starting in the 1960s. Increasing the availability of qualified birth attendants did not gain much attention until the 1960s because more urgent epidemics such as malaria needed the immediate attention of public health workers during the late 1940s and 1950s. Starting in the mid-1960s, the government not only eliminated lay birth attendants through legal enforcement, but offered a plan to encourage licensed midwives to practice in rural areas to "provide every woman with a safe childbirth and reduce the maternal death rate" (see Taiwansheng zhengfu, *Taiwan guangfu sanshi nian*, 14:19). With government subsidies—two years' free rent, a bicycle, and a birth pack—licensed midwives established 360 clinics in remote areas between 1966 and 1982. At their peak in 1970, 206 government-subsidized midwives' clinics delivered almost 16,000 babies, about 4 percent of the country's total births (see Taiwansheng fuyou weisheng yanjiusuo, *Fuyou weisheng zhuyao tongji*). Officials claim that this was the key to the government's success in reducing births attended by unlicensed birth attendants from 27 percent to 1 percent between 1966 and 1982.

45. Author's interview with Yuzhi, June 30, 2005, Hualien.

46. Author's interview with Chaodi, March 28, 2005, Taipei.

47. Author's interview with Aluan, December 7, 2003, Taipei.

48. Fan Yen-chiou, *Riben diguo fazhan xia zhimin Taiwan de renzhong weisheng*, 238–40.

49. Yasui and Sakai, *Taiwan ni okeru ikuji sōdan*, 317.

50. Ibid., 314–15.

51. Author's interview with Ade, March 13, 2005, Taipei. Ade gave birth to her first daughter in Chia-Yi in 1938.

52. Nakayama, "Nihon no boshiseisaku no rekishi," 42–43.

53. You, "Riju shiqi Taiwan de zhiye funü," 135. Also see Hong Y. and Chen, *Xianshengma, chanpo, yu fuchanke yishi*, 32–33.

54. The length and quality of education differed by race as well: while most Japanese midwifery students received two years of training at Taipei Hospital, most Taiwanese entered half-year rush courses. Additionally, since the language of instruction was initially Japanese, some Taiwanese faced learning problems (see You, "Riju shiqi Taiwan de zhiye funü," 136).

55. Mary Helen Mackay was listed as the first of eleven graduates on the graduation list for that year ("Josanpu sotsugyo shiki," 376). According to Hong and Chen, Taiwanese women were reluctant to receive the formal midwifery education, and it was Mary Helen Mackay's example that convinced some women to attend the program (Hong Y. and Chen, *Xianshengma, chanpo, yu fuchanke yishi*, 53).

56. The educational requirement for a midwifery program in Taipei Hospital was extended from three years in 1907 to six or even eight years in 1922. See Wu Chia-Ling, "Yiliao zhuanye, xingbie, yu guojia," 208.

57. To move away from the debate over whether colonial health policy was either hegemonic or beneficial, Margaret Jones proposes judging effectiveness by the extent and timing of policy transfer from the center to the periphery, as well as by the results of such policies in terms of "whether they improved health and autonomy" ("Infant and Maternal Health Services in Ceylon, 1900–1948," 264). If we adopt such criteria, compared to the cases of Ceylon and the United Kingdom that Jones analyzes, midwifery programs were transferred from Japan to Taiwan within an even shorter time. However, Jones neglects the fact that such transfer might create an ethnographic divide within a colony, particularly where migration from the imperial center was encouraged. In terms of the quality of midwifery education and the number of midwives trained, the colonizer developed more resources of modernized birth attendants for Japanese women in Taiwan than for Taiwanese women. The racial difference in midwifery education was officially lifted as a result of the so-called equal education policy in the early 1920s (see Hong Y. and Chen, *Xianshengma, Chanpo, yu fuchanke yishi*, 37). Still, the number of trained Taiwanese midwives remained considerably less than that of Japanese midwives.

58. Taiwan shakai jigyōsha, "Jinteki shigen jūjitsu to jidōhogo," 78.

59. Author's interview with Huamei, December 14, 2005, Kaohsiung.

60. Author's interview with Aying, September 20, 2005, Kaohsiung.

61. Author's interview with Afang, September 16, 2005, Taipei. Afang gave birth to her first child in a newly industrialized sugar town in 1939.

62. See also Lin, "Transforming Patriarchal Kinship Relations," 71–77.

63. Hong Y. and Chen, *Xianshengma, chanpo, yu fuchanke yishi*, chapter 6.

64. Davis-Floyd and Sargent, *Childbirth and Authoritative Knowledge*, 6.

65. Fu D., *Yaxiya de xin shenti*, 93–94.

66. Lo, *Doctors within Borders*, 4–24.

67. Wu Chia-Ling, and Fu, Daiwei, "Research Agenda, Public Policy, and the Social Construction of Cesarean Sections in Taiwan."

Part III

Campaigns for Epidemic Control

A Forgotten War

Malaria Eradication in Taiwan, 1905–65

Lin Yi-ping and Liu Shiyung

> The microbe is nothing; the terrain, everything.
> —Louis Pasteur, 1822–1895[1]

On November 1, 1965, Taiwan was officially entered in the World Health Organization (WHO) registry of areas where malaria had been eradicated. The event was a major success of WHO's Global Malaria Eradication Program, and a very happy ending to the American-funded war against mosquitoes in Taiwan. The intensive, island-wide war against malaria was carried out over fifteen years, between 1951 and 1965. Although sixty-six countries participated in the worldwide spraying campaign of dichlorodiphenyltrichloroethane (DDT) in the late 1950s and 1960s, Taiwan was one of the first to join the program, and one of the very few island countries that were selected as a showcase for the scheme. Taiwan has largely held onto its eradication record, unlike many other sites that experienced a resurgence of the disease beginning in the 1980s. Currently, 40 percent of the world's population, mostly those living in the world's poorest countries, is at risk of malaria. According to WHO estimates, more than 500 million people become severely ill with malaria every year.[2]

In this chapter, we examine the rise and fall of public health campaigns against malaria in Taiwan in the twentieth century and explore the social and historical contexts that shaped their outcomes. Before the 1950s war on mosquitoes, Japanese in Taiwan experimented with very different and more labor-intensive strategies for controlling malaria during their fifty years of colonial rule. Like the Guomindang (Kuomintang, or KMT) government and WHO in the 1950s, Japanese policymakers claimed that the reduction in malaria mortality achieved under their rule was the result of an enlightened government using the best modern scientific technology available.

Politically, public health was promoted before the Second World War under Tokyo's imperial mission much as it was in America's free world alliance system during the cold war. In fact, a long-term overview of malaria control efforts in Taiwan shows how prewar Japanese policies played an unacknowledged role in the postwar story. Technologically, the contrast between these two public health regimes reveals the influence of socioeconomic factors on technical choices, and the way outcomes are constrained by the methods selected. The changing historical specificities of the public health programs that have attempted to deal with the complex problem of malaria in Taiwan, as elsewhere, show the difficulty of evaluating the precise contribution of public health policies to outcomes.

The long-term overview also shows that the degree of virulence of malaria outbreaks should be correlated with economic activities like colonization, urbanization, industrialization, and migration, as well as agricultural development and ecological change. In conclusion, we suggest that twentieth-century socioeconomic development in Taiwan, quite apart from public health policies, has played an important role in making Taiwan virtually malaria-free today.

Parasites, Mosquitoes, and Human Beings

Malaria is a parasitic infection that is transmitted by certain species of mosquito. The disease it causes is among the most difficult to tackle. Of the three elements involved in human malaria—parasites, mosquitoes, and human beings—the human element has generally received the least attention, time, and resources.[3] The human factors in antimalaria programs in various parts of the world have included population distribution, patterns of settlement, the types of dwellings, administrative and social organization, and the range of economic activities.

Anopheles minimus, the major vector that transmitted malaria in Taiwan, is a kind of domestic mosquito, interacting with and living very close to human beings. Though it breeds in rivers and irrigation systems (preferably in clear, moving water), it lives solely on human blood, bites at night, and rests in the house (especially on bedroom walls or under beds) during the day. Not only does it need proper environments to live and reproduce, it also needs human beings to transport it over any great distance. Anopheles minimus does not travel far on its own; it moves with humans today by train, boat, or car and in the past by ox wagon.

Malaria is a very old disease. The parasite and the mosquito have co-evolved with human beings over time. In terms of human cultural evolution, malaria most likely became widespread only after the invention of agriculture, about ten thousand years ago.[4] Frank Livingstone demonstrated in 1958 how people in West Africa transformed the environment through slash-and-burn agriculture during the Iron Age.[5] This practice resulted in an increase in the density of *Anopheles gambiae* mosquitoes, which subsequently turned to humans for their primary source of blood feasts, thereby spreading malaria. Peter Brown indicated that the spontaneous decline of malaria in northern Europe in the late nineteenth century was highly correlated with changing agricultural crop choices and housing patterns.[6] Timothy Mitchell, however, told an interconnected story of war, agriculture, and the malaria epidemic in Egypt.[7] He suggested that it was through the circuits of dams, irrigation, and sugar cultivation that *Anopheles gambiae* invaded Egypt in 1942.

Our story of malaria control and eradication in Taiwan starts with some major ecological changes and population movements in the seventeenth century, when the name "island of miasma" was first coined by early Chinese settlers. These early immigrants used Chinese medical terms evoking miasma (*zhang, zhangqi,* or *zhangli*) to describe the diseases they encountered, and attributed their own suffering to their maladjustment to the water and soil (*shuitu bufu*). The diseases these early immigrants described were possibly malaria; from an ecological perspective, the epidemics of malaria were indeed due to the explorers' maladjustment to the water and soil of a new territory.[8] After all, there should not have been a large population of mosquitoes waiting on a sparsely populated island covered with camphor trees. It was more likely that these explorers were involved in the dangerous jobs of deforesting and constructing irrigation systems, which created perfect breeding spots for the mosquitoes and guaranteed an abundance of human blood for them to feed on.[9] Among the endemic diseases of Taiwan between the seventeenth and the early twentieth centuries, malaria—locally referred to as the disease of wind and soil (*fengtubing*)—proved a major hazard for all invaders, from General Koxinga's soldiers to Dutch priests, Qing government officials, and Japanese colonists.

Japanese Efforts to Control Malaria

In 1895, Taiwan became the first colony in the new Japanese Empire. The endemic disease malaria and the epidemics of infectious diseases (plague,

cholera, and smallpox) immediately challenged the new colonial government. At first, malaria mortality was higher for the Japanese immigrants
in Taiwan (116.24 per 10,000 in 1899) than it was for the local Taiwanese
(17.69 per 10,000).[10] Improving public health in Taiwan and controlling the
transmission of infectious disease became the most important missions of
the new colonial government.[11]

In 1902, malaria mortality for Japanese immigrants had decreased to
52.27 per 10,000, but mortality for the native Taiwanese had increased to
46.23 per 10,000. Malaria was the top cause of death in Taiwan before 1911
(see figure 1).[12] By 1911, plague was generally under control in Taiwan, and
the Japanese colonial government had started an islandwide malaria control program.[13] From 1912 to 1921, malaria was one of the top three causes
of death, along with pneumonia and diarrhea. In 1920, cholera and smallpox were both brought under control, and by 1923, malaria had reached the
same status. After 1925, malaria ceased to be one of the top four killers, and
in 1935 it was the tenth leading cause of death in Taiwan.[14] These statistics
show real improvement in public health, which validated to the Japanese
what they saw as scientifically enlightened imperial governance.

In 1906, after a serious malaria epidemic at a camphor company in southern Taiwan, the Japanese colonial government began to plan an antimalaria strategy. In 1910, a pilot program began to apply the Koch method
in controlling malaria. This method involved screening all residents in an
area to identify those carrying the parasite, and administering antimalarial
drugs, based on quinine, to the identified carriers.[15] The method had first
been tested in the German colony of New Guinea by Robert Koch in 1900.
Beginning in 1911, Japanese public health authorities established malarial
control districts of approximately 2,000 inhabitants each. Using the basic
grassroots administrative structure of the hokō,[16] supplemented by the labor
power of their corps of imported Japanese sanitary police, the Japanese
authorities gradually expanded the network of malarial control districts—
beginning with locales where Japanese colonists lived and adding natural
resource development sites and highly malarious areas.[17] In 1932, there were
208 malarial control districts, and by the end of the 1930s, more than three
million people were undergoing annual routine blood examinations.[18] This
last development was made possible by a newer, more accurate method
of blood sampling developed by Morishita, which could be conveniently
used on schoolchildren.[19] By the end of the 1930s, malaria carriers identified through this method and chronic sufferers identified by their enlarged

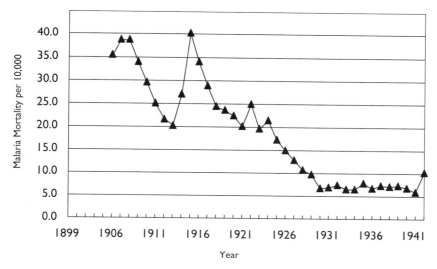

Figure 1. Malaria mortality of Taiwan, 1899–1941.
Sources: Chen Shaoxin, *Taiwan de renkou bianqian yu shehui bianqian* and Department of Health,
Malaria Eradication in Taiwan (Taipei: The Executive Yuan, 1993).

spleens (splenomegaly) were expected to report to a local hospital, and their
families would receive free follow-up exams for three to five years.[20]

From its early stages, this labor-intensive strategy of malaria control,
focused on identifying and curing malaria carriers, was admired in the colonial world. In 1916, a delegate of the Imperial Council of India argued for a
similar malaria prevention program for his own colony:

> They [the colonial government of Taiwan] set about doing this in
> a very business-like fashion. By way of experiment certain districts
> were selected and on a certain day all the inhabitants were made to
> appear at an appointed time to have their blood examined microscopi-
> cally with a view to finding out if they were malaria carriers. Those in
> whom the malaria parasites were found were placed under treatment
> for 30 days in order that the parasites may be exterminated.[21]

Identifying and treating the human carriers was the foundation of Japanese antimalaria efforts, but these measures were complemented by initiatives in public education and environmental management. Schools and
clinics educated the public about mosquito control and promoted the use
of screens, bed nets, and mosquito coils.[22] Films, newspapers, and exhibi-

tions were also used to inform the public.[23] In line with the practice in many other countries before the development of effective chemical insecticides, Japanese public health experts emphasized ecological changes like swamp drainage, improvements in housing, and landscape design for malaria prevention.[24] The Japanese public health officers also imported larvae-eating angelfish from Hawaii to the rivers of rural Taiwan, and water-absorbing eucalyptus trees from Australia to the city streets.[25]

Urbanization and rising living standards in the cities were important in reducing mosquito populations there, but the countryside lagged behind. The most massive control initiatives in the rural lowlands of western Taiwan came with the construction of the Great Jia'nan Irrigation System and Wushantou Dam in the 1930s. To build this system, the authorities invested in a comprehensive antimalarial program for the region, involving contributions from malariologists, entomologists, biologists, and engineers, who worked together to construct a permanent drainage system for the surrounding wetlands.[26] Villagers were enlisted to clear brush, spread larvae-killing oil on standing water, and destroy containers that might hold rainwater.[27] But along Taiwan's less developed eastern coast, where there was little colonial government infrastructure, new Japanese colonists suffered greatly, and many returned to their previous homes.[28] In this region, malaria eradication was largely deemed a failure.

Supporting these policies was the work of Japanese scientific experts from a variety of fields. Some entomologists who worked on collecting and identifying Taiwanese species of mosquitoes eventually found out that out of the fifteen indigenous species of mosquito, only *Anopheles minimus* and *Anopheles sinensis* were carriers of the malaria plasmodium.[29] Some physicians experimented with different formulas and dosing schedules for quinine therapy, and they arrived at a protocol that paralleled the one later used in the Japanese military.[30] A few experts carried out laboratory tests on herbs used in Chinese medicine which were reputed to have antimalarial effects, particularly *changshan* (*Dichroa febrifuga*) and *chaihu* (*Bupleurum*). However, these experiments did not stimulate great enthusiasm or lead to the widespread production or clinical use of Chinese *materia medica*.[31]

Throughout, the Japanese judged their programs against standards of Western science and biomedicine. They worked to learn and retest the latest research results from abroad and were proud of their independent contributions to scientific knowledge.[32] The colonial bias of the operation is clear. Districts inhabited by Japanese colonists had top priority, and only Japanese were eligible for public doses of quinine as prophylaxis (for prevention rather than cure). Still, by the 1920s and 1930s, Taiwanese exposed to the broadening program seemed to trust scientific malariology and most were willing to follow preventive rules. One of our interviewees observed:

> In school we had routine blood tests and physical examinations every semester . . . At home the sanitary policeman was rigid in environmental cleanliness and clearing . . . From newspapers I gained a lot of knowledge about malaria and . . . when I was infected I believed the doctor would give me proper medicine.[33]

Malariology became popularized and rooted in at least one generation of Taiwanese—including A-nan, who was a schoolboy in the mid-1930s.

The Resurgence of Malaria after the Second World War

The Second World War brought this period of public health under Japanese colonialism to an end. The infrastructure of public health systems in Taiwan collapsed during the war, and by 1942 malaria reemerged as a major cause of death. The immediate postwar years in Taiwan were chaotic. After fifty years of Japanese colonization, the island was returned to Chinese rule. Change of government, inflation, economic depression, population movement, shortage of medication, and neglect of public health infrastructure all contributed to the resurgence of infectious diseases in 1946 and 1947. Cases of cholera, smallpox, and plague were reported on the island, and it was estimated that more than one million people were infected with malaria during these years.[34]

With financial support from the U.S. government and the Rockefeller Foundation, the Joint Commission for Rural Reconstruction (JCRR) started to rebuild the health stations in every township in 1945. It also reestablished the formerly Japanese-led malaria research center (the Taiwan Provincial Malaria Research Institute, or TAMRI) as the scientific arm of control efforts. By the end of 1952, all 155 of the prewar malaria stations had reopened. TAMRI held seven four-week intensive training courses for the 227 former malaria technicians of the stations. The practice of "island-wide simultaneous malaria parasite surveys among preschool-age children"[35] was resumed in 1950 and lasted for ten years. To organize this extensive survey, TAMRI convened a series of meetings with the technicians of the antimalaria stations. At these meetings, clean slides, antimalaria drugs, report forms, and all other necessary supplies were provided. On December 17, 1951, the first postwar survey was carried out, and 13,885 blood smears were taken and examined. Among the 13,885 children examined in the survey, 1,198 (8.63 percent) tested positive for malaria.

In addition to reestablishing the antimalaria stations, the JCRR also supported the building and establishment of local health centers in every town. There were only fifty-six local health centers and 775 public health personnel in place between 1946 and 1949. With the financial support from the JCRR, the numbers increased to 252 centers and 1,486 personnel in 1950, 356 centers and 2,208 personnel in 1951, and 367 centers in 1954—one in every town on the island. Each health center had at least three fulltime personnel: a doctor, nurse, and midwife. The JCRR provided the centers with bicycles, medical supplies, and free medications. It even provided monthly financial support of $30 to $60 to cover the traveling expenses of the public health workers' home and school visits. Essentially, JCRR sponsorship made it possible for Taiwan to restore a functioning public health infrastructure within ten years of the war's end.

DDT: A New Chemical Weapon

Also under JCRR sponsorship, TAMRI resumed the formerly Japanese-led research program in 1946 and initiated a series of new investigations that built on colonial knowledge, but emphasized new medicines and technologies rather than prevention through public health infrastructure. TAMRI planned the environmental engineering of mosquito-breeding streams, particularly around the coal-mining towns of Jilong. It tracked the geography and seasonality of mosquito habitats in rice farming areas, and the relationship between mosquito prevalence and the growing seasons for rice. In addition, it conducted clinical trials for the new antimalarial drug chloroquine, both as prophylaxis and cure. Most importantly, it experimented with new pesticides. Finding that spraying DDT on rice fields was ineffective—it was both laborious and inefficient in reaching mosquito larvae in paddy water—TAMRI concluded that spraying of houses was the best option.

The DDT program launched in 1951 directly linked antimalarial activities in Taiwan to a global effort in partnership with WHO. With the aid of the new chemical weapon—the effective, long-lasting, and inexpensive pesticide DDT—the ambitious Global Malaria Eradication Program aimed to eliminate the parasite-carrying mosquitoes within every household. The eradication method developed by Dr. Fred Soper, the world's most influential malaria expert after the Second World War, was based on modern warfare, in which task forces of uniformed men armed with spray guns went on search-and-destroy missions.[36] Taiwan was one of the first countries to embark on this war on mosquitoes, four years before the U.S.-funded eradication program was announced at the eighth World Health Congress in 1955.

The 1951 agreement between the KMT government of Taiwan and WHO was called an "Expanded Program of Technical Assistance for Economic Development." The first objective of this agreement was to assist the government in "the control of malaria and eventually the eradication of this disease in the whole island of Taiwan, with modern methods at the lowest feasible cost."[37] The project aimed to control malaria and other insect-borne diseases and to improve the general health of the population, agricultural production, and the general economy of Taiwan.

The eradication program was preceded by experiments for two years, to ensure that it would be evidence-based. There were scientific studies on the effectiveness of DDT spraying on different walls, field research into mosquito habitats, and cost-effectiveness studies of different eradication procedures.[38] Even the operation models of the house-spraying teams were experimentally verified. The successful program benefited from generous financial and technical support from the United States, excellent Japanese-trained local malariologists, well-trained house-spraying teams, and highly cooperative Taiwanese residents.

Using the scientific evidence collected between 1952 and 1954, an island-wide antimalaria DDT-spraying operation was finally undertaken in 1954. News coverage of the planned malaria eradication program had begun as early as July 13, 1952. In a series of newspaper interviews, TAMRI's director, Dr. Kuang-Chi Liang, explained the details of the program to the general public.[39] On the eve of operations, in a letter to all county and city governments, Liang outlined the "principles of the publicity campaign for anti-malaria DDT-spraying operation." He wrote that the operation was "an enterprise unprecedented in Taiwan" and that "for this reason the understanding and enthusiastic support of the people at all social levels are indispensable for the success of the operation, and a publicity campaign for the operation is of considerable importance accordingly."[40]

TAMRI made handbills and posters for the campaign and suggested several actions, including attending villagers' meetings, asking for the support of schoolmasters and local opinion leaders, putting up posters along main streets, using loudspeakers for local propaganda, and showing related slides at cinemas. It also suggested that local governments ask for news reporters' support.

A colorful poster announcing the arrival of the DDT-spraying team instructed residents to cover food, remove bedding, look out for children, and confine pets and livestock (see figures 2 and 3). A poster and warning sign with the text "please do not wipe off DDT" was to be pasted on the door of each house after spraying was finished. While the sanitary policemen of the Japanese colonial period had disappeared after the Second World War, there is some evidence that Taiwanese police forces were involved in the malaria eradication program. An "Order to Prohibit Wiping Off DDT after Being Sprayed" issued by the governor of Taiwan in 1953 stated that wiping off DDT in the course of general housecleaning was a "serious mistake" and that doing so "not only nullified the great amount of insecticides and manpower used in the DDT spraying completely, but also greatly hampered the four years of malaria control in this project."[41]

The DDT house-spraying campaign turned out to be a big success and was heartily welcomed by most residents of the island. "Who wouldn't have liked DDT house-spraying back then?" asked a Mrs. Cheng, who was recently married in 1954 and living in central Taiwan.[42] A follow-up study in central Taiwan indicated that after a single spraying of DDT, a residence could stay mosquito-free for a whole year. Some Taiwanese citizens, however, concluded that malaria had disappeared when the Japanese left Taiwan and that the spraying was simply aimed at insect pests in general.[43]

Following the conclusion of the Second Asian Malaria Conference for the Western Pacific and South-East Asia Regions in 1954, it was decided to extend the malaria eradication program in Taiwan for another two years in order to spray the whole island. The extended plan was to include the nonendemic metropolitan area in 1956, and spraying in 1957 would be limited to high-endemic areas and the aboriginal villages. The budget of the extended program was provided by the Council for United States Aid and Foreign Operations Administration. In May 1958, the government of Taiwan again signed a "Plan of Operations for Malaria Eradication in Taiwan, China, FY-1959–FY-1963."[44] The term "eradication" was widely used in the document prepared by TAMRI.

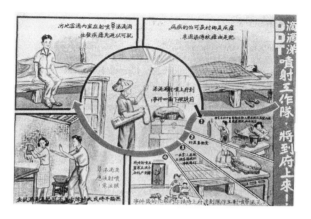

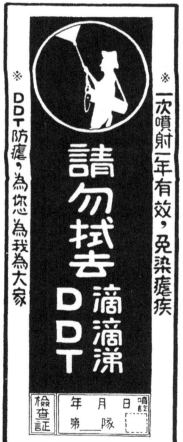

Figures 2 and 3.
Poster and stickers used by the DDT house-spraying team to inform residents to prepare for the spraying and not to wipe DDT off the wall.
Source: Department of Health, Malaria Eradication in Taiwan (Taipei: The Executive Yuan, 1993), pp. 99, 172.

Final Victory

The final victory of the Taiwanese war against malaria came in 1965, when Taiwan was entered in WHO's Official Register of Malaria Eradication. The official malaria-free designation was not an easy goal to achieve and was even more difficult to maintain. To stay in the register, a country must have the financial resources and operational facilities to prevent the reintroduction of the disease. How did Taiwan reach the goal of eradication so soon and maintain its malaria-free status for so long? According to Andrew Spielman and Michael D'Antonio, all successful malaria eradication programs either occurred in island countries or were directed against easy-to-kill mosquito species.[45] It could very well be the case that Taiwan was the perfect size for an island and that *Anopheles minimus*, the major parasite-carrying mosquito in Taiwan, was an easily killed species. Further, the strict border controls enforced by martial law from 1949 to 1987 also made Taiwan an unusually restricted area for immigration and travel.[46] Nevertheless, the true story in Taiwan behind the simple metaphor of the war against malaria may be more complex than Spielman and D'Antonio suggest.

As the DDT program was so powerful and easy to implement, the functions of antimalaria stations in collecting blood samples and providing necessary preventive education to the public eventually became unimportant. American aid to rebuild the colonial antimalaria infrastructure was redirected to train more spraying teams and produce more DDT powder. The DDT program seemed so promising that the demand for preventive public education waned. Even the medicines for active malaria patients were neglected in all government reports.

Medication for treatment was not included in the long list of equipment, supplies, and technical literature to be provided by WHO in 1952.[47] A 1956 document titled "Instructions to be Followed in Dealing with Malaria Patients" from the governor of Taiwan to all local governments, private and public hospitals, and clinics stated that "all malaria patients and carriers should be treated" and "no fee should be charged to the patients."[48] There were, however, only 437 cases reported in 1956 (see figure 4). In the five-year malaria eradication program signed in 1958, there were some descriptions of antiparasite measures as well as antimosquito measures and case detection measures. As it later turned out, only 199 parasite carriers were detected from November 1957 to June 1958.[49]

Where did the 1.2 million active carriers of malaria go? The answer is

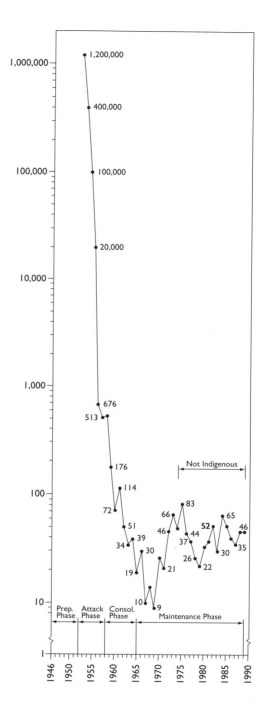

Figure 4.
Malaria prevalence and the phases of malaria eradication program in Taiwan, 1950–1990 (in log scale).
Source: Department of Health, Malaria Eradication in Taiwan (Taipei: The Executive Yuan, 1993), p. iii.

probably found in the 155 antimalaria stations originally established during the Japanese occupation period and rebuilt after the war, and in the 367 postwar local health centers. The technicians in the areas where malaria was endemic, the public health workers in every township, and country and city doctors were probably the ones who found and cured these millions of malaria patients. They are the hidden heroes of the war against malaria.

The reasons behind the American financial support for the eradication programs are clearly economical and political.[50] The reasons why the KMT government in Taiwan entered the world war against mosquitoes at such an early stage, however, have never been explored. The official reason was to free Taiwan from serious malaria epidemics.[51] Nevertheless, it should be remembered that malaria had been well controlled and was only the tenth leading cause of death in Taiwan right before the Second World War. While malaria prevalence in the chaotic postwar years was estimated to have reached levels as high as 1.2 million cases per year, malaria mortality is unlikely to have been very high. As a matter of fact, malaria had not been the most serious health threat in Taiwan since the late 1930s.

We speculate that with sufficient supplies of antimalaria medication, a functioning public health system, and improved nutrition, malaria prevalence would have most likely dropped to prewar levels on its own. Ironically, the best evidence to support our speculation comes from the celebrated statistics of the eradication program. As shown in figure 4 (notice the deceptive "log scale" of the number of cases), the period of dramatic decline of malaria prevalence in Taiwan after the Second World War was from 1950 (1.2 million cases per year) to 1953 (20,000 cases per year). At this time, the malaria eradication program was only in its preparatory phase—training, experimenting, and preparing for the major attack. When the DDT house-spraying teams searched up and down to destroy mosquitoes in every house on the island between 1955 and 1957, yearly malaria cases in Taiwan were only in the hundreds. The mosquito, supposedly man's deadly foe, was possibly just a scapegoat in this war.

Why did the KMT government decide to turn their DDT-spraying guns against mosquitoes? An interesting coincidence was the parallel between the war plan of the malaria eradication program to Chiang Kai-shek's plan to fight Communist China. In 1950, Chiang retreated to Taiwan and announced his war plan as "one year to prepare, two years to attack, three years to sweep, and five years to success."[52] In the malaria eradication program, the four phases were preparation, attack, consolidation, and maintenance. Chiang's plan to defeat the Communists was criticized as "impossible and a lie to the people" as early as 1951 by the renowned intellectual Yin Haiguang.[53] As it turned out years later, it was indeed an unrealized dream for Chiang, residing in a small island, to fight the big mainland next door. It was an intriguing turn for the KMT government in Taiwan to dedicate their efforts to fighting the little mosquitoes in every household in 1952. After all, the war against mosquitoes was waged with the best American weapons, sophisticated Japanese-trained experts, and a well-trained army. It was a winnable war in the 1950s, which could further solidify the military-base image of Taiwan.

Conclusion

Malaria was considered one of the major health problems facing colonial Taiwan from the beginning of the Japanese occupation.[54] Fighting malaria certainly required significant financial and organizational resources. As this chapter has illustrated, the scientific ambitions of colonial malariologists and officials, the demands of colonial economic development, and the social realities of the Taiwanese countryside all came together to make the anti-malaria campaign in social medicalization an extremely complex process.[55] The theoretical and laboratory research on malariology gave Japanese ma-larial experts and the colonial government confidence. With their mastery of contemporary biomedical science, colonial officials introduced measures to promote the prevention and cure of malaria in the cities and Japanese settlements. However, the effectiveness of rural antimalaria campaigns was not actually determined by better theories or available methods, but rather by which strategies best met the developmental needs of the colonial state.

Nonetheless, the key Japanese claim—that better science would produce improved control methods and guarantee a healthier environment—was successful propaganda, clearly reflected in the example of the background music in a 1939 informational film. The film producers of *Mararia* (malaria) used a classical symphony for the introduction to modern malariology, light jazz to highlight promising treatments, and finally a pastorale to evoke the improvement of the rural environment.[56] For Taiwanese citizens, the les-son of the Japanese antimalaria program was probably "confidence in mod-ern medicine,"[57] while "integration to local context" remained only a minor afterthought.[58]

Postwar malaria eradication depended on three new elements: foreign aid, military-like promotion, and DDT. Throughout the 1950s and 1960s, WHO was involved in planning and carrying out eradication activities in the western Pacific region, including Taiwan, Hong Kong, Japan, Singapore, and Vietnam. Between 1960 and 1965, the malaria eradication program in most of the region was vibrant, active, and optimistic, with the eradication certificate in 1965 attesting to the success of the antimalaria war in Taiwan. In comparing the colonial period to the postwar KMT regime, it is evident that the main focus of antimalaria activities switched from early-modern naturalist to modern technical pursuits. Entomological efforts to study *anopheles* mosquitoes became the biologists' work, while the chemists applied DDT to eradicate insect pests and other animals. After the 1950s, when DDT joined the war on mosquitoes in Taiwan, the music of this antimalaria campaign sounded more like a military marching band.

This study of malaria eradication efforts in Taiwan is situated at the crossroad of medical and political history. Discussions of the discourse of political history often neglect the power of technological development, and the study of technology can overlook the socioeconomic framework over time. With this issue in mind, we have framed our story as one about the history of colonial and postcolonial politics, but we have centered our narrative on the ever-changing ways in which modern medicine has been articulated and applied, bringing technical systems and institutions of medical history into the foreground.[59]

Finally, the power of global capitalism cannot be neglected in describing the ups and downs of malaria in the history of Taiwan. In this larger framework, human actions to control and eradicate the disease are minimal as compared to the political, economic, and environmental factors that increased or suppressed the disease. Wars have had a major impact on malaria, and so have meteorological events. Increased malaria mortality and morbidity were highly correlated with the two world wars (1914–18 and 1938–45), and small malaria epidemics broke out after earthquakes and typhoons. The last malaria epidemic recorded in the colonial period followed the 1935 earthquake in Hsinchu County.[60]

In addition to wars, earthquakes, and typhoons, economic activities were an underlying factor in the rise and fall of malaria epidemics in both the colonial period and the postwar period. Around the world, agricultural practices, including irrigation, have played a central role in historical and contemporary outbreaks, as have developmental projects like transportation works, power plants, and dams. We suggest that activities of the Japanese colonizers stimulated the malaria epidemics in the late nineteenth century and the early twentieth. Japanese colonists came to Taiwan for rice and sugar, and the year-round irrigation technology that they brought to Taiwan for producing them were prone to malaria infection. The Japanese colonists were also busy constructing roads and railroads. From 1898 to 1905, the number of railroad stations increased from eleven to sixty-five, and the length of railroads from 209 kilometers in 1900 to 924 in 1905.[61]

The industrialization and urbanization of colonial Taiwan started in the 1930s. The first hydraulic power plant was built in 1934, and the first modern, mechanized coal mine reached full operation in 1937. The year 1935 marked the beginning of the so-called industrial movement and was also when malaria fell to tenth place among leading causes of death for the Taiwanese population. Replacing it at the top were pneumonia and diarrhea, diseases that Chen Shaoxin described as "the products of crowded urban life."[62] This decline of malaria mortality signaled the beginning of Taiwan's "epidemiological transition."[63] From 1910 to 1930, the death rate decreased from 28.5 per 1,000 to 20.0, and average life expectancy increased from 29.3 to 42.6 for males, and from 32.3 to 47.7 for females.[64]

The process of industrialization and urbanization in Taiwan continued in the postcolonial period. After the Second World War, the agricultural economy of Taiwan transitioned to manufacturing and then to the chemical and electronic industries.[65] Gone were the days of tea, camphor, rice, and sugar. In 1980, Taiwan's major export was light chemical industrial products; by 2001, it was heavy chemical industrial products. The proportion of Taiwanese who made their living from farming declined from 58 percent in 1956 to 42 percent in 1970, and to 17 percent in 2000. The per capita GNP was $217 in 1965, $2,344 in 1980, and $14,188 in 2000. This growth was the so-called economic miracle of Taiwan.[66]

The decline of overall mortality in Taiwan continued from the 1950s through the 1990s.[67] This demographic transition included a change in dominant causes of mortality from infectious to chronic diseases, prolonged life expectancy, and a decline in fertility. In modern, industrialized Taiwan, the miasma is no longer the infectious malaria. Taiwanese factory workers and the general population as well are now worried about their exposure to chemicals at work and about chemical pollution in their daily lives.[68] Cancer has been the major cause of death in Taiwan since the 1980s.[69]

Gone is malaria, and almost gone is *Anopheles minimus*. The mosquito's population was reduced by DDT in the 1950s and continues to decline each year.[70] With the disappearance of their favorite habitat—agricultural villages close to clear, moving water—the malaria-transmitting *Anopheles minimus* can be found in only nineteen Taiwanese towns today, the majority of which are inhabited by aborigines of southern and eastern Taiwan.

It is no surprise that the headline-making news of the first locally transmitted malaria case in Taiwan after thirty-eight years of eradication came from a mountainous aboriginal village in eastern Taiwan.[71] In recent years, many young aborigine men have been hired as loggers in the Solomon Islands, a malarious area in the western Pacific. One of the Taiwanese loggers brought back malaria parasites and infected his uncle, a local janitor. This sad story of imported disease, exported labor, racial discrimination, unemployment, and poverty underlies the economic miracle of Taiwan. Clearly, parasites and mosquitoes always lurk in the shadows waiting to pounce, and stories of war between human beings and infectious diseases will continue.

NOTES

1. Farmer, *Infections and Inequalities: The Modern Plagues*. Berkeley: University of California Press, 1999: 37. Louis Pasteur was said to have reversed all his earlier arguments with his old adversary on his deathbed by declaring, "Bernard avait raison. Le germe n'est rien, c'est le terrain qui est tout."
2. World Health Organization, "Malaria."
3. Prothero, "Foreword."
4. Brown, "Culture and the Global Resurgence of Malaria."
5. Livingstone, "Anthropological Implications of Sickle Cell Gene Distribution in West Africa."
6. Brown, "Culture and the Global Resurgence of Malaria."
7. Mitchell, *Rule of Experts*, chapter 1.
8. Liu Cuirong and Liu, "Taiwan lishishang de jibing yu siwang."
9. House, *Japanese Expedition to Formosa*, 53.
10. Chen Shaoxin, *Taiwan de renkou bianqian yu shehui bianqian*, 81.
11. Fan Yen-chiou, "Yixue yu zhiming kuozhang."
12. Chen Shaoxin, *Taiwan de renkou bianqian yu shehui bianqian*, 82–83.
13. Fan Yen-chiou, "Yixue yu zhiming kuozhang," 134.
14. Chen Shaoxin, *Taiwan de renkou bianqian yu shehui bianqian*, 138.
15. Fan Yen-chiou, "Nueji fangzhishuo."
16. The Japanese adopted the *hokō* system established during the Qing dynasty in Taiwan, adapting it to better address crime and epidemics. The *hokō* system in colonial Taiwan was supported and financed by local police departments who executed

governmental orders. The *hokō* system had its origins as a system of criminal discipline. This was quickly replaced with its use as a system to organize social activity for Japanese colonial purposes. The *hokō* system and the organizations that developed around it were involved in the vast number of social and health reforms implemented by the Japanese including anti-malaria campaigns since the 1920s.

17. Barclay, *From Far Formosa*, 136; Liu Cuirong and Liu, "Taiwan lishishang de jibing yu siwang," 92–106.

18. Taiwansheng wenxian weiyuanhui, *Taiwansheng tongzhi gao*, 198–200; Weishengshu, *Taiwan diqu gongkong weisheng fazhanshi*, 216–17.

19. Zeigler, "Editorial."

20. C. T. Chen, Wu, and Hsieh, "Differences in Detectability of Minor Splenomegaly through Variation in the Recumbent Position of the Patient," 561, 566–67.

21. Farid, "Views and Reflections on Anti-Malaria Programs in the World," 244.

22. See, for example, an advertisement posted by Shinogi seiyaku kabushikikaisha (Shinogi Pharmaceutical Company, Ltd.), in Shimizu, *Jiyō eiseikowa*, the back cover of the book.

23. Newspapers such as *Taiwan nichinichi shinpō* 台灣日日新報 were a powerful tool to educate people and raise alarm about the crisis. See, for example, "Shakoku 社說 [Editorial announcement]," November 16, 1919. According to a public announcement in the same newspaper, circulating antimalaria films were a welcome form of urban entertainment (see "Kōku 公告 [Public announcement]" August 13, 1939). Exhibitions were another popular channel to promote preventive knowledge. And Zhuang Yongming has studied how folk songs in Taiwan were revised to educate people on various topics, including hygiene. For examples of folk songs, see also Zhuang's *Taiwan geyao zhuixiangqu*.

24. "Mararia yobōhō ni tsuite" 麻剌利亞預防法について [About methods to prevent malaria], *Taiwan shinpō* 台灣新報, October 1898; and "Mararia netsu yobōhō taii 麻剌利亞預防法大意 [The general concept of malaria prevention]," *Taiwan shinpō*, April 1897.

25. Tsukiyama, "Mararia yobōhō."

26. Morishita et al., "Wusandōni okeru mararia ryukō kyūsono bōatsuni All Quinization no kōkoni tsuite," 713.

27. Hitōgawa, "Tainanshōshita niokeru 'mararia bōatsusagyō no jisai to sono seiseki."

28. Taiwan Sōtokufu eiseika, *Taiwan mararia gaikyō*, 8–9.

29. Omori, "Kotoshu no anofielishu ni tsuite"; Omori and Noda, "On an Anopheline Mosquito, *Anopheles Arbumbrosus*, Newly Found in Taiwan," 920.

30. Kobayashi Hiroshi, *Hikone shi no mararia taisaku*, 152–53.

31. Morishita and Nabika, "Mararia chiryō kansuru kenkyū 5"; and Ōda, Morishita, and Nabika, "Mararia chiryo kansuru kenkyu 3."

32. Regarding malariotherapy, Japanese physicians would have known about such treatments from the League of Nations' promotion thereof after the 1920s and

would also have worked on their own experiments. See Wada, "Mahisei chihō no mararia ryohō."

33. Authors' interview with A-nan (pseudonym), July 27, 2002, in Baiho, Tainan
County. A-nan was born in 1929 and became a member of the local DDT spraying
team in 1956.

34. Republic of China (Taiwan), Executive Yuan, Department of Health. *Malaria
Eradication in Taiwan*, 35.

35. Taiwan Malaria Research Institute, *Annexes to the Plan of Operations*, Document 2023, 51.

36. Spielman and D'Antonio, *Mosquito*, 135.

37. Taiwan Malaria Research Institute, *Annexes to the Plan of Operations for Malaria Eradication in China (Taiwan)*, Document 2025, 69.

38. See R. B. Watson and Liang, "Seasonal Prevalence of Malaria in Southern For-
mosa"; and R. B. Watson, Paul, and Liang, "A Report on One Year's Field Trial of
Chlorguanide (Paludrine) as a Suppressive and as a Therapeutic Agent in Southern
Taiwan (Formosa)."

39. See, for example, anonymous writer, "Bensheng sinian punue jihua," *Lianhe
Bao*, July 14, 1952, and "Fangnuezhidao shouchong miewen," ibid., July 17, 1952.

40. "Fangnuezhidao shouchong miewen," *Lianhe Bao*, July 17, 1952.

41. Taiwan Malaria Research Institute, *Annexes to the Plan of Operations for Malaria Eradication in China (Taiwan)*, Document 2004, 14.

42. Authors' interview December 20, 2003, in Taichung. Mrs. Cheng was born in
1931.

43. Authors' interview with Mrs. Wang, September 21, 2004, in Kaohsiung.

44. Taiwan Malaria Research Institute, *Annexes to the Plan of Operations for Malaria Eradication in China (Taiwan)*, Document 2025, 69; Document 2023, 46.

45. Spielman and D'Antonio, *Mosquito*, 162.

46. Martial law was imposed by Chiang Kai-shek in May of 1949 and was not lifted
until 1987. It is the longest period of martial law in modern history. The travel ban to
mainland China was not lifted until a few months after the lifting of martial law.

47. Taiwan Malaria Research Institute, *Annexes to the Plan of Operations for Malaria Eradication in China (Taiwan)*, Document 2026, 79.

48. Ibid., Document 2027, 81.

49. Ibid., 171.

50. Spielman and D'Antonio, *Mosquito*, 155–56.

51. Republic of China (Taiwan), Executive Yuan, Department of Health, *Malaria
Eradication in Taiwan*, 71.

52. Chiang Kai-shek announced that slogan at the monthly assembly of the Central Committee of Mobilization. Speech has quote from Guoshiguan (Academia Historica) ed., *Taiwan zhuquan yu yige zhongkuo lunshu dashiji*, 16.

53. Yin, "Fangong dalu wenti," 3.

54. Liu S., "Differential Mortality in Colonial Taiwan," 231–32.

55. Birn and Solorzano, "Public Health Policy Paradoxes."

56. Morishita Kaoru and Ōda Junro, *Mararia* (Taiwan Sōtokufu, 1939) (film).

57. Interview with A-nan (pseudonym), July 27, 2002, in Baiho, Tainan County.

58. The KMT government after the Second World War also realized that "an impressive sequence of directors had both administrative and technical talent and shared field-oriented skills and capabilities with personnel at all staff levels, many of whom had developed innovative methods of overcoming many obstacles quite commonly found in a truly 'grass-roots' campaign." Republic of China (Taiwan), Executive Yuan, Department of Health, *Malaria Eradication in Taiwan*, 271.

59. W. Anderson, "Where Is the Postcolonial History of Medicine?" 526.

60. Morishita, Sugida, and Hitōgawa, "Shinchikushōshita shisaichihō ni botsuhatsu seru ryukosei mararia ni tsuite."

61. Taiwansheng jiaotongbu, *Taiwansheng jiaotong jianshe*, 7–8.

62. Chen Shaoxin, "Taiwan de renkou bianqian *yu shehui bianqian*," 96–97.

63. For the definition of "epidemiological transition," see McKeown, *The Role of Medicine*, 29–65, and 91–113.

64. Mirzaee, "Trends and Determinants of Mortality in Taiwan," 191–94.

65. Republic of China (Taiwan), Executive Yuan, Council for Economic Planning and Development, *Taiwan Statistical Data Book*.

66. All numbers are extracted and recalculated from Wang Z., *Women ruhe chuangzaole jingji qiji*, 9.

67. Republic of China (Taiwan), Executive Yuan, Department of Health, *Health Statistics in Taiwan*.

68. M. S. Chen and Huang, "Industrial Workers' Health and Environmental Pollution under the New International Division of Labor," 1229.

69. Republic of China (Taiwan), Executive Yuan, Department of Health, *Health Statistics in Taiwan*.

70. Department of Health. *Health Statistics in Taiwan*, 2005.

71. "Chunüe 38 nian Taiwan shoujian nüeji jieru ganran," *Zhongguo Shibao*, September 8, 2003.

The Elimination of Schistosomiasis in Jiaxing and Haining Counties, 1948–58

Public Health as Political Movement

Li Yushang

Schistosomiasis, also known as bilharzia, is a severe, infectious parasitic disease that has long been endemic in China's Jiangnan region.[1] Mentions of the disease in the modern period are frequent. During the second Sino-Japanese War (1937–45), Huang Shaohong, the provincial administrator of Zhejiang, pointed out in the context of comparing the different diseases faced by the provincial government that acute infectious diseases usually had only a short-term impact and were easily prevented or eliminated. Chronic infectious diseases such as schistosomiasis, by contrast, were more harmful in the long run, as effective preventive measures were not understood and often neglected by the population. Such diseases actually brought more harm to the region.[2] In the 1950s, the early years of the People's Republic of China, senior residents of the area recalled that the "big belly disease" (the local term for schistosomiasis) had been widespread back in the late imperial period.[3] This statement is confirmed by clinical cases recorded by medical doctors of the region in the Qing dynasty.[4] Surveys undertaken in the 1950s and 1960s show infection rates of 56.9 percent, 64.66 percent, 29.32 percent, 26.5 percent, and 19.99 percent respectively for Jiaxing, Jiashan, Pinghu, Haiyan, and Tongxiang Counties in the northern Zhejiang Plain, with total infected populations of 354,625; 245,774; 239,082; 101,638; and 183,126, respectively.[5]

The spread of schistosomiasis is closely related to environmental and social factors. With its high infection rate and long-term impact on the population, schistosomiasis is at least as important as the plague or cholera for modern China. However, scholars have focused more on acute diseases, and relatively little research has been done on the history of this chronic disease.[6] This chapter is a preliminary survey on the control of the disease both as a public health issue and as a political movement in the first decade of Communist rule. Located in the northern part of Zhejiang Province, Jiaxing and Haining are well known as a watery region, a land flowing with milk and honey, but also as an area impacted by schistosomiasis. In 1949, Jiaxing Region administered two cities and ten counties, which included Jiaxing City, Jiaxing County, and Haining County. Because of the high rate of infection in these areas, the Nationalists and Communists focused on the prevention and cure of this disease, and records of their attempts are well preserved.

The Republican government, in charge of China from 1911 to 1949 and dominated by the Nationalists for much of that time, had been informed of the problem of schistosomiasis some time before, but the first institute dedicated to schistosomiasis control was not established until 1948, three years after the end of the second Sino-Japanese War and in the middle of the civil war with the Communists.[7] After the Communist victory in 1949, the first priority of the PRC in Jiaxing and Haining was the establishment of organizations and control centers to combat schistosomiasis at certain test points. From 1956 to 1958, schistosomiasis control quickly became a mass political movement, which made it possible for the first time in history for the local people to create a better environment and eliminate snails, a necessary host for the parasite that causes the disease. It was also during this period that the government and the rural population established direct contact. In this chapter, I would like to present a picture of schistosomiasis control up through 1958, the year of the Great Leap Forward. In 1956, the government initiated a political mass movement for both treatment and prevention, hoping for total eradication of the disease. The results were limited. I will not go much beyond the 1950s, but it is perhaps useful to mention here that the control program emphasized the elimination of snails only after 1964, and it was soon thereafter interrupted by the Cultural Revolution. Decisive action against the disease took place relatively late, in the 1970s. In other words, in this chapter I am dealing only with the earliest stage of the PRC's public health program against schistosomiasis, a program that was much colored by political movements.

Schistosomiasis as an Environmental Disease

Schistosomiasis is a disease caused by parasitic worms. Infection occurs when a person's skin comes in contact with contaminated fresh water in which certain types of snails that carry schistosomes are living. The fresh water is usually contaminated by human urine or excrement that contains schistosoma eggs. The eggs hatch, and if certain types of snails are present in the water, the parasites grow, enter the snails by penetrating their feet, and multiply inside the snails. The new parasites, known as *cercariae*, leave the host snail after seven to eleven weeks and enter the water, where they can survive for about forty-eight hours. Penetration of the human skin occurs after the cercaria have attached to and explored the skin. The parasite secretes enzymes that break down the skin's protein to enable the cercarial head to penetrate the skin. As the cercaria penetrates the skin, it transforms into a migrating schistosomulum.

Parasites reach maturity in six to eight weeks, at which time they begin to produce eggs. Some of these eggs pass through the walls of the blood vessels of the human host and travel to the bladder or intestines, from where they are excreted through the urine or stool. Up to half the eggs released by the worm become trapped in the mesenteric veins or are washed back into the liver. Worm pairs can live in the body for an average of four to five years, but they may remain for up to twenty years. Trapped eggs mature normally, secreting antigens that elicit a vigorous immune response. The eggs themselves do not damage the body. Rather, it is the cellular infiltration resulting from the immune response that causes the classic pathology. Patients usually show the following symptoms: abdominal pain, cough, diarrhea, eosinophilia (extremely high white blood cell count), fever, fatigue, and hepatosplenomegaly (enlargement of both the liver and the spleen).[8]

Waterways in the northern Zhejiang Plain form extensive networks, and residents of this area often built their houses along these watercourses. Open toilets were often located just next to them, and women cleaned their families' chamber pots in the same waterways.[9] As a result, schistosoma eggs contained in human excrement easily entered the water. Furthermore, local peasants used a mixture of river mud, green manure, and human excrement as fertilizer, as noted in the Jiaxing City archives in the case of Dongzha Village, for example.[10] To make things worse, some of the boatmen and fishermen of the region—including 1,260 people in Xiashi, in Haining County—actually resided on boats, on which there were no toilets at all.

Table 1. Schistosomiasis Infection of Livestock in Jiaxing County, 1959

	Buffalos	Yellow cattle	Goats	Pigs	Dogs	Rabbits
Number inspected	4,663	2,891	128	444	32	65
Number of positive reactions	559	919	12	25	11	4
Original infection rate (%) in this report	11.90	31.80	9.37	5.63	34.37	6.10
Corrected infection rate (%)	11.99	31.79	9.38	5.63	34.38	6.15

Source: "Inspection on Schistosomiasis in Livestock," in Jiaxingshi dang'anguan, no. 53-1-326, 64.

These fishermen simply urinated and excreted directly into the waterways. With 60 percent of the fishermen infected with schistosomiasis, their excrement turned out to be a major source of infection.[11]

In this region, livestock was another primary host of schistosomes. The rate of infection of livestock in Jiaxing County in 1959 is shown in table 1.

As this table shows, the infection rate for yellow cattle was the highest, with the exception of dogs, whose high rates were probably a result of poor sampling in 1959 (infection rates of dogs in 1955 were 10.34 percent).[12] Yellow cattle, unlike buffalos, had poor immunity against schistosomes, thus had high infection rates. Both animals were nonetheless major sources of infection of the disease because they were usually pulled into the watercourses and often excreted on the spot.[13] It was also a common practice in the northern Zhejiang Plain to make yellow cattle bathe in the rivers, and waterwheels of the area were powered by man, wind, or yellow cattle. Places that utilized the strength of the yellow cattle for this purpose had a higher infection rate. In Jiaxing County, the utilization of buffalos and yellow cattle for the purpose of bailing out the rice fields was relatively widespread. Irrigation canals where buffalos and yellow cattle were utilized were therefore a serious source of infection, though in places that relied solely on machines and manpower, irrigation canals did not pose as great a threat in terms of infection.[14] However, in the 1950s, experts and authorities concerned with the control of schistosomiasis did not place much importance on prevention of the disease in livestock. It was only much later that they realized the significance of controlling schistosomiasis in livestock and consequently made it a priority.

In Zhejiang, snails thrived in rivers (7.21 percent), other waterways (11.65

percent), ponds (2.93 percent), and paddy fields (74.70 percent).[15] Jiaxing served as a hub for the Taihu basin, and due to the existence of networks of slow-moving waterways around it, snails spread to every corner of the area.[16] It is thus not surprising that schistosomiasis was prevalent. However, the distribution of snails differed from town to town because of different ecological settings. For example, in Baoshan, where the current in the Huangpu River runs faster than elsewhere, snails were not common in the waterways but were found mainly in rice fields,[17] while snails were not found in some fields of Suzhou because the surface of the fields was four to six feet higher than that of the canals.[18] As for Haining, snails were found mostly along riverbanks and in ditches and rice fields.[19] According to a survey from 1949 in Jiaxing County, snails there lived mostly in riverbanks and the ditches in rice fields.[20] A survey from 1950 in the area of Dongzha Village of Jiaxing County showed that while no snails were found in the paddy fields, 43.6 percent, 33 percent, and 23.4 percent of the snails there were found in waterways, on riverbanks, and in irrigation ditches, respectively.[21] Nevertheless, such figures do not mean that rice fields in Jiaxing were free of snails. They were definitely present in fields below the water level, but only rarely in higher ground. However, in the 1950s, the government encouraged draining flooded paddy fields to create more dry rice fields, for the purpose of increasing rice productivity. This move changed the outlook of rice cultivation in this region and should have provided favorable conditions for the reduction of snails in paddies.

It was, however, still extremely difficult to exterminate snails, since they were a part of the region's natural ecosystem.[22] Back in 1958, residents in Haining questioned whether the methods they were taught to use in killing snails were effective, since even after repeating four or five times the process of ridding the ditches of snails and burying them underground, snails were still prevalent.[23]

The last stage in the cycle of infectious schistosomiasis takes place in human hosts after contact with the larvae in the water. In Zhejiang Province, local residents got infected by frequent contact with water for their daily activities and chores (cleaning, swimming, bathing, and work such as farming, fishing, and flood mitigation).[24] In Pinghu County, local people obtained their drinking water from the same rivers that they swam, fished, and bathed in. Furthermore, farming, which increased contact with water, was the most important economic activity in the area.[25] To make matters worse, some towns in Jiaxing County developed a tradition of bathing newborns in

Table 2. The Relationship between Occupation and Infection Rate in Jiaxing County, 1956

	Factory workers	Peasants	Students	Officials	Fisher-men	Other residents	Military
Number inspected	3,239	590	11,757	6,836	903	23,468	136
Number of positive reactions	1,056	305	1,815	2,659	598	5,172	6
Original infection rate (%) in this report	32.60	51.69	15.44	38.90	66.22	22.04	4.41
Corrected infection rate (%)	32.60	51.69	15.44	39.90	66.22	22.04	4.41

Source: "The Relationship between Infection Rate and Occupation," in Jiaxingshi dang'anguan, no. 53-1-326, 56.

rivers as a ritual to pray for the baby's good health. And when parents went to work, their children played in the vicinity of the house and got infected from dew tainted by snails.[26] In fact, people of different walks of life had different levels of exposure to polluted water and thus had different rates of infection. The relationship between occupation and infection rate in Jiaxing County in 1956 is shown in table 2.

According to the table, fishermen and peasants suffered from the highest infection rates, due to their frequent exposure to water. According to surveys by agricultural cooperatives in some villages in Jiaxing County, a greater number of positive cases were found among those who had contact with water in their professional work, such as farmers toiling in paddy fields. Among males, individuals who bathed in rivers had a higher infection rate; and among females, individuals who cleaned their hands and feet in the rivers or canals suffered from a higher infection rate than those who came in contact with water only while performing house chores.[27]

Schistosomiasis was indeed an environmental disease that required much more than providing treatment to infected patients. As we shall see in the following sections of this chapter, in the early 1950s, the government assigned medical teams to villages and towns throughout Jiaxing County to provide treatment for patients, but it did not pay enough attention to preventive measures, which consisted of improving the environment. As a result, reinfection was a serious problem, with a rate of about 40 percent.[28] Although molluscicides were already commonly accepted internationally as the only effective measure to control schistosomiasis,[29] this approach was not effectively and systematically practiced in China until the 1970s, after the Cultural Revolution. This failure was partially of a political nature.

1948–55: A Difficult Beginning

Before the onset of the second Sino-Japanese War in 1937, public health in Xinsheng Town of Jiaxing County was a matter left to the town administration.[30] A county public health office was established only after the war, in 1945. This offered mobile medical services to implement disease control and help residents improve sanitary conditions.[31] At the same time, sanitary police were dispatched to conduct surveys and improve local hygiene.[32] During this period, the Nationalist government focused on sanitary issues, including improving cleanliness in the urban environment and preventing epidemics of acute diseases. However, many towns remained dissatisfied with the work of the sanitary police and asked for the establishment of better equipped and more sophisticated public health organizations at the local level.

Public health in rural villages was largely neglected. In general, sanitary conditions remained poor in both urban and rural areas. In 1946, a survey by the Jiaxing County government on local health and hygiene revealed the problem was a lack of resources. Table 3 shows the data collected by the survey for Caopu Town and Longnan Village.

Neither Caopu nor Longnan reported any cases of schistosomiasis, malaria, or fasciolopsiasis, probably because the interviewers did not include questions regarding such issues in this survey. In surveys from the 1950s, however, schistosomiasis was clearly an important issue. Hence we know that in addition to the poor sanitary conditions shown in these simple reports, underreporting of diseases and poor surveying were a problem in the period after the second Sino-Japanese War. This report also confirms the well-known fact that most medical practitioners in small towns and villages of China were traditional Chinese doctors instead of MDs, despite the Nationalist regime's harsh attitude toward traditional Chinese medicine in the 1920s and 1930s.[33] As a result, doctors trained in Western medicine were basically unavailable.

The postwar Nationalist government did eventually begin to pay attention to the schistosomiasis problem. A program to control the disease began in Zhejiang in 1948, when a prevention center for endemic diseases in the province was established. In Zhejiang Province, a research institute on en-

Table 3. Data from Caopu Town and Longnan Village from 1946 Survey

	Caopu	Longnan
Number of Chinese doctors or Western MDs, and if they are registered	2 Chinese, not registered; no Western MDs	1 Chinese doctor, registered; no Western MDs
If customary, midwives are trained in Western obstetrics and gynecology	No	No
Inoculation of children against smallpox	Free vaccines provided	All children inoculated
Local epidemics (such as schistosomiasis, malaria, or fasciolopsiasis)	None mentioned; however, a few cases of smallpox found	None
General environment, including the cleaning of roads, ditches, and toilets, and the presence of trashcans along with proper management of garbage	8 trashcans set up, which were cleaned once daily; ditches were excavated	No toilets or trashcans; roads in the village are small paths in the farms; ditches taken care of by peasants
General condition and cleanliness of wells	NA	No wells found
Presence of public toilets, and if they are well maintained	NA	No public toilets found
School environment	Not perfect	Roughly acceptable

Source: "Hygiene Survey at Caopu Town and Longnan Village, Jiaxing County in 1946," in Jiaxingshi dang'anguan, no. 304-5-139.

demics—located in the southern part of Jiaxing County, with a branch in Buyun Town—was set up under the direction of Chen Chaochang, a parasitologist. The institute provided treatments and carried out surveys. However, only 1,000 outpatients were treated there in 1948, and the effect of disease control was obviously limited.[34]

In brief, from 1945 to 1949, during the civil war between the Nationalists and the Communists, the general condition of public health in China's rural areas remained largely unchanged. Public health units established by the government did not have the necessary resources to improve conditions, given the unstable political situation and short time span. While prevention centers were established, they could not meet local needs, and the problem of schistosomiasis inevitably persisted into the Communist era, after 1949.

Thus the Communist local government in Zhejiang inherited the problematic public health situation of the Nationalist regime. In the ten counties of Jiaxing Region, college-trained medical doctors were few in the early 1950s, and in Jiaxing City, which had a population of 40,000 in 1916,[35] only about a dozen such doctors were in practice.[36] Up to 1955, Jiaxing Hospital had insufficient professional staff formally trained in Western medicine. As a splenectomy usually took five to six hours, and the number of patients was great, many patients had no chance to be operated on.[37] The situation was definitely even worse in rural areas.[38] The primary medical force to rely on in the fight against any disease was still practitioners of traditional Chinese medicine (TCM). In view of this problem, the PRC government began to do two things: it recruited students to receive basic medical training for the implementation of disease control measures, and it mobilized TCM doctors to participate in the control project.[39] In 1954, for instance, the Jiaxing Schistosomiasis Control Center trained 342 health assistants to help professional MDs to organize propaganda and implement control measures.[40] These locally trained health assistants were to become the most important personnel in implementing the schistosomiasis control program from 1956 to 1958.[41]

Nevertheless, I must point out here that this lack of biomedical resources was partly compensated for by the accessibility of TCM in the early 1950s. The authorities often claimed that Chinese medicine made impressive progress in the treatment of schistosomiasis. For example, a local doctor called Xu Bihui disclosed a special formula that had been kept secret in his family for generations, known to be effective in treating the disease. Several more formulas were discovered and publicized subsequently.[42] By the end of 1956, more than a dozen new herbs or drugs were claimed to be effective treatments for schistosomiasis by TCM doctors and the population of Zhejiang Province.[43] Similar discoveries were witnessed in Haining as well. For example, a peasant from Huangwan Village proposed that a herb called *huoxuelong* (blood-vitalizing dragon), long used in a secret prescription transmitted in his family, was effective for the treatment of what was called the swell—a popular name for schistosomiasis.[44] However, despite the growing euphoria, most experts admitted that TCM was useful only in the treatment of patients in the late stages of an illness and was not effective with early symptoms.[45] Chinese doctors essentially applied drugs to do two things: to eliminate stagnating fluids inside the body and to reinforce the patient's physical resistance. Drugs were used to discharge fluids from the body, while replenishing herbs were prescribed to enhance the functions of the spleen and kidney, and to ease the liver and facilitate digestion.[46] However, it was still Western medicine that produced the fastest and most obvious results.

Despite moderate progress in the training of medical personnel and growing public interest in medicine, schistosomiasis control was not thought out or implemented wholeheartedly by local authorities before 1956. The main problem was, in fact, the lack of understanding of the schistosomiasis situation by leading political cadres, as most of them were from urban areas where the disease was rare. Moreover, they did not consider the prevention of schistosomiasis their responsibility. In Zhongdai Village of Jiaxing County, for example, party cadres were not aware of the gravity of the schistosomiasis problem and did not take any action before 1953. Hence only 3,808 patients, or 2.34 percent of the total number of cases, received treatment from 1952 to 1955. Most of the infected individuals were not treated, and preventive measures (proper management of excrement, cleaning of waterways, and extermination of snails) were simply ignored.[47] As a result, no fundamental measures were taken in the region before 1955; in fact, the first time the problem was given serious thought on a high political level was as late as 1953.

In May 1953, when Shen Junru, chairman of the Democratic League— a party of senior and middle academic rank in culture, education, science, and technology in China—returned to his native area of Jiaxing, he realized the gravity of the schistosomiasis problem and appealed to Beijing for assistance. Mao Zedong responded enthusiastically and indicated that control measures must be strengthened.[48] In August 1954, a trial project was implemented in Jingxiang Village of Jiaxing County.[49] However, the project was aborted after a series of political purges of important cadres in the remaining months of the year.[50] The launch of a persistent schistosomiasis control program only began after the end of this purge, in 1955.

1956–58: A Health Issue or a Political Issue?

Mao Zedong became more focused on schistosomiasis in 1955, when the party was considered purified after several years of political purges. Professor Su Delong, a renowned researcher on the disease, recalled that Mao "had to face so many infected peasants and soldiers."[51] In the winter of 1955, the central government issued the slogan "We must exterminate schisto-somiasis!"—which became the central directive. A central task force with nine members was set up in Beijing, and special regional teams dedicated to this objective were formed at all administrative levels of the provinces. In the same year, the central government ordered the formation of a new task force for schistosomiasis control with five members in Jiaxing County, below which related offices were also set up by local government bureau-crats.[52] In the same year, a Schistosomiasis Control Committee was set up in Haining.[53] Schistosomiasis control had finally become a central issue on the formal agendas of the national party and the government.

The national Agricultural Development Plan drafted in 1956 included a twelve-year schistosomiasis control program aimed at eradicating the disease. By this time, the local bureaucratic structure was organized to facilitate mass movements directed from the center. The vertical structure built at the county level since 1949 to quicken the implementation of orders down to the lowest village levels had become much more streamlined by 1958, with central commands coming directly from the Communist Party to the production teams that had replaced traditional villages. In addition, the inhabitants of Zhejiang had already gained some experience in controlling the disease using new knowledge brought by foreign experts in the early 1950s. The residents of Jiaxing and Haining, for example, were encouraged to eliminate snails by cleaning the waterways and burying the snails,[54] a lesson that Chinese doctors had learned from Japanese experts in the early 1950s.[55] The people of these regions seemed to be politically and technically ready to try something more ambitious and radical.

When Mao went to Shanghai in 1957, he asked Su for his opinion on the feasibility of eliminating the disease within the targeted time limit, but met with a negative response.[56] The central government thus adjusted its goal and declared that the disease must be eliminated within seven years by combining all the resources of Chinese and Western medicine. Given this official objective, party cadres of Zhejiang Province, in great political fervor, reduced the number of years to five,[57] and some counties in the province even cut it down to three.[58] In 1956, the government of Haining County assigned half of its medical staff to work on schistosomiasis control and established disease control units in some of the villages and towns.[59] However, for the most politically fervent cadres of the time, the project was not fully integrated into the production plans of the communes and production teams as expected, in the sense that it did not provoke a truly general mass movement.[60] Initial popular reaction to the project was lukewarm, and the whole project came to a halt in 1957.[61] This shows that the responsibility for schistosomiasis control was still largely left to the less politicized public health units. The only progress made in 1956–57 was the above-mentioned fact that more human resources in the form of locally trained health assistants were now available in the control program. But events quickly took yet another decisive turn in the following year.

In 1958, the year of the Great Leap Forward, schistosomiasis control became a central issue for the Communist Party and the government. The head of party propaganda in Haining County declared that schistosomiasis would be eliminated in the area within one year.[62] As a consequence, all party and government cadres and officials were mobilized to fight the disease until its ultimate eradication.[63] The vertical bureaucratic structure of disease control that had been set up a few years earlier became a key factor in this program. In the words of active cadres, disease control measures could now be implemented quickly and with vitality in the form of political movements or raids, often as part of the national Patriotic Hygiene Movement. As had been pointed out in a 1956 health report in Haining, "the key to success lies in the mobilization of the young, women, and students, under the leadership of the party and the government."[64] This bureaucratic structure was in full force in 1958, essentially for the dual purpose of exterminating the snails and instructing the peasants. In Haining County, for example, eight to twelve active young people from each commune were selected to form a shock team to remove snails from the neighborhoods. Altogether, 5,355 people of the county were assigned to 308 such youth teams.[65] Students were mobilized to help search out and exterminate snails during their winter break.[66] Teachers, health assistants, party cadres, and commune accountants were also asked to prepare propaganda for the various movements.[67]

In Xieqiao Village, a task force was set up under the direct command of the local party secretary to make sure that control measures were integrated into the general production plan of the newly formed commune.[68] Lai Guangxing, the deputy director of the health department of Zhejiang Province, aptly stated that the extermination of schistosomes was not merely a medical issue but also an important political mission.[69] The urge for a Great Leap Forward in public health and the pressure to achieve this important political mission drove all towns and villages in Haining County to accelerate their efforts in order to meet the official goal of eliminating schistosomes in one year.[70]

Meanwhile, on top of the existing health assistants, the Communist Party attempted to foster a bigger group of professionals. In 1958, training programs were organized at the village level in the Haining area, aimed at producing more doctors, midwives, and health assistants to deal with the disease.[71] While the extermination of snails was a good test for the efficacy of mass mobilization during this period, the treatment of patients with the disease lay at the center of the medical program. The work of many more medical personnel at different administrative levels, rural and urban doctors, and local health assistants, was coordinated to treat patients.[72]

According to available statistics, infection rates for rural villages in Jiaxing County had reached 71.6 percent in the 1950s; in other words, 350,000 people were infected. The only biomedical treatment used at that time was injections of antimony potassium tartrate, which took twenty days for each course of treatment. Thus, it would have taken the local hospitals a full hundred years to complete treating all patients, given their limited capacity.[73] As a political mission, the elimination of the disease was urgent. In view of the large number of untreated patients, innovation was needed badly. Jin Yuehua, a doctor in Jiaxing, recalled that "the so-called three-day, seven-day, or 24-hour antimony therapies were the product of this era. All task forces were pressed to follow suit. Individuals who did not act accordingly would be 'showing the white flag,' meaning that they were labeled as having committed a political error."[74] In Xiashi Town of Haining County, all medical teams shortened the therapy from three to two days, and from six injections to four. The treatment was also shifted from being applied in the daytime to the nighttime, and from hospitalization to outpatient service.[75] In fact, the three-day therapy was finally implemented in the whole of Haining County.[76] Obviously, medical teams did everything they could to avoid being accused of lagging behind in this mass political movement.

Most experts at that time considered that schistosomiasis could not be eliminated, especially within a short period of time. They were convinced that controlling the disease required a high level of technology and could not be achieved through mass movements or a Great Leap Forward. Many doctors objected to the three-day therapy, including a Dr. Feng Heling in Xiashi, who said: "Side effects have been serious even for a twenty-day therapy. A three-day course is even more risky."[77] However, since the priority lay in achieving the political mission within a short period, medical teams modified the doses of the drugs in order to meet the prescribed goal. To avoid the death of patients, some reduced the dose to a level that could not

effectively kill schistosomes, while others increased the dose disproportion-
ately to cut the course to two days or even one.[78] Despite all the undesirable
results, a large proportion of patients were treated with shortened courses
of therapy. From 1952 to 1958, 80.92 percent of treated patients in Jiaxing
County accepted a three-day or two-day course, while only 14.57 percent
had the traditional twenty-day therapy.[79] In other words, while the twenty-
day therapy had been mainstream from 1952 to 1957, shortened therapies
had become the norm in 1958. Meanwhile, false reports were made. Under
constant pressure from the government, some medical teams took in new
patients before they finished treating previous ones, so that the latter never
finished their treatments. There were also teams that allowed health assistants to treat patients in the place of doctors, naturally with little success.[80]

Another problem was the implementation of control measures. Before
1958, the emphasis was on treating outpatients, and teams were encouraged to go out and search for new patients. One good illustration would be
the way in which the agricultural cooperative in Shuangshan Village in Haining County worked with the control station in Xiashi Town. The cooperative signed a contract with the station in April 1956, specifying that while
patients from Shuangshan would go to Xiashi for treatment and the Shuangshan cooperative would pay for all fees, the Xiashi control station would
actively improve the treatment to make it shorter.[81] However, in reality the
cooperative was afraid of the negative impact of treatment on its agriculture
productivity and could not honor the contract, and the station consequently
did not get paid for enough patients and accumulated bad debts.[82] The treatment of patients in other places was sometimes described as similar to that
of guerrilla warfare: "We went to one place to treat patients, and then we
quickly moved to another. We were on the move all the time."[83] To achieve
their goal, a large number of medical staff moved from cities to villages and
established quite a few makeshift hospitals and clinics in 1958.[84]

When urban medical personnel treated patients in rural villages, different strategies were employed. For example, in Shenshu Village of Haining
County, the medical team was split into five small units, each with one doctor and one assistant. These units were dispatched at night to deliver treatments to individual homes in the five different areas of the village. They
were to "'attack' in different directions but [follow the orders from] a central core."[85] Such proactive measures were supported by cooperatives. In
the village of Xiashi, for instance, cooperatives and medical teams agreed to
work together to make sure that the latter would receive patients sent by the

former to be treated. In this way, the medical personnel were guaranteed a treatment quota.[86] However, since the whole project was implemented in the form of a top-down political movement, with preconceived rigid time-tables and spatial organization and little flexibility, many patients were not treated properly.

Worse still, after the initial enthusiasm of the movement cooled off, medical help once again became out of reach for the masses of peasants.[87] In fact, the top-down, vertical bureaucratic structure that had helped to mobilize large masses of peasants in no time had a potential weakness: enthusiasm quickly ebbed when political movements subsided.[88] Nonetheless, on August 12, 1958, the party and government of Zhejiang Province declared that schistosomiasis in Haining County was basically eliminated.[89]

The Masses and the Weight of Tradition

The traditional popular view of schistosomiasis was different from modern scientific knowledge and hence constituted a big obstacle to modern control measures. Most locals thought that schistosomiasis was caused by bad *fengshui* (geomancy),[90] or that to get sick was "foreordained."[91] In the 1950s, residents of the region called the disease *guzhang* (the swell), *huangbing* (the yellow disease), *shang* (damage), *masha* (dysentery), and so on. Symptoms like diarrhea, fever, and fatigue were commonplace, and peasants generally thought that the disease was a result of overwork.[92] Some people considered the presence of blood in the stool to be simply a result of exhaustion and did not associate this symptom with being infected with schistosomiasis.[93]

Popular attitudes in the 1950s also made treatment more complicated because female peasants in particular were reluctant to hand over stool samples, as they regarded such an action as embarrassing. To avoid embarrassment, many handed over the stool of other people or even of animals,[94] while some families gave the stool of one member divided into as many bags as there were family members or simply refused to hand in any samples at all.[95] Unpopular inspectors, sometimes nicknamed "Mr. Stool," encountered constant quiet resistance from the peasants.[96]

There was a popular saying in Jiaxing that "even with a doctor father, the swell is incurable." "The swell" or "big belly" were signs of death, and people considered the advanced stage of schistosomiasis as hopeless. This belief persisted until the late 1950s.[97] However, it did not encourage patients to seek medical help in the early stage of the disease. In the early 1950s, many peasants of Jiaxing Region did not accept therapy until they were forced to by the authorities, and they remained reluctant to take injections and medicine.[98] Some patients were as much concerned about the side effects of antimony as they were about the disease.[99]

Furthermore, the treatment of schistosomiasis greatly affected the productivity of the patients. Sick leaves interrupted the general production plan and reduced the income of the communes.[100] In 1956, some local cadres in Xiashi Town, for instance, opposed treatment on the basis of such concerns. In Xieqiao Village in the same year, cadres could not even send the previously promised thirty patients to receive treatment for fear of a labor shortage during the peak season.[101] In order to force peasants to undergo treatment, the authorities resorted to the work grading system (in which peasants got points or scores after a day's work, which determined the grain ration they could get at the end of the year): those who did not go for treatment as scheduled would have points deducted. Even though this measure was effective, production leaders and other peasants greatly resented it because "we were very busy in the second peak season of 1958, and strong bodies had to leave for injections for fear of having their points taken away, leaving the fields unattended. Members of the commune were very critical of this!"[102] To fit in the agricultural calendar was indeed one key in the success of the treatment program, as providing treatment in the slack season would be much more effective.[103] To be more specific, if the local party units and government promoted control measures from May to September, they usually achieved bad results.[104] This was an experience that cadres in Jiaxing and Haining learned after 1956.[105]

It was as difficult to persuade peasants to accept treatment as it was to convince them of the importance of prevention. A key issue in prevention was the cleaning of toilets for the purpose of eliminating snails in the waterways. To change the peasants' toilet habits proved difficult. The recommended new way of organizing toilets was that all vats for excrement were to be concentrated and grouped into one public, closed area, so that the stool could be treated at once in an enclosed spot that was well separated from water sources. However, in the rural villages of Jiangnan, peasants were reluctant to "break ground" (*potu*)[106] and believed that moving outhouses was unlucky.[107] Some elderly peasants did not consider open toilets a cause of "the swell" and claimed it was unnecessary to change or move the toilets.[108]

Moreover, new ideas about toilets conflicted with the peasants' tradi-

tional habits and economic interests. Toilets of the Jiaxing region were traditionally set up in the back of the home and were used by every member of
the family—men, women, and children. However, the new, public toilets,
often located at a distance from the homes, created great inconvenience
for everyone, and some simply resorted to "peeing wherever they liked," as
some senior residents of Zhongdai Village complained.[109] According to Shi
Youquan, who from 1954 to 1958 was in charge of the toilet control project
in Jingxiang, Jiaxing County, these attempts led to a series of failures and
demanded tremendous perseverance.[110] In Haining County, another person
in charge of a similar program from 1955 to 1968 in another rural village,
reported that all trials failed in the end:

> People in the village were quite used to sitting on their own toilets in-
> stead of going to the public ones. Local residents considered it handy
> to clean their own excrement basin, which was commonly placed in
> the back of their own houses. The public grouped toilets were hard to
> clean, especially on rainy days. Thus, when the task force left, local
> people immediately moved the excrement basins back to their houses
> and stole the bricks and wood materials of the public toilets for other
> uses. Not long afterwards, even the wooden lids of the public toilets
> were taken away.[111]

In terms of people's livelihood, human manure served as a primary
source of fertilizer in the Jiangnan region (along with the excrement of
livestock) and was considered a valuable commodity,[112] as shown in Yu Xinzhong's chapter in this volume. As the popular saying goes: "A basin of night
soil is worth a basin of gold." In 1953, when production was first organized
in mutual aid teams and private property was still maintained, the Communist Party in Zhongdai Village of Jiaxing County attempted to group private toilets in one place, but the trial soon failed because, according to Yao
Hubao, a local peasant woman, peasants were afraid their own stool would
be taken for "public uses."[113] After 1956, agricultural land in the villages
was largely collectivized, with only small plots reserved for private use.
The "incomplete collectivization of human manure resulted in the fact that
cabbages on private plots were two-thirds larger than those on collective
land."[114] The same happened to the Baihua production team in Jiaxing: "In
the winter, [the party] gave directives; in the spring, things got loose; and
in the summer, things collapsed. In the fall, the cycle began all over again."
The conflict over the public use of private manure remained unsolved.[115]

The management of water and the extermination of snails naturally remained problematic under these conditions. The people of the Jiangnan region traditionally cleaned their toilets in the waterways, and repeated propaganda did not change this behavior.[116] Similarly, burying snails as a required task was carried out only halfheartedly by the peasants and did not meet the technical standards.[117] This is best illustrated by what some peasants in Zhouzhen Town said: "We can eat a dozen such small animals without getting sick. Why bother wasting our time and energy on burying them?" Hence, even after the specification of what was supposed to be done, some communes simply could not achieve their goals.[118] In general, the elimination of snails received only lip service.[119] Peasants were unenthusiastic about policies considered to be essentially political missions contradictory to their traditional habits and livelihood.[120]

In the 1950s, when the political priority was economic production, control measures that were aligned with the production cycle met with the least resistance. All other attempts proved to be failures. In 1956, Zhongdai Village successfully combined the construction of irrigation channels with the burying of snails.[121] Similarly, Xinmin Village made snail burying a part of its electric irrigation works.[122] Both cases were enlightening, and party cadres in Haining stated that "prevention work could go along with production activities such as irrigation or manure gathering. This makes prevention much easier."[123] However, as we have seen earlier, most other control measures, especially the treatment programs, went against the immediate interest and tradition of the peasants and proved to be failures in the 1950s.

Conclusion

From 1948 to 1958, the Nationalist Party and the Communist Party both faced innumerable challenges in rural Jiangnan, with schistosomiasis control being a major one. Compared to other diseases endemic to the Jiangnan region, schistosomiasis was intimately related to the environment and certain occupations. While a large number of people were infected, no perfect remedy emerged before the end of the 1970s. In fact, to eliminate such a disease, nonmedical measures such as large-scale community efforts were required to break the life cycle of the schistosomes.

To change the environment required tremendous human and material resources, which were impossible to organize before 1956. The socialist reform implemented by the PRC after 1956 had a strong impact on the rural world and turned peasants into members of communes and production teams. From 1956 to 1958, this revolution intensified, and it became possible for the central government to rouse the masses into collective actions against schistosomiasis. Because Chairman Mao himself emphasized the question of schistosomiasis control, it immediately became a political issue of top priority from 1956 to 1958, and a key program in the Great Leap Forward.

Nevertheless, as control measures ran against both the habits of the populace and the production requirements of the Great Leap Forward, they were doomed to failure. The 1959–63 famine caused a further setback, and the infection rate increased. From 1964 to 1966, efforts resumed with a new emphasis on prevention—that is, the elimination of snails. However, the Cultural Revolution put a halt to such attempts from 1966 to 1969. It was only in the post–Cultural Revolution era of the 1970s that the government could at last fully implement control measures by both improving treatment of patients with the use of Praziquentel, a new drug, and by systematically clearing the water channels of snails.[124] In the 1980s, schistosomiasis was only found in a small proportion of rural areas where the water level was hard to control, and in mountainous areas where the population was relatively small, such as Hunan and Jiangxi.[125]

Since 1980, a new political climate and the resulting new production mode have diminished the government's ability to mobilize the peasants. The large-scale reconstruction of farms and irrigation systems and resulting ecological changes; industrialization and urbanization; the change in peasants' lifestyle, occupation, and production; along with a new remedy for schistosomiasis have all resulted in an environment where schistosomes do not survive easily. As infection rates have decreased, the natural habitat of schistosomiasis has gradually disappeared.

NOTES

All translations are mine, unless otherwise indicated.

1. Given the high rate of infection, local residents' height, weight, productivity, and household income, as well as birth and death rates, were affected by the prevalence of the disease. Detailed figures can be found in the research report on schistosomiasis in Jiaxing City Archives (Jiaxing dang'anguan, no. 53-1-10, 49–51).

2. Huang Shaohong, *Wushi huiyi*, 455.

3. Xiao Rongwei and Ye Jiafu, *Xuexichongbing*, 1.

4. On the basis of clinical cases noted by doctors of the Qing dynasty, Li Weipu ("Lei xuexicongbing de zhongyi wenxian ziliao") found that many eminent doctors of the Jiangnan region observed cases highly suggestive of schistosomiasis; this suggests that schistosomiasis was prevalent during the imperial period.

5. Qian, *Zhonghua Renmin Gongheguo xuexichong dituji*, 1.

6. For notable exceptions, see Zhejiangsheng xuexichongbing fangzhi bianweihui, *Zhejiang xuexichongbing fangzhi shi*, and Wang X., *Shanghai xiaomie xuexichongbing de huigu*. These books present brief histories of prevention and cure in Zhejiang and Shanghai, respectively, but do not provide details on specific counties.

7. Officials in charge of the public health administration of Zhejiang Province reported the issue of parasitic diseases in their reports as early as 1937, the year when the second Sino-Japanese War broke out. See, for example, Chen W. and Pu, "Zhejiangsheng fangzhi jiangpianchongbing chubu gongzuo baogao."

8. For more information, see Huang Y., *Shiyong linchuang chuanranbing xue*, 469–70.

9. Because of the value of excrement as agricultural fertilizer, the contents of chamber pots were often composted before the emptied basins were cleaned in the waterways. See "Zhonggong Zhouzhen xiangwei guangyu quanxiang yi jibenshang xiaomie xuexichongbing de jingyan baogao," *Haining Ribao*, April 19, 1958, and Jiaxingshi dang'anguan, no. 53–1–181, 129.

10. Jiaxingshi dang'anguan, no. 53–1–10, 46.

11. Zhonggong Zhejiang shengwei chusihai jiang weisheng bangongshi, *Zhejiangsheng Hainingxian fangzhi xuexichongbing de zhongda shengli*, 47.

12. Zhejiang Jiashanxian difangbing fangzhi xiaozu lingdao bangongshi (Supervising office of the Group for Prevention and Control of Endemics of Xiashan county of Zhejiang Province) 浙江嘉善縣地方病防治小組領導辦公室, ed., *Zhejiang sheng Jiashanxian xuexichong bing liuxing qingkuang he fangzhi gongzuo ziliao huibian* 1949–1985 (Compiled data on the epidemic situation of schistosomiasis in Jiashan County of Zhejiang Province 1949–1985) 浙江省嘉善縣血吸虫病流行情况和防治工作資料滙編 1949–1985). Jiashan: Internal Documents, 1985, p. 42.

13. Zheng W., Lin, and Zhong "Riben zhuxuexichongbing zhi linchuangguan."

14. *Jiaxingshi dang'anguan*, no. 53–1–10, 2.

15. Zhejiangsheng xuexichongbing fangzhi bianweihui, *Zhejiang xuexichongbing fangzhi shi*, 20.

16. Chen Chaochang, Yuan, and Ye, "Yinian lai Jiaxing dingluoshi tianran ganran zhuxuexichongbing weiyou zhi diaocha."

17. *Baoshanqu dang'anguan*, no. 145–3–14, 40.

18. Meleney and Faust, "The Intermediate Host of Schistosome Japonicum in China."

19. Fou Shanyong, *Hainingshi weisheng zhi*, 76.

20. Chen Chaochang, Yuan, and Ye, "Yinian lai Jiaxing dingluoshi tianran ganran zhuxuexichongbing weiyou zhi diaocha."

21. Jiaxingshi dang'anguan, no. 53–1–10, 53.

22. Jiaxingshi zhengxie wenshi ziliao weiyuanhui, *Song wenshen*, 33 and 74.

23. "Zhonggong Zhouzhen xiangwei guangyu quanxiang yi jibenshang xiaomie Xuexichongbing de jingyan baogao," *Haining Ribao*, April 19, 1958.

24. Zhejiangsheng xuexichongbing fangzhi bianweihui, *Zhejiang xuexichongbing fangzhi shi*, 22.

25. Jiaxingshi dang'anguan, no. 53–1–10, 12.

26. Jiaxingshi zhengxie wenshi ziliao weiyuanhui, *Song wenshen*, 91.

27. Jiaxingshi dang'anguan, no. 53–1–10, 46.

28. Jiaxingshi zhengxie wenshi ziliao weiyuanhui, *Song wenshen*, 33.

29. World Health Organization, *Epidemiology and Control of Schistosomiasis*, 57.

30. *Jiaxing difang jianshe xiehui xianzheng jianshe kaochatuan baogaoshu ji fulu*, 37.

31. Jiaxingshi zhi bianzuan weiyuanhui, *Jiaxingshi zhi*, 1675.

32. Xinshenzhen zhi bianzuan weiyuanhui, *Xinshengzhen zhi*, 210.

33. *Huzhoushi dang'anguan*, no. 107–4–4, 55–76. On the attitude of the Nationalists toward traditional Chinese medicine, see Lei, "When Chinese Medicine Encountered the State."

34. Jiaxingshi zhengxie wenshi ziliao weiyuanhui, *Song wenshen*, 229 and 112.

35. Li G., *Zhongguo xiandaihua de quyu yanjiu*, 441.

36. Ibid., 43.

37. Ibid., 100.

38. Ibid., 95.

39. Ibid., 28–29 and 77, respectively.

40. Jiaxingshi dang'anguan, no. 53–1–5, 2–3.

41. Ibid., 88.

42. Jiaxingshi zhengxie wenshi ziliao weiyuanhui, *Song wenshen*, 79.

43. Ibid., 6.

44. Ibid., 224.

45. Ibid., 84.

46. Jiaxingshi dang'anguan, no. 53–1–181, 61.

47. Ibid., 53–1–21, 29.

48. Jiaxingshi zhengxie wenshi ziliao weiyuanhui, *Song wenshen*, 464.

49. Jiaxingshi dang'anguan, no. 53–1–5, 81.

50. Jiaxingshi zhengxie wenshi ziliao weiyuanhui, *Song wenshen*, 72.

51. Warren, "Farewell to the Plague Spirit," 124–25.

52. Jiaxingshi zhengxie wenshi ziliao weiyuanhui, *Song wenshen*, 231.

53. Hainingshi dang'anguan, no. 102–1–8, 14.

54. Mao, *Jianguo yilai Mao Zedong wengao*, 75.

55. See Warren, "Farewell to the Plague Spirit," 128–30, and Yoshitaka, "Guanyu xuexichongbing fangzhi gongzuo de yijianshu," 297–302.

56. Yu Shunzhang, "Yi Su Delong jiaoshou," *Wenhui Bao*, August 14, 2004.

57. Jiaxingshi dang'anguan, no. 53–1–5, 79.

58. Ibid., 81.

59. "Quanxian xuexichongbing fangzhi gongzuo guihua caoan," *Haining Ribao*, March 10, 1956.

60. Hainingshi dang'anguan, no. 102–1–8, 11–12.

61. Zhonggong Zhejiang shengwei chusihai jiang weisheng bangongshi, *Zhejiangsheng Hainingxian fangzhi xuexichongbing de zhongda shengli*, 14–15.

62. "Quanxian xuefang xianchang huiyi chuixiang jinjunhao," *Haining Ribao*, March 16, 1958.

63. "Rang gengduo de laodongli touru chungeng shengchan," *Haining Ribao*, March 28, 1958.

64. Hainingshi dang'anguan, no. 102–1–8, 8–9.

65. Zhonggong Zhejiang shengwei chusihai jiang weisheng bangongshi, *Zhejiangsheng Hainingxian fangzhi xuexichongbing de zhongda shengli*, 14.

66. Hainingshi dang'anguan, no. 102–1–28, 100.

67. Jiaxingshi dang'anguan, no. 53–1–5, 81–82.

68. Hainingshi dang'anguan, no. 102–1–70, 40.

69. Jiaxingshi zhengxie wenshi ziliao weiyuanhui, *Song wenshen*, 18.

70. "Zhuchangxiang xuefang gongzuo shengli zaiwang," *Haining Ribao*, April 26, 1958.

71. In 1957, Dingqiao Village had thirteen people trained. In Shijing Village, four medical professionals (one doctor, one midwife, and two health assistants) were trained in 1958. See Hainingshi dang'anguan, no. 102–1–18, 1, and no. 102–1–29, 1–43. Also see "Benxian xunlian xuefang yiwu renyuan," *Haining Ribao*, April 19, 1956.

72. Zhonggong Zhejiang shengwei chusihai jiang weisheng bangongshi, *Zhejiangsheng Hainingxian fangzhi xuexichongbing de zhongda shengli*, 17–19 and 31.

73. Jiaxingshi zhengxie wenshi ziliao weiyuanhui, *Song wenshen*, 42–43.

74. Ibid., 134–35.

75. Zhonggong Zhejiang shengwei chusihai jiang weisheng bangongshi, *Zhejiangsheng Hainingxian fangzhi xuexichongbing de zhongda shengli*, 40.

76. "Yong Sanri liaofa yizhi xuexichongbing chengji lianghao," *Haining Ribao*, February 13, 1957.

77. Zhonggong Zhejiang shengwei chusihai jiang weisheng bangongshi, *Zhejiangsheng Hainingxian fangzhi xuexichongbing de zhongda shengli*, 4 and 38.

78. Jiaxingshi zhengxie wenshi ziliao weiyuanhui, *Song wenshen*, 45.

79. Jiaxingshi dang'anguan, no. 53–1–81, 59.

80. Ibid., 53–1–265, 40–41.

81. Hainingshi dang'anguan, no. 102–1–16, 16–17.

82. Ibid., 102–1–8, 7.

83. Jiaxingshi zhengxie wenshi ziliao weiyuanhui, *Song wenshen*, 193.

84. For example, party cadres in Haining County changed clinics into local hospitals and health centers and staffed them with many local people. As a result, Xiashi Village of Haining had seventy-one medical staff in 1958, thirty-two of whom had been assigned by the county government to offer aid, and twenty-one of whom were

local people, while the rest were the staff of the local clinic. See Zhonggong Zhejiang shengwei chusihai jiang weisheng bangongshi, *Zhejiangsheng Hainingxian fangzhi xuexichongbing de zhongda shengli*, 17–19 and 31.

85. Ibid., 51.

86. Ibid., 29.

87. Jiaxingshi zhengxie wenshi ziliao weiyuanhui, *Song wenshen*, 75.

88. Ibid., 43.

89. "Xuanbu benxian jiben xiaomie xuexichongbing," *Haining Ribao*, August 13, 1958.

90. Jiaxingshi zhengxie wenshi ziliao weiyuanhui, *Song wenshen*, 156.

91. Jiaxingshi dang'anguan, no. 53–1–336, 62.

92. Baoshanqu dang'anguan, no. 145–3–14, 35.

93. Jiaxingshi dang'anguan, no. 53–1–336, 62.

94. Jiaxingshi zhengxie wenshi ziliao weiyuanhui, *Song wenshen*, 75.

95. Ibid., 144.

96. Ibid., 164–65.

97. Jiaxingshi dang'anguan, no. 53–1–336, 62.

98. Jiaxingshi zhengxie wenshi ziliao weiyuanhui, *Song wenshen*, 138.

99. "Zhiliao xuexichongbing de qianhou," *Haining Ribao*, July 13, 1956.

100. Jiaxingshi dang'anguan, no. 53–1–336, 86.

101. Hainingshi dang'anguan, no. 102–1–8, 7.

102. Jiaxingshi dang'anguan, no. 53–1–336, 86.

103. "Zhengqu jinkuai de xiaomie xuexichonging," *Haining Ribao*, March 10, 1956.

104. "Dagao weisheng yingjie guoqing," *Haining Ribao*, May 8, 1959.

105. Jiaxingshi dang'anguan, no. 53–1–265, 7. Zhonggong Zhejiang shengwei chusihai jiang weisheng bangongshi, *Zhejiangsheng Hainingxian fangzhi xuexichongbing de zhongda shengli*, 5.

106. Jiaxingshi zhengxie wenshi ziliao weiyuanhui, *Song wenshen*, 164–65.

107. Jiaxingshi dang'anguan, no. 53–1–336, 62.

108. Zhonggong Zhejiang shengwei chusihai jiang weisheng bangongshi, *Zhejiangsheng Hainingxian fangzhi xuexichongbing de zhongda shengli*, 63.

109. Jiaxingshi dang'anguan, no. 53–1–21, 26–27.

110. Jiaxingshi zhengxie wenshi ziliao weiyuanhui, *Song wenshen*, 151.

111. Quoted in Cao, Zhang, and Chen, *Dangdai Zhebei xiangcun de shehui wenhua bianqian*, 314–15.

112. Jiaxingshi zhengxie wenshi ziliao weiyuanhui, *Song wenshen*, 151.

113. Jiaxingshi dang'anguan, no. 53–1–21, 29.

114. Hainingshi dang'anguan, no. 102–1–70, 40.

115. Jiaxingshi dang'anguan, no. 53–1–336, 87–88.

116. Jiaxingshi zhengxie wenshi ziliao weiyuanhui, *Song wenshen*, 5.

117. Jiaxingshi dang'anguan, no. 53–1–181, 91.

118. "Zhongguo Zhouzhen xiangwei guanyu quanxiang yi jibenshang xiaomie xuexichongbing de jingyan baogao," *Haining Ribao*, April 19, 1958.

119. Jiaxingshi dang'anguan, no. 53–1–10, 86.

120. On the contrary, policies in accordance with tradition usually worked much better. For example, the fourth day of the second lunar month was the day before the beginning of spring, the most auspicious day in the whole year. It was believed that moving anything on this specific day wouldn't cause any bad luck. Party cadres of Shidai and Sandai Villages of Jiaxing were said to have successfully moved the local toilets on that day. However, we do not know if they were later moved back to their original places. See Jiaxingshi dang'anguan, no. 53–1–21, 27.

121. Ibid., 20.

122. "Jieshao Xinminshishe tumai dingluo gongzuo," *Haining Ribao*, December 4, 1957.

123. Zhonggong Zhejiang shengwei chusihai jiang weisheng bangongshi, *Zhejiangsheng Hainingxian fangzhi xuexichongbing de zhongda shengli*, 6.

124. Zhejiangsheng xuexichongbing fangzhi bianweihui, *Zhejiang xuexichongbing fangzhi shi*, 30–32.

125. Yuan, Zhang, and Jiang, *Xuexichongbing fangzhi lilun yu shijian*, 10.

Conceptual Blind Spots, Media Blindfolds

The Case of SARS and Traditional Chinese Medicine

Marta E. Hanson

Despite its near daily coverage of the epidemic of severe acute respiratory syndrome (SARS) from mid-March to the end of June 2003, the U.S. media were silent about one key phenomenon in mainland China. The Chinese media, and English versions of Chinese news from agencies such as the Xinhua News Service told a different story. But outside of mainland China to this day, the untold narrative is of the central role that Chinese medicine played from the initial outbreak in Guangdong Province in November 2002 through the epidemic's denouement in June 2003. I do not refer to the mad rush to buy the latest preventive Chinese SARS drug of the week, nor to the fact that there was a subsequent boom in traditional Chinese pharmaceuticals while the larger economies in East Asia suffered. These two angles were well covered. Rather, I mean the fact that doctors trained in traditional Chinese medicine (TCM) treated more than half of the SARS patients in the hospitals of mainland China with Chinese herbal medicines. They made that choice neither because they did not know any better nor because they had limited access to biomedical therapies. These same physicians also drew simultaneously from the biomedical repertoire of antibiotics, steroids, antivirals, and respirators.

Why did the media in the United States and, for the most part, in Europe ignore this dimension of the SARS epidemic? Conversely, what conceptual frame, therapeutic rationale, and integrative approach did physicians trained in Chinese medicine use to respond to SARS in mainland China? How has science since the epidemic evaluated the SARS herbal formulas and translated their use into a new biomedical framework? The following analysis responds to these questions.

SARS in the Western Media

The World Health Organization (WHO) issued the first global alert for cases of atypical pneumonia in China's Guangdong Province, Hong Kong, Vietnam, and Canada on March 12, 2003.[1] Just three days later, the first news of SARS appeared in the *New York Times*.[2] Several days later, Dr. Lawrence K. Altman, a *Times* medical reporter who coauthored the first article, compared the new disease to other diseases considered new to human experience—which were, more accurately in most cases, diseases newly identified and defined. Altman mentioned the spread of AIDS around the world, Legionnaires' disease, and Lyme disease among others in the United States.[3] He also discussed the Hendra virus that had killed horses and two people in Australia in 1994; Hong Kong's avian flu of 1997, which had led to the deaths of thousands of chickens but not yet humans; and Singapore's and Malaysia's Nipah virus of 1999, which had destroyed Malaysia's pig industry and killed over a hundred people.[4]

Since the first week, coverage in the *New York Times* and other English-language newspapers focused on the following topics: epidemiology and virology, the disease's global spread and mortality, and the politics of control and subsequent public-health failures to prevent the spread of SARS in China. Historians contrasted current responses to SARS to comparable situations during the 1832 cholera epidemic in Britain, the Montreal smallpox epidemic of the 1880s, and especially the 1918–19 influenza pandemic, which during the SARS epidemic became the historical experience most feared as a modern possibility.[5] When people ceased to eat out in the Chinatowns of San Francisco, Honolulu, Toronto, and New York, the history of prejudice in San Francisco toward Chinese in the name of public health returned to haunt media coverage.[6] In contrast to the history of racist public-health policies toward Chinese in the United States, however, the false rumors of SARS cases in Chinatowns in the United States had spread through Chinese-language networks and contributed to a psychology of fear within Asian immigrant communities. The people in these Asian communities quarantined themselves and contributed most to the precipitous drop in revenue in the Chinatowns of New York and San Francisco.[7] Nevertheless, when the University of California, Berkeley, chose to err on the side of caution by prohibiting students from SARS regions in Asia from attending the university's summer session, accusations of the return of anti-Chinese prejudice appeared on the op-ed page of the *New York Times*.[8] Berkeley based restricted access to its campus that summer, however, on WHO-designated SARS regions and not on the racial categories Asian American or Chinese, as the author of the opinion piece suggested. Although overreaction cannot be discounted, prudence rather than prejudice informed Berkeley's decision.[9] Television commentators, journalists, physicians, and academics daily voiced their opinions, policy suggestions, and history lessons as news of the outbreak hit the newspapers in mid-March, spread dramatically throughout the world during the spring, and finally subsided with the end of summer.

Despite such extensive daily coverage of the SARS epidemic in the English-language media, the involvement of doctors trained in TCM remained hidden behind a screen of other news angles of greater interest, understanding, and relevance to a Western audience. From March 15 to mid-October 2003, the *New York Times* published only two articles about Chinese medicine and SARS. Both reports focused on what was happening in the streets, but not in the hospitals, of SARS regions. According to an article published on April 4, a rumor had circulated online and through the local Chinese press that SARS had arrived in New York's Chinatown. Although the rumored SARS death of a prominent restaurant owner proved false, locals and visitors alike deserted the businesses along Canal Street. Pharmacies in the neighborhood, however, could not keep enough supplies of the Chinese medicines believed to support the immune system and prevent pneumonia.[10] The second *Times* article, from May 10,[11] followed through on an earlier *Times* story that pharmacies in Guangdong Province were selling out not only of antibiotics, but also of traditional Chinese medicines and ordinary salt.[12] The unprecedented sale of salt was based on a rumor that salt baths could prevent pneumonia. SARS may have put a dent in the economies of East Asia, but sales of traditional medicines as well as of bleach, masks, and antibiotics thrived. Two months later in Beijing, when most other businesses were suffering losses, Chinese pharmacies continued to rack up sales of these and other newly tailored SARS prevention products. Provincial and municipal governments even approved of regionally appropriate herbal formulas for SARS prevention.[13]

The enormous Chinese pharmaceutical industry certainly took advantage of people's fears of SARS contagion to make a quick yuan. There is no doubt that there was a buying frenzy for any defense from the Chinese medical arsenal. Many of the therapeutic weapons of fashion may have been more effective as psychological palliatives than as physiological interventions. Aware of this situation, Elisabeth Rosenthal of the *Times* dismissed as unscientific the proclamation of acting health minister Wu Yi that "Chinese medicine is an important force in the fight against SARS."[14] With this dismissal, the journalist both legitimated the gap in coverage and marked a boundary beyond which her colleagues need not go. By playing this rhetorical card, she missed the far more complex and potentially interesting story for *Times* readers that mainland physicians advocated Chinese medicine not only to prevent its spread in the streets, but also to treat SARS patients in their hospitals.[15]

Blind Spots and Blindfolds

The metaphor of a conceptual blind spot captures the phenomenon of not knowing what one does not know, a profound epistemological problem yet a situation that is both philosophically well known and ethically justifiable. The media-blindfold metaphor, however, refers to the more problematic choice authors make to overlook, ignore, or consciously disregard facts, situations, and even histories that do not fit their dominant narrative of what is true, relevant, and newsworthy. The following account attempts to remedy the former with a mirror on how the past is embedded in the present, and to correct the latter by calling attention to the complexity lost through acts of blindfolding, or the self-deprivation of sight and insight. These are not new phenomena special to the European and American encounter with Chinese medicine at the opening of the twenty-first century: other chapters in this book refer to comparable examples of blind spots and blindfolds among the Japanese residents of Shanghai, for example, who looked down on Chinese night-soil practices without understanding their complex economic and agricultural contributions; the European and American observers of the Manchurian plague who discounted all Chinese medical interventions before there was any better biomedical option; and those who blamed indigenous lay midwifery for high infant mortality rates in Taiwan in the 1940s, when many other factors were at play.

Although it received some cursory coverage in the European media, the significant role that practitioners of TCM played in treating SARS patients in the hospitals of the People's Republic of China was ignored in all major U.S. media. Yet from the beginning, physicians in the Guangzhou Hospital of Traditional Chinese Medicine treated their SARS patients with a combination of injected Chinese formulas, Western steroids, and antibiotics. Their hybrid approach has a specific political and economic history unique to the PRC. Although Western-trained Chinese physicians attempted to abolish Chinese medical practices during the first National Public Health Conference in 1929, they separated out Chinese drugs for further study in a new research program called Scientific Research on Nationally Produced Drugs (*guochan yaowu kexue yanjiu*). This marked the beginning of scientific research on Chinese drugs independent of TCM theories—research that was carried out exclusively by Western-trained Chinese scientists. This research may best be understood as a process of extracting Chinese drugs from their traditional social and technical network of Chinese-style pharmacists and doctors and assimilating them into the new biomedical social and technical network of Western-trained doctors, which explicitly excluded practitioners of TCM.[16]

During the Chinese civil war (1945–49), however, when Chinese Communist Party policy explicitly encouraged the cooperation of Chinese and Western medicine (*zhong xi yi hezuo*), a shift occurred toward a state-enforced cooperation between the two sides. Since the First and Second National Health Conferences in the PRC in 1950 and 1951, a vision to unify Chinese and Western medicine (*zhong xi yi tuanjie*) has guided state policy toward healthcare. The intent was to maximize the resources of traditional Chinese physicians while gradually adopting the new technologies of Western medicine, which were more expensive, rarer, less developed, and largely concentrated in urban hospitals. Both early policies of cooperation and unification aimed to use Western medicine to make Chinese medicine more scientific and systematic. By 1956, Mao Zedong had developed the idea of the integration of Chinese and Western medicine (*zhong xi yi jiehe*).[17] This new policy placed Chinese medicine for the first time on equal footing with Western medicine and gave practitioners of TCM more professional autonomy. In the same year, the PRC established four Chinese medicine colleges spread across the new communist state: in Chengdu in the southwest, Guangzhou in the south, Beijing in the north, and Shanghai in central China. With the government's establishment of separate TCM colleges and of required TCM courses in biomedical colleges, integration became built into medical institutions. All students of TCM study modern biomedical topics like anatomy, physiology, virology, and epidemiology, as well as Chinese medicine. Here the distinction between the classical Chinese medicine of China's past and the new, state-created hybrid called Traditional Chinese Medicine of the present is relevant. Although their training is in separate colleges, the curricula overlap, and doctors of TCM and biomedical doctors upon graduation receive the same MD degree with the same legal status. The difference is in their chosen specialties and postgraduate training. Graduates of a TCM college, for example, sometimes use their training as a steppingstone to become biomedical doctors, or they may take postgraduate courses that qualify them to practice biomedicine, perform surgery, or prescribe Western drugs. The result is that TCM doctors may work side by side with their biomedical colleagues and may themselves be qualified to use biomedicine in a variety of medical settings beyond a Chinese medical hospital, such as a department of Chinese medicine in a Western-style hospital.[18]

It was within this context of state-sponsored medical integration that physicians in the Hospital of the Guangzhou College of TCM in Canton used both Chinese herbs and Western drugs to treat their SARS patients. The Chinese herbs were from the class that clear heat and resolve toxins (*qingre jiedu*) and functioned to reduce inflammation in the lungs and expel the invading pathogen.[19] In the context of a century of experimenting with integrated medicine in modern China, the "clearing heat and resolving toxins" strategy that dominated during the SARS epidemic is best understood as a contemporary instantiation of Chinese-biomedical integration, and not as an unchanged traditional therapeutic strategy from the classical Chinese medicine of antiquity. After SARS spread globally, Chinese physicians in the Guangdong Provincial Hospital of TCM continued to experiment with combinations of TCM drugs and biomedical methods including oxygen inhalation, respirators, corticosteroids, the broad spectrum antiviral drug ribavirin, and, in one case, the serum extracted from SARS survivors for their antibodies.[20] Outside hospitals, practitioners of TCM also played significant roles along with biomedical doctors, public-health professionals, and government officials in implementing public-health initiatives and especially in recommending preventive medicines to the public—first in mainland China, and later in Hong Kong, Taiwan, Singapore, and Vietnam. Shortly after the epidemic subsided, for example, World Scientific published a book in English edited by Dr. Ooi Eng Eong, a medical microbiologist who heads the Environmental Health Institute in Singapore, and Professor Leung Ping Chung, who is a practitioner of Chinese medicine at the Institute of Chinese Medicine at the Chinese University of Hong Kong, as well as an expert in orthopedics and osteoporosis.[21] Although predominantly covering biomedical knowledge and preventive methods, the book also included a chapter titled "Use of Herbal Medicines" that gave four prescriptions recommended for preventing SARS. The sources of these prescriptions were TCM practitioners and professors from a Chinese medical college in Shenzhen, the Beijing University of Chinese Medicine, Singapore's ECM Chinese Medical Center, and the Hong Kong Baptist University. Furthermore, the School of Chinese Medicine at Hong Kong Baptist University held meetings in the spring of 2003 on TCM methods to both treat and prevent SARS and published the proceedings later that year.[22] Practitioners of Chinese medicine in Taiwan also summarized their interpretations of and recommendations for treating and preventing SARS.[23]

The integrated treatments used in mainland China, however, were not used to treat any SARS patients in any hospitals outside the country.[24] Hong Kong differed from all the other East Asian SARS regions, however, in its greater social networks with traditional Chinese medical institutions and physicians. Although Hong Kong has no formal infrastructure in the public hospitals for Chinese medical practitioners and biomedically trained physicians to work together that compares to the situation in mainland China, in the past two decades various institutions have formalized education in Chinese medicine, and Donghua (Tung Wah) Hospital (established in 1872) continues to provide some Chinese medicine to its patients. The Hong Kong Baptist University, for example, started a full-time bachelor's course in Chinese medicine in 1998 and a year later established a School of Chinese Medicine.[25] This school was the most actively involved in issues regarding the role of practitioners of TCM during the Hong Kong SARS epidemic. University leaders proposed the use of Chinese medicine as early as March 2003, set up an anti-SARS university committee to establish guidelines for citizens to use Chinese medicinal SARS preventives, and began a public discussion of how to treat SARS with Chinese medicine. Even the Hong Kong Hospital Authority convened a meeting on May 30 with mainland Chinese physicians to discuss the use of integrated treatments of SARS patients.[26] When the Hong Kong Baptist University held a meeting on the role Chinese medicine could play in controlling the epidemic, the participants also discussed working in the future with mainland Chinese physicians to analyze the efficacy of the therapies they used.[27]

People who cannot read Chinese or who do not read the English-language papers in East Asia remained unaware of these initiatives. Biomedicine dominates the hospitals, clinics, health insurance policies, and public-health initiatives of the world's modern nation-states to such an extent that anything outside its purview is, at best, considered complementary or marginalized as alternative—or simply written off as superstitious quackery. The biomedical model has become so powerful and pervasive that it prevents nonallopathic treatments from being seen as realities that can matter in clinical medicine. Further veiling occurs when the alternative is expressed both in a non-European language and through the lexicon of a medical system as fundamentally different as Chinese medicine is to biomedicine. Three factors—linguistic barriers in the media, the biomedical dominance in modern healthcare, and the perceived incommensurability of Chinese medicine and biomedicine—produced a conceptual blind spot in the Western media that prevented journalists and readers alike from seeing the fuller, more compelling story of the interactions between biomedical and traditional Chinese medical institutions, researchers, and practitioners.

SARS, TCM, and the WHO

A review of the integrated SARS treatments in mainland China entered the Anglophone media when medical experts from the WHO attended a three-day international meeting in Beijing from October 8 to 10, 2003. Officials in China's State Administration of Traditional Chinese Medicine had requested guidance from the WHO to help them evaluate thirteen clinical trials that had been conducted on integrated TCM and biomedical treatment of SARS patients. The WHO organized the resulting international meeting with financial backing from the Nippon Foundation. There were sixty-eight participants: four members of the WHO Secretariat[28] and fifty-one official representatives and seventeen observers from mainland China, Hong Kong, Japan, Vietnam, Thailand, and the Netherlands, who gathered to evaluate evidence on integrated SARS treatments from clinical trials conducted in mainland China.[29] Although the majority of those from mainland China came from TCM institutions and hospitals, most had titles indicating that they were physicians, and at least those from Hong Kong's Guanghua (Kwong Wah) Hospital had been trained in biomedicine. Of the 195 SARS-designated hospitals, 102 had TCM professionals helping with the treatment of SARS patients. It is not clear if these professionals were already working at these hospitals, sent as additional staff from other hospitals, or hired to help just during the epidemic. The WHO report states that ninety-six TCM hospitals sent 2,163 members of their medical staff to ninety-three of the hospitals. During the course of the epidemic then 47.7 percent of the SARS-designated hospitals received help from the medical staff of TCM-designated hospitals. The State Administration of TCM established twenty-one research projects, and local governments in Beijing, Tianjin, and Shanghai carried out comparable research on integrated TCM and biomedical treatments for SARS. The report states: "Among the 5,327 confirmed SARS cases, 3,104 (58.3 percent of the total SARS patients in China) received TCM intervention."[30] Regrettably, the report did not clarify what percentage of these TCM treatments took place in the ninety-six TCM hospitals or in the ninety-three SARS-specific hospitals that accepted the help of medical staff sent from TCM hospitals.

These general figures roughly sketch the contours of institutional collaboration in mainland China between TCM hospitals and the predominantly biomedical SARS-designated hospitals, as well as of state and local government initiatives for medical research on integrated TCM-biomedical treatments. The WHO experts concluded that "integrated treatment by TCM and Western medicine for SARS is generally safe," listed its potential benefits, and provided seven recommendations related to TCM, biomedicine, and SARS treatment and prevention. Zhang Xiaorui, the coordinator of the WHO's office on traditional medicine, remarked that although Chinese clinical studies so far had revealed no known severe side effects of TCM in SARS patients, comparable good reports for treating SARS patients with only Western medicine had yet to be published.[31] That 58.3 percent of the SARS patients in China received some kind of TCM treatment deserves serious reflection and analysis, even if this fact did not result in any Anglophone media coverage beyond summaries of this international meeting in Beijing, and current evaluations of their integrated treatments do not end up measuring up to the criteria of evidence-based medical research.[32]

From October 20 to 21, the WHO hosted a meeting in Geneva of the WHO Scientific Research Advisory Committee on Severe Acute Respiratory Syndrome (SARS). In contrast to the international WHO meeting in Beijing earlier in October, there were only two representatives from mainland China on the advisory committee, Dr. Xu Jianguo, of the National Center of Communicable Diseases, and Dr. Dong Xiaoping, of the National Institute of Virology—both of whom had been trained in biomedicine, and neither of whom had attended the earlier meeting. Of the thirteen Asian committee members (from China, Singapore, Malaysia, the Philippines, Japan, and Bangladesh), six came from the Hong Kong SAR (Special Administrative Region) government and hospitals. None of these members had been to the earlier meeting. Of the four WHO representatives who had, only the medical officer, Dr. Simon Nicholas Mardel, also attended the Geneva meeting. His role in the second meeting was a ten-minute briefing on "clinical issues, including blood safety and treatment."[33] Although what he said in those ten minutes was not recorded in the summary of the meeting, a published interview with him on October 24 provides some details. He acknowledged that Chinese medicine had been used along with Western drugs and respiratory assistance, but he concluded that "in analyzing those treatments, because of the emergency situation, we were unable to say with any certainty whether any of those treatments definitely work." He continued: "If SARS was to re-emerge we would still not know what the best treatment to recommend is."[34]

Given the diversity of approaches used to treat SARS patients and the lack of any systematic clinical trials, the medical experts gathered in Geneva could not form a consensus on the best way to treat SARS. The WHO experts, including Mardel, did concur, however, in the final report for the October 10–12 WHO meeting in Beijing that the three most important methods used during the SARS outbreak—Western drugs (i.e., the antiviral ribavirin and anti-inflammatory steroids), respiratory assistance, and Chinese herbal formulas—should all be systematically tested in clinical trials during the next comparable epidemic. They also agreed on the protocols for clinical trials on these three possibilities and their combinations.[35] The WHO's *Essential Medicines Annual Report of 2004* even featured this report in its summary of highlights of the past year: "A very special piece of work was a report on clinical trials on the treatment of SARS with a combination of traditional Chinese medicine and Western medicine."[36] Despite this official WHO recognition of the significant role that Chinese medicine had played during the epidemic, one fundamental question remains: What exactly did TCM physicians prescribe to their SARS patients?

SARS and Wenbing

An interview published at the peak of the epidemic in China in the *Shanghai Youth Journal* offers an entry into this question. Ma Xiaonan, a journalist, interviewed Dr. Shen Qingfa, a senior professor at the Shanghai University of Traditional Chinese Medicine, one of the four TCM colleges established in 1956.[37] Just a week before, on April 17, 2003, Shanghai had established two SARS advisory groups of experts: one containing twenty virology specialists; the other, ten experts in TCM. Dr. Wu Yingen, one of Shen's colleagues, had been chosen to head the ten-member TCM group.[38] As a member of this group, Shen became one of the most prominent Shanghai physicians dealing with SARS. He was also director of the Research Institute of Warm Diseases (*wenbing*) at the Shanghai University of TCM and coauthor of two clinical texts, one on the understanding of acute infectious diseases in Chinese medicine and one entitled *Studies on Warm Diseases* (*Wenbing xue*). In contrast to the biomedical definition of SARS as the first newly emergent disease of the twenty-first century, the definition used by the biomedically trained professionals involved in researching, tracking, and controlling it in 2003 (see the chapter in this volume by Tseng and Wu), for Shen and other Chinese physicians thinking within the TCM framework, SARS was a familiar hot-wind disorder within the broader Warm disease category.[39] In mainland China, and to a very limited extent in Hong Kong,[40] the medical response to SARS patients in the hospitals relied on *wenbing* diagnostic methods and treatments for acute infectious diseases. The following translation of the *Shanghai Youth Journal* interview with Shen casts light on both the meaning of these terms within a TCM framework and the consensus about SARS in the TCM community of mainland China.

Reporter Ma Xiaonan Interviews *Wenbing* Doctor Shen Qingfa

Ma: What is the most important function of the group of TCM experts?

Shen: Currently, we are responsible for devising a prevention plan and examining trends in a timely manner. Moreover, we are examining the clinical diagnosis and treatment of SARS from the perspective of TCM. Presently, we have already established most of the plan for preventing SARS in Shanghai.

Ma: According to TCM doctrine, what is SARS?

Shen: It is a type of epidemic warm disease [*wenbing*]. More precisely, one can place SARS in the group of heat-wind epidemics [*refeng yi*]. Heat-wind epidemics occur most often in the spring and manifest symptoms similar to SARS.

Ma: Everyone says now that TCM drugs are most effective for preventing SARS, but not for treating it. What do you think of this issue?

Shen: It is true that prevention is most important; however, from our current perspective, Chinese drugs can also be very effective for treatment and are especially effective during the recovery stage. On April 10, I went to investigate the situation in Guangdong. At the No. 1 Hospital of the Guangzhou College of TCM, there were thirty-three SARS patients. After receiving a combination of Chinese and

Western treatments, the rates of fever dropped and recovery times quickened. Soon there were no longer any patients who had used TCM treatments [left in the hospital wards]. This hospital had more than 800 beds and more than 1,000 medical personnel. Because they had paid attention to the appropriate preventive effects of Chinese drugs, there was not one medical personnel infected by SARS. Concurrently, the hospitals in Hong Kong are now already beginning to emphasize using Chinese medicine along with Western treatment methods.

Ma: Is there any useful outcome of taking *banlangen* (isatis root) to treat SARS?[41]

Shen: The preference for *banlangen* among Shanghai natives is related to prevention efforts during the Hepatitis A epidemic in 1989. *Banlangen* is known without doubt to clear heat and resolve poison. However, is this appropriate for SARS? Since we have not scientifically followed it closely and compared the two [epidemics with each other], it is very difficult to be sure.[42]

SARS in the above interview is *feidianxing feiyan*, which is translated into English as atypical pneumonia. Common Chinese usage shortens this name to *feidian* (atypical). Under the system of integrated Chinese and Western medicine, TCM practitioners use biomedical disease nomenclature with the understanding that any biomedical diagnosis can then be broken down into a larger number of discrete Chinese medical syndromes and patterns of illness. Yet, as can be seen from Angela K. C. Leung's and Sean Hsiang-lin Lei's chapters in the present volume, the traditional category of *chuanran* (contagious) could not have taken on the meaning of infection implied in infectious disease until after the arrival of the germ theory, the microscope, and the entirely new intellectual space of the laboratory, in which scientists could isolate, analyze, and distinguish discrete microorganisms for the first time.[43] The Chinese medical neologism *feidianxing feiyan* avoids the kind of complex change over time that the old Chinese phrase *chuanran* underwent in the twentieth century by its straightforward translation of a one-to-one correspondence with a biomedical category. It does not raise eyebrows. From a biomedical perspective, however, the concepts of Warm disease and heat-wind epidemics raise more doubts than eyebrows. The terms are conceptually opaque and linguistically unintelligible. They represent disease concepts from another time, place, and culture, of interest perhaps to medi-

cal anthropologists but antithetical to the basic premises of modern epidemiology, virology, and pharmacology that framed nearly all medical accounts of the SARS epidemic in the Western media, as well as the biomedical
response to it.

In the case of SARS in modern China, however, people fell deathly ill with
wenbing, were treated for *wenbing*, and either recovered and died from *wenbing*. Today the Chinese category of Warm diseases includes the afflictions
that biomedicine classes as acute infectious diseases. Although before the
modern thermometer there was no concept of a measurable fever in Chinese
medicine, now *wenbing* are equated with febrile diseases due to a climate-
sensitive external pathogen, which causes one's temperature to rise and
fever symptoms to set in. Diseases that become epidemic (*wenyi*) are the
most virulent and contagious forms of Warm diseases.

The class of *wenbing* epidemics within which Chinese physicians placed
SARS has a well-known history within the TCM world. This history began
with the very ancient medical category of Cold Damage (*shanghan*)—externally caused disorders associated with unseasonable weather and treated
most often with prescriptions based upon the classic work of pharmacy by
the Eastern Han official and physician Zhang Ji (second century CE). Over
time, Cold Damage nosology branched into types associated with different
seasonal configurations, including distinct regional variants. A divergence
between Cold Damage and Warm disease began to appear in the seventeenth century, and in the nineteenth century the separate Warm diseases
medical "current of learning" (*xuepai*) emerged. It identified the disease
pattern with the warm, damp southeastern coast; used distinct diagnostic
methods and herbal remedies based on four factors, or stages; and developed a coherent group of texts. In the early years of the PRC, this *wenbing*
current of learning became formally institutionalized into a medical discipline (*ke*) that is taught as part of the TCM core curriculum and is recognized in every hospital where TCM is practiced. In addition to the volu-
minous *wenbing* literature in Chinese written by doctors like Wu Yingen
and Shen Qingfa,[44] several publications on the *wenbing* discipline have been
written in English for clinicians.[45] My own work has examined its historical
origins, conceptual transformations, and social foundations.[46]

This history is taken for granted by Shen in his interview for *Shanghai
Youth Journal*. By placing SARS in the group of "heat-wind epidemics" that
"occur most often in the spring and manifest symptoms similar to SARS,"
Shen emphasizes the role seasonal change plays in epidemic outbreaks of

this type. Modern epidemiology also considers seasonal change to be a factor in the emergence and spread of epidemics such as malaria, dysentery, dengue fever, and influenzas similar to SARS. The modifier "heat-wind," however, is not equally familiar. What Shen means by "heat" and "wind" is neither the sensation of the sun's heat nor the brush of a cool breeze, but rather two pathogenic climatic factors characteristic of spring. In Chinese medicine, the combination of heat and wind can enter a vulnerable human body and suddenly destabilize the person's health; these pathogenic climatic factors are conceptually analogous to the viruses, bacteria, and parasites of biomedicine, although they nonetheless remain linguistically incommensurable.

Comparing Biomedicine and Chinese Medicine

This point raises the complex issue of how biomedicine differs from Chinese medicine as practiced today. This difference has occupied the minds of both Westerners and Chinese since the Jesuits arrived in China in the late sixteenth century, and its complicated history cannot be summarized here. More recently, theoretical, historical, and anthropological studies of Chinese medicine have also wrestled with the issue. Other scholarship focuses on medicine in Greek and Chinese antiquity to understand the historical contexts of a conceptual divergence that persists to the present.[47] A common modern formulation of this divergence holds that while Western biomedicine emphasizes structure and organs, Chinese medicine stresses function and movement; the former is more reductionist and atomistic, and the latter is more holistic and system oriented. The most common perception in China is that Western medicine is fast and best for acute diseases, while Chinese medicine is slow and better suited to chronic cases.[48] These operative binaries of acute and chronic depend on biomedical assumptions that present themselves today as fact but that are best understood as historical constructs active in the present, which emphasize the temporality of a disease over the spatiality of the inner-outer dyad of classical Chinese medical thinking.[49]

In the colleges and hospitals of TCM in China, however, acute infectious diseases are well within the TCM doctor's expertise. A biomedical disease is often refined into numerous TCM patterns and syndromes. Their acuity in time does not bracket them off from TCM expertise. Rather, the important distinction for TCM doctors who treat infectious diseases is that between organic illnesses and seasonal disorders. This contrasting operative dyad of organ-based and environmental disease arguably updates the more spatial emphasis of orthodox medical learning on whether the cause of an illness is due to an inner imbalance or an external invasion—or, more likely than not, a combination of both. In this organ-environmental dyad, biomedicine excels at organ- or tissue-centered problems, such as traumatic injuries requiring surgery, damaged organs for which a transplant would save a life, and malignant cancer cells that only tailored pharmaceuticals and radiation can control. By contrast, seasonal disorders are those triggered by obvious external pathogens; they range from the common cold and influenza to cholera and bubonic plague.[50] Although in biomedicine these are examples of infectious diseases, in Chinese medicine their emergence is also correlated with a body compromised by either the cold of the previous winter or unseasonably cold weather during the spring, or a combination of the two. The human body is a microclimate, potentially as susceptible to pathogenic climatic factors as it is to virulent microorganisms. Whenever people do not properly maintain their bodies' natural defenses through healthy diet, exercise, sexual moderation, and adequate sleep, they become more vulnerable to any of these external pathogens.

According to the TCM doctrines called upon to explain the eruption of SARS in late 2002 and spring 2003, the warm and damp climate in southernmost China, combined with a sudden cold snap in early spring, made the local population constitutionally more susceptible to the external pathogens that contributed to the outbreak in viral pneumonia. According to some TCM physicians, this susceptibility was increased by the allegedly sedentary habits and rich diet of Guangdong's modern urbanites. TCM doctors did not deny that bacteria and viruses exist; nor did they ignore the roles played by the civet cat and coronavirus once a consensus had formed around their causal role in the epidemic. The TCM doctors simply chose to focus on other factors, arguing that the combination of an internal bodily imbalance and an external environmental irregularity made infection more likely. Prevent the internal imbalance, and the coronavirus cannot enter the body and wreak havoc. The doctors did not deny the reality of the infectious disease pathogens identified by germ theory over the past century; they simply pointed to the larger role of climates and constitutions in any outbreak.

Treating SARS

Near the end of his interview, Ma asked Shen whether TCM drugs were effective beyond the prevention of SARS. This question expressed another common perception that Chinese medicine is good for strengthening the body's defenses against epidemics, but once someone has contracted an infectious disease, he or she should check into a Western hospital. Shen represented an alternative perspective, shared by his colleagues at the No. 1 Hospital of the Guangzhou College of TCM, whom he had visited just two weeks before the interview on April 10, 2003. Also in Canton on April 7, WHO officials had visited the Guangdong Provincial Hospital of TCM to evaluate the hospital's effectiveness of treating more than a hundred cases of atypical pneumonia with traditional Chinese herbal medicine.

Dr. Lin Lin, then director of the provincial hospital's respiratory department, explained that they divided the cases of atypical pneumonia into four levels (*sifen*)—the early, middle, climax, and late phases. Lin and his staff gave their SARS patients different herbal formulas according to each one of the four levels of symptoms their patients manifested.[51] WHO officials would have seen this four-level method of diagnosis practiced when they visited the hospital on April 7, though none commented on it. An article published the next day in the Hong Kong paper *Dagong Bao* further elaborated on the four-level approach to treating SARS.[52]

The *wenbing* approach breaks down the course of the infectious disease according to four levels of penetration into the body. The four levels are named defensive (*wei*), *qi*, constructive (*ying*), and Blood (*xue*). The initial, or defensive, level refers to the onset of the disease when the patient first has feverish symptoms, a cough, and dryness in the mouth and feels aversion to cold. The second, or *qi*, level marks deeper penetration of the pathogen and a more serious turn in the illness. The lungs become more congested, and the patient has a high fever, thick and yellow phlegm that comes up with coughing, and heat in the lungs. The third, or constructive, level (sometimes called the climax level) signifies a further worsening of the condition. The patient has a persistently high fever, goes in and out of consciousness, and has such difficulty breathing that oxygen must be delivered through a mask or respirator. The fourth, or Blood, level is the most serious, final phase of the illness. The stage is called Blood because the patient begins to cough up blood, passes blood in the urine, bleeds through the gums, and can have a significantly reduced—even fatally low—platelet count.[53]

The Guangdong physicians did not use one standard cocktail of drugs for the entire course of SARS in their patients. This is where the Chinese medical treatment of SARS differed most significantly from biomedicine. Instead of relying on steroids to control the inflammation and ribavirin to control the virus, they adjusted herbal formulas to four possible levels of penetration into the patient's body. When Shen remarked that "hospitals in Hong Kong are now already beginning to emphasize using Chinese medicine along with Western treatment," he referred to this *wenbing* method of diagnosing four levels of increasing severity of SARS and adjusting herbal formulas accordingly. The SARS experience in mainland China, in fact, resulted in a new focus on the TCM approach to toxins, epidemics, and Warm diseases, which despite having a long established history in classical Chinese medicine (see the chapter in this volume by Leung) also opened up unresolved clinical debates artificially closed in the standardization of the curriculum in the 1950s and 1960s.[54] These debates have continued long after the epidemic subsided. This experience not only encouraged new histories of epidemics in China's past and in global medical history, but it has also reinforced the Chinese government's patronage of TCM as an integral aspect of the nation's healthcare system—and the government has financially supported it since, in preparation for the next pandemic. Yet what remained a powerful echo from the past during the 2003 SARS epidemic in mainland China was an old emphasis on regional variations in climates and constitutions.

SARS Climates and Constitutions

Chinese physicians adapted herbal formulas not only to changes in their patients' conditions, but also to obvious differences in regional climates. In mid-April 2003, for example, two doctors of the Cui Yueli Center for Traditional Medicine Research in Beijing distributed a pamphlet through their clinic that recommended adjusting SARS herbal formulas to climatic differences. Their summary of the causes of SARS also demonstrates the persistence of a key concept in classical Chinese medicine: differences in climates correlate to discernible variations in human constitutions. The following explanation reflects the logic of the doctors' reasoning:

> Chinese doctors have long believed that "if essence is not stored in the winter, then spring will bring warm diseases." An understanding of the application of this concept to the various climatic regions of China helps us to begin to understand SARS through the prism of Chinese

science. In southern China, a warm damp climate keeps the defensive and constructive qi of the local population on the surface. There is little opportunity for the storage of essence on the inside. Therefore, in most years, the combination of a warm climate with relatively little storage of essence in the winter creates heat in the body. In south China, this is generally not a problem and actually represents the normal situation . . . This year, however, a relatively cold winter in southern China was followed by a sudden cold snap in early spring, giving rise to the unusual situation of internal heat and external cold. The general warmth of the internal constitutions of the local population was out of step with the unusually cold weather. This is a situation conducive to invasion by external pathogens and brings to mind the saying "excessively cold winters lead to heat diseases in the spring."[55]

The concept of the body as microclimate is central in this passage. The idea of building up one's defenses to withstand external pathogens is also obvious through the agricultural metaphor of "storage of essence in the winter." The binary *yin-yang* also comes to the fore in the conflict between internal heat and external cold. The meaning of the statement "in southern China, a warm damp climate keeps the defensive and constructive *qi* of the local population on the surface," however, is not readily apparent to a lay audience. The four levels refer simultaneously to the four main stages of the progression of an infectious disease and the four levels of defense within the human body—defensive, *qi*, constructive, and Blood. Just as sensitive people are said to wear their emotions on their sleeve or even have thin skin in colloquial English, in Chinese medicine, Cantonese are thought to wear their most protective *qi* on the outer surface of their bodies. Doctors in the Far South were further advised to modify formulas, taking into account the greater dampness in the region: "Chinese doctors have utilized the primary approach of 'clearing heat' [*qingre*] and a secondary goal of 'resolving toxins' [*jiedu*] in the treatment of SARS. In southern China, doctors have also been modifying formulas to dry the dampness [in their patients]."[56]

These two passages illustrate how place matters in TCM interpretations of SARS. First, the warm and damp climate of southern China, combined with an unseasonable cold snap in the spring, created conditions ripe for vulnerability to an external pathogen: in a biomedical frame, the first known transference of a coronavirus from the civet cat to humans; in a TCM frame, pathogenic climatic *qi*. The authors also argued that comparable seasonal irregularities around Beijing made people vulnerable as well when

SARS spread north. Conversely, they explained the odd absence of SARS cases in Shanghai to normal weather patterns. Within the TCM framework, there was no one set treatment for all patients with SARS, which was the goal of biomedical research and WHO guidelines. Doctors in different regions were expected to adapt formulas according to not only the four stages of development of SARS in each patient, but also to local climatic conditions and constitutional predispositions. In southernmost Guangdong and Guangxi Provinces, TCM doctors therefore added to the standard *wenbing* formulas herbs intended to dry out the damper local type of constitutions of their SARS patients. Far to the north in Beijing, in contrast, doctors added moistening herbs to help lubricate the dryer local constitutions and lungs of their SARS patients. Although no longer central to biomedicine in either the West or China, the resonance of regional climates and individual constitutions nonetheless persists in present-day interpretations of Chinese traditional medicine and, in the case of SARS in mainland China, in the hybrid integrated medical treatments used to treat a majority of SARS patients.

Scientific (Lost in) Translation

The rationale of climates and constitutions prevalent in Chinese medical articles published during and after the SARS crisis in mainland China, however, disappears from the medical discourse when researchers analyze the same Chinese herbs in clinical trials and translate their efficacy into the language of science and measurable results. This translation process for the case of SARS and TCM began with the October 8–10 international meeting when the Chinese State Administration of Traditional Chinese Medicine requested WHO guidance to assess clinical trials of integrated treatment of SARS patients. The participants at the WHO meeting summarized their conclusions according to three levels of assessment. First, "there were sufficient data in the clinical reports to show that integrated treatment with TCM and Western medicine for patients with SARS is safe." Second, the basic problem of the clinical trials was that only two included randomly selected patients, whereas the remaining eleven were either prospective cohort or retrospective studies. Although the participants thought that the data from the clinical trials were insufficient, they nevertheless concluded that the data suggested potential benefits that would require further study. These included the alleviation of fatigue and shortness of breath, facilitation of lung inflammation absorption, reduction of the risk of oxygen desaturation, stabilization of abnormal fluctuation of oxygen saturation in the blood, reduction in the dosage of glucocorticoids and antiviral agents, and reduction of overall healthcare costs. The participants also concluded, however, that the data in the clinical reports were inconclusive in three important ways. First, although Chinese clinicians claimed that the mortality rate was lower for the patients who received integrated treatment than for those who received only Western medicine, misdiagnosis of SARS may have contributed to the lower recorded mortality rate. Second, the finding on prevention was also flawed by the fact that only 40 percent of the subjects who had taken TCM formulas to prevent SARS had returned the questionnaires. Third, the study on convalescence compared only one group treated with TCM and one that followed an exercise program, without a control group that received neither treatment nor exercise.

Despite these considerable shortcomings in the clinical trials on combined TCM and Western treatments for SARS, which Dr. Simon Mandel mentioned in his October 24 interview with *Agence France Presse*, the WHO panel in Beijing concluded that these initial studies should nevertheless be made available as reference material for future treatment of SARS. The participants also argued that a clinical protocol should be established so that if SARS were to return, clinicians could scientifically evaluate the efficacy of integrated treatment compared with biomedical treatment.[57]

Five physicians from the Chinese Cochrane Center at the West China Hospital of Sichuan University followed up the final recommendation of the WHO report in 2006. This Sichuan group is the officially designated Cochrane Center for all of China.[58] The group includes Li Youping, then director of the Cochrane Acute Respiratory Infections Group within the Chinese Cochrane Center. Although the report did not provide any information on the members' medical training or expertise in either Chinese medicine or biomedicine, they wrote a systematic review for the Cochrane Library of SARS-TCM studies according to the protocols of evidence-based medicine without any mention of four-level analysis, regional variations in formulas, or individual constitutions.[59] They reviewed eleven randomized and one quasi-randomized controlled trial (RCTs) of treatments for diagnosed SARS patients using either Chinese herbs combined with Western medicines or Western medicines alone. They controlled for the problem of misdiagnosis mentioned in the earlier WHO report by excluding all patients who did not meet the WHO diagnostic criteria for SARS. They also excluded all SARS cases complicated by other illnesses. For the 654 SARS patients treated in the RCTs and one quasi-RCT that they evaluated, they found that a total of twelve Chinese herbs had been used. Of these, the members of the group concluded that two might improve symptoms, five might improve lung infiltrate absorption, four might decrease the dosage of corticosteroids, three might improve the quality of life, and one might shorten the length of stay in the hospital. Contrary to TCM claims, the members of the group did not find that the combination of Chinese herbs with Western drugs decreased morbidity compared to the use of Western medicine alone. Only two of the trials reported adverse events. The group concluded that the quality of the evidence in the trials was weak and recommended long-term follow up.[60]

This 2005 analysis is the only systematic review to date of the empirical evidence of the benefits and risks of TCM combined with biomedicine for treating SARS. As such, it represents the beginning of the process of evaluating Chinese herbs for SARS according to the standard criteria of evidence-based medicine. The conceptions of climates and constitutions, heat-cold, damp-dry, and regional variation central to classical Chinese medicine and even today's TCM practice, all of which were invoked during the SARS epidemic in mainland China, have been systematically edited out in the process of scientific evaluation. As Sean Hsiang-lin Lei has previously argued, this process of scientific translation reorganizes the social and technical networks in which the drugs will be used shedding in the process what is newly considered obsolete. Socially, the process of extracting Chinese drugs from their social and technical network of doctors trained in Chinese medicine in mainland China and assimilating them into the new network of international biomedicine socially excludes Chinese-style practitioners from these international networks. Intellectually, it also leaves untranslated their explanatory models and therapeutic rationales—based on variable climates and constitutions—as if they were not only incommensurable but also irrelevant.[61] Mainland TCM doctors, however, practice a kind of medical bilingualism. While they accepted the biomedical nosology of SARS as atypical pneumonia and even acknowledged the role of the coronavirus from the Civet cat, they nonetheless followed standard practices of integrated Chinese TCM, which conceptually still rely on nonbiomedical diagnostic categories and therapeutic rationales. Yet practitioners of integrated medicine in China are diverse. What we see in the Chinese Cochrane Center at the West China Hospital of Sichuan University is another approach to integration in Chinese medical culture today that attempts to redefine Chinese medicines according to the protocols of standardized clinical trials of modern pharmaceuticals and evidence-based medicine. The process essentially strips the original products of their history, culture, and rationales of use, in order to prepare them for global export. Within China, there are thus several medical cultures of integration.[62]

Illusory Divisions

That classical Chinese medicine correlated climates and constitutions may be unremarkable. Comparable views were recorded in the *Hippocratic Writings*[63] of Greek antiquity (circa the fifth century BCE), the earliest Sanskrit treatises of classical Indian medicine (circa the first century CE), and Islamic medicine. Ideas that climate and geography determined racial differences legitimated much of Europe's colonial expansion and domination through the beginning of the twentieth century. The development of tropical medicine cannot be disentangled from either European imperialism or the concept of climates and constitutions. Within this book, Angela K. C. Leung's chapter shows, and Sean Hsiang-lin Lei's chapter reemphasizes, that by the mid-seventeenth century, the Chinese concept of *chuanran* contained two contradictory meanings: one concept, closer to the idea of indirect infection (via air or water), referred to epidemic diseases as caused by a local environmental *qi*; the other meaning, comparable to direct contagion (person to person), referred more often to nonepidemic and even chronic diseases understood to be passed from person to person. Lei argues that only with the 1910 Manchurian experience with pneumonic plague did the Chinese medical discourse combine these two meanings of *chuanran* into a new conceptualization of *chuanranbing* as "an acute and widespread epidemic that was transmitted by direct and intimate human interaction." Despite this early and successful integration of germ theory and contagion into the Chinese medical definition of *chuanranbing* in the early twentieth century, however, the old conceptions of regional climates and constitutions still prevails in mainland Chinese medical practice. A version of geographical determinism continues to hold sway even in the West, most notably in the genre of comparative history of science and civilizations—of which Jared Diamond's *Guns, Steel, and Germs* is a classic example. What is remarkable about Chinese medical concepts of climates and constitutions is not so much their existence, but rather their persistence into the present. This persistence breaks down the illusion of a barrier between past ways of knowing and present modus operandi, between so-called traditional and modern medicine—as if the two sides do not interact today in clinical medical practice, when in medical practices both within mainland China and globally the barrier has become more porous than solid. This persistence of older concepts is a form of resistance to the teleological assumptions of the inevitability of their modern replacements.

Over fifty years of Chinese national policy to integrate Chinese and Western medicine, however, have created a state-mandated medical pluralism, which the medical anthropologist Volker Scheid aptly calls "hegemonic pluralism."[64] Linguistic barriers, biomedical bias, and conceptual incommensurability, however, all contribute to the ignorance of this history, bias against the logic of such medical concepts and therapies, and their dismissal as clinically, socially, and politically irrelevant in the modern world outside of mainland China. Not news, in other words, considered fit to print. This regional revision of the global SARS story contributes at least one constructive corrective. To understand fully the contemporary Chinese practice of integrative medicine, one must untie multiple blindfolds in the media, recognize the conceptual blind spots that block individual awareness and thus collective vision, and attempt to transcend the problems of incommensurability through both translation and historically informed contextual explanation. Perhaps these conceptual strategies will also open up a new realm of clinical possibilities beyond mainland China. This process of untying, unveiling, translating, and situating, for now at least, provides the clarity to permit what are far more interesting, complex, and revealing questions about what mainland Chinese physicians were thinking when they administered integrated treatments to their SARS patients, and about how historically, sociologically, and politically they came to think and practice that way.

NOTES

I would like to acknowledge the insightful comments and suggestions of the two readers for this essay, as well as the confident editorial minds of both Angela K. C. Leung and Charlotte Furth. Early on in the project, Judith Farquhar and her research collaborator, Zhang Qicheng, kindly asked one of their research assistants to compile a CD of Chinese publications on SARS and TCM for me. Their collective efforts have significantly improved the original draft. All translations are mine, unless otherwise indicated.

1. P. Leung and Ooi, eds. SARS War, 18–19, 59.

2. Lawrence K. Altman and Keith Bradsher, "Mysterious Respiratory Illness Afflicts Hundreds Globally," *New York Times*, March 15, 2003.

3. For an argument that Lyme disease may not have been new to human experience even in the 1970s, see Aronowitz, "Lyme Disease." Evidence of the HIV/AIDS virus dates back to at least the 1930s.

4. Lawrence K. Altman, "The Doctor's World: In New Outbreak, Eerie Reminders of Other Epidemics," *New York Times*, March 18, 2003. For explanations of the Paramyxoviruses blamed for the Hendra and Nipah epidemics, as well as the influenza viruses related to the Asian avian flu of 1997 and February 2003, see P. Leung and Ooi, *SARS War*, 27–33.

5. The report "The Long View" on BBC Radio 4, April 14, 2003, compared SARS to the 1832 cholera epidemic in Britain. In a CBC radio interview, Michael Bliss compared SARS to the Montreal smallpox epidemic of the 1880s and 1918–19 influenza pandemic.

6. Calvin Sims, "A Respiratory Disease: California; In Asian American Neighborhoods, Fear and Precaution Are Spreading," *New York Times*, April 5, 2003. For the history of these prejudices in public health, see Shah, *Contagious Divides*.

7. Jennifer Lee, Dean E. Murphy, and Yilu Zhao, "The SARS Epidemic: Asian-Americans; In U.S., Fear Is Spreading Faster than SARS," *New York Times*, April 17, 2003.

8. Iris Chang, "Fear of SARS, Fear of Strangers," *New York Times*, May 21, 2003.

9. Two letters to the editor immediately dismissed Chang's accusation, under the heading "Prejudice or Prudence on SARS," in *New York Times* of May 23, 2003. The letters were by Garry Perkins, from Chicago, and Gerald N. Rosenberg, writing from Xiamen, China, where much more Draconian measures were taken.

10. Susan Saulny, "In Chinatown, an Outbreak of Fear: Herb Shops and Rumors Thrive on Virus Panic," *New York Times*, April 4, 2003.

11. Elisabeth Rosenthal, "Herbs? Bull Thymus? Beijing Leaps at Anti-SARS Potions," *New York Times*, May 10, 2003.

12. Lawrence K. Altman and Elisabeth Rosenthal, "Health Organization Stepping Up Efforts to Find Cause of Mysterious Pneumonia," *New York Times*, March 18, 2003.

13. See Rosenthal, "Herbs?"

14. Ibid.

15. For one of the earliest special issues of a TCM journal devoted to clinical studies of the integration of Chinese and biomedicine to treat SARS patients, see the special issue on SARS in *Tianjin zhongyiyao*.

16. See Lei, "From *Changshan* to a New Anti-malarial Drug," 324.

17. See the summary of the history of Chinese government policy toward integrated medicine in Scheid, *Chinese Medicine in Contemporary China*, 69–72. For an extended discussion of the politics of these changes in policy toward Chinese medicine, see Taylor, *Chinese Medicine in Early Communist China*.

18. This summary of the current situation of integrated medicine in mainland China draws on Scheid, *Chinese Medicine in Contemporary China*, 85–86.

19. Zhu M., "Guangzhou zhongyiyao daxue yifuyuan jizhen ke shou zhi Feidian 37 li linchuang zongjie."

20. For a study of the integrated treatment of 103 SARS cases at the Guangdong Provincial Hospital of TCM from January to April 2003, see Hai Xia, "Guangdong sheng zhongyiyuan zhiliao Feidianxing feiyan linchuang jingyan." Ninety-six patients were cured, and seven died. For a summary of experiments with the serum method in Hong Kong, see interview with P. Leung in P. Leung and Ooi, eds. "Never Too Old a Remedy."

21. P. Leung and Ooi, eds. SARS War.

22. See Hong Kong Baptist University, School of Chinese Medicine, Xianggang jinhui daxue Zhongyi xueyuan kang yanxing dong shilu.

23. For a synthesis of SARS and TCM research in Taiwan, see Huang P. et al., 2004 Nian Wenbing guoji xueshu yantaohui, 553–68.

24. See "Use of Herbal Medicines," 103–9. Considerable coverage about the roles of TCM doctors and medicines also appeared in the mainland Chinese media and on SARS Web sites. The comparable situation in Vietnam is not as clear.

25. For a good summary of Chinese medicine in Hong Kong, see the section on "Traditional Chinese Medical Practice" in Hong Kong Museum of Medical Sciences Society, Plague, SARS and the Story of Medicine in Hong Kong, 248–51.

26. "Chinese Medicine Better Used in HK to treat SARS," Xinhua Economic News Service, June 26, 2003.

27. See Hong Kong Baptist University, School of Chinese Medicine, Xianggang jinhui daxue Zhongyi xueyuan kang yanxing dong shilu.

28. The four WHO representatives were Dr. Hendrik Bekedam, the WHO's representative in the PRC; Dr. Seung-Hoon Choi, an expert on traditional medicine in the WHO's Regional Office for the Western Pacific, in Manila, the Philippines; Dr. Simon Nicholas Mardel, medical officer, SARS Clinical Group, Global Alert and Response, Department of Communicable Disease Surveillance and Response, the WHO; and Dr. Zhang Xiaorui, coordinator, Traditional Medicine, Essential Drugs and Medicines Policy, the WHO.

29. For a full list of the participants, see the annex of World Health Organization, SARS, 192–95.

30. For the statistics, see ibid., 5–6.

31. For the conclusions, see ibid., 7–8.

32. Several sources announced the results of this international meeting: BBC Monitoring International Reports ("China: Combined Western and Chinese Medicine Said Safe in SARS Treatment," October 10, 2003); Business Daily Update ("Integrated Treatment Benefits Highlighted," October 13, 2003); and World News ("TCM Safe in SARS Treatment," October 13, 2003). The New York Times, however, did not cover the story, focusing instead on the new regulations for SARS laboratories after a Singaporean postdoctoral student contracted SARS from a medical lab he visited (Lawrence K. Altman, "Experts Urge Tightening of Safeguards in SARS Labs," New York Times, October 22, 2003).

33. *WHO Scientific Research Advisory Committee on Severe Acute Respiratory Syndrome (SARS)*, Geneva 20–21 October 2003, Department of Communicable Disease Surveillance and Response, WHO/CDS/CSR/GAR/2004.16, 10. For a list of the participants, see 14–15.

34. "Experts Fail to Identify Best Way to Treat SARS," *Agence France Presse*, October 24, 2003.

35. World Health Organization, *SARS*.

36. See the section "Traditional Medicine: Many Innovative Materials," World Health Organization, *Essential Medicines Annual Report 2004* (2005): 1.

37. Ma, "Zhongyi zhuanjia."

38. "Shanghai Mobilizes Traditional Chinese Medicine to Curb SARS," *Xinhua General News Service*, April 17, 2003.

39. See Peng S. et al., *Wenbingxue*.

40. See "Doctors in HK Hospitals Softening Stance Against Chinese Medicine" and "Use of Chinese Medicine for SARS Treatment Urged in HK," *Xinhua General News Service*, April 18 and 22, 2003, respectively.

41. The botanical name for *banlangen* is *Isatis tinctoria* L., or *Isatis indigotica* Fort. Its pharmaceutical name is *Radix isatidis*. Commonly referred to as isatis root, it is credited with antimicrobial, antiparasitic, and antiviral effects. In addition to its use in Shanghai, it was one of the most popular Chinese SARS drugs sold throughout Asia, the United States, and Canada. For the situation in Canada, see Ricky Leong, "Rush Is on for Root in Chinese Treatment: SARS 'Prevention,' Doctors Skeptical but Herbalists Busy," *The Gazette* (Montreal), April 4, 2003.

42. Ma, "Zhongyi zhuanjia."

43. See the chapters in this book by Angela K. C. Leung and Sean Hsiang-lin Lei.

44. In addition to Wu and Shen, *Zhongyi waigan rebingxue*, see also the most important textbooks of the mid- and late 1980s by Meng Shujiang, *Wenbing xue*. See also the two-volume compilation of fifty *wenbing* texts from the Ming dynasty through the Republican period, edited by Li Shunbao, *Wenbingxue quanshu*. These are only some of the major publications in the field. There have been hundreds of publications on *wenbing* in the PRC, Hong Kong, and Taiwan in the past century.

45. See Hsu and Wang, *The Theory of Feverish Diseases and Its Clinical Applications*, and the more up-to-date and complete Liu G., *Warm Diseases*.

46. In addition to my Ph.D. dissertation, "Inventing a Tradition in Chinese Medicine," see Hanson, "Robust Northerners and Delicate Southerners" and *Speaking of Epidemics in Chinese Medicine: Disease and the Geographic Imagination in Late Imperial China*, forthcoming.

47. See Kuriyama, *The Expressiveness of the Body and the Divergence of Greek and Chinese Medicine*, and Lloyd and Sivin, *The Way and the Word*.

48. I borrow the distinctions between fast and slow, and acute and chronic, from Volker Scheid's excellent assessment in Foreword to Liu G., vii.

49. Charlotte Furth deserves credit for this insight on operative medical dyads.

50. For the distinction between organic illness and seasonal diseases, and a dis-

cussion of the centrality of seasonal diseases in the work of the early Chinese medical pioneers of the Republican era, see Scheid, Foreword, vii.

51. "WHO Experts Examining Ability of Traditional Chinese Medicine to Treat SARS," New China News Agency, *Beijing Xinhua in English*, April 7, 2003. James Maguire, one of the members of the WHO medical team present that day, noted that "patients in the hospital have more rapidly recovered from the disease." He also commented that "they need to further study and keep a close watch with this information about the effect of Chinese medicine on atypical pneumonia treatment."

52. "Yong wenbing de guandian lai zhiliao Feidian," *Dagong Bao*, April 8, 2003.

53. For a clinical example of the four-stage diagnosis used for SARS patients in Guangdong, see Hai, "Guangdong sheng zhongyiyuan zhiliao Feidianxing feiyan linchuang jingyan."

54. I thank the first reader of the original draft of this chapter for bringing this important point to my attention. Because of the constraints of space and time, I was unable to provide illustrative examples.

55. Fan Z. and Zhang, "Zhongyi bu pa Feidian." I thank Jason Robertson for sending this source to me from Beijing.

56. Ibid.

57. These paragraphs are summarized from the introduction to World Health Organization, *SARS*, 2–3, 7–9.

58. Liu, X., et al., "Chinese Herbs Combined with Western Medicine for Severe Acute Respiratory Syndrome (SARS)," The Cochrane Collaboration (2), 2006, 1–68. See the list on the Cochrane Collaboration Web site for centers, http://www.cochrane.org/contact/centres. The Web site address for the center in China is: www.ebm.org.cn. It does not provide, however, information on the reviewers' credentials.

59. For a brief history and explanation of the Cochrane Collaboration project for evaluating clinical medicine, see Dickersin and Manheimer, "The Cochrane Collaboration." For a thorough description of the criteria of systematic reviews applied to Complementary and Alternative Medicine (CAM) therapies, see Manheimer and Berman, "The Cochrane Column."

60. Liu, X., et al., "Chinese Herbs Combined with Western Medicine for Severe Acute Respiratory Syndrome (SARS)," 1–2.

61. See Lei's account of an earlier example of this process in "From *Changshan* to a New Anti-malarial Drug."

62. Again, I would like to acknowledge Charlotte Furth for this insight.

63. Lloyd, *Hippocratic Writings*.

64. See chapter 3 in Scheid, *Chinese Medicine in Contemporary China*.

Governing Germs from Outside and Within Borders

Controlling the 2003 SARS Risk in Taiwan

Tseng Yen-fen and Wu Chia-Ling

"SARS needs to be regarded as a particularly serious threat for several reasons. The disease has no vaccine and no treatment, forcing health authorities to *resort to control tools dating back to the earliest days of empirical microbiology: isolation and quarantine.*"
—World Health Organization, "SARS"

The outbreak of severe acute respiratory syndrome (SARS) in 2003 was characterized by several novelties that worried health experts and the public. SARS was described as a "new, unpredictable, and particularly dangerous" disease because it was found to have the following biomedical characteristics:[1] even though doctors of traditional Chinese medicine (TCM) consider it as yet another *wenbing* epidemic (see Hanson's chapter in this volume), biomedical doctors perceive it as a novel disease whose source and mechanisms of transmission are unknown; it is difficult to diagnose clinically, and no effective way has been developed to identify the virus in the laboratory; and lastly, medicines and vaccines available for the effective cure or prevention of SARS are absent and difficult to develop in the short term. From our point of view, it is true that SARS is a novel disease, but the response of contemporary society has been informed partly by hygienic modernity—a particular set of understandings of how modern people should and can control health hazards. The SARS outbreak revealed the evolving governing framework for controlling infectious disease by public health authorities at the nation-state and transnational levels, at a time when emerging globalization discourse on the spread of disease had been dominating public health ideology.[2] This chapter analyzes the decision-making processes of health authorities responding to new health risks and uncertainties, as exemplified by the emergence of SARS in the twenty-first century.

Many social scientists have called for a model to analyze expert responses to risk that goes beyond technical matters. We will follow this line of inquiry by viewing health policies as much more than just scientific, technical decisions. In this context, we see a need to incorporate subjective risk perceptions into the analysis. Many authors comparing regulatory policies in different countries emphasize the subjective nature of risk perceptions.[3] They offer examples to show how differences in risk regulation policies between countries reflect subjective interpretations stemming from technical assumptions, political priorities, and cultural expectations. Our analysis in this chapter emphasizes the interests of politics. Health authorities make their decisions based on their risk perception frameworks, whether cautious or neutral, and based on politically compelling reasons. According to Anthony Giddens, modern people increasingly live in a risk society that is "a high technological frontier which absolutely no one completely understands and which generates a diversity of possible futures."[4] In governing such a risk society, Giddens argues, there is a new moral climate of politics. In our view, this new moral climate is what David Fidler referred to as "good governance," which is one that enhances the capacity to control health hazards.[5] In such a political climate, health authorities are increasingly afraid of being accused of covering up risks and not responding to potential hazards.

The outline of this chapter is as follows. We first introduce the context of creating borders for guarding against the SARS virus, a process that presented tremendous challenges for health authorities. We then uncover the process of policy formation in two radical germ governance measures regulating people's mobility between and within state borders: the travel advisory issued by the WHO and the home quarantine implemented by the government in Taiwan. These two policy measures represent dramatic changes in the prevention of global infectious diseases, in terms of the risk control scale.

The first part of our analysis discusses the travel advisory issued by the WHO to control the global spread of SARS. The WHO first designated SARS-affected areas and then issued a travel advisory against all but essential trips to such areas, the harshest warning ever issued by the WHO, which resulted in a dramatic decrease in the number of travelers to SARS-affected areas, including some of the world's busiest transportation hubs. Fidler has argued that issuing the travel advisory radically changed the WHO's previous policy of "germ governance" in controlling global infectious diseases.[6] In preventing the spread of SARS internationally, the WHO's first action was to define the SARS risk as a global danger. Next, it moved to communicate the risks not only to member states, but also to nonstate actors such as travelers.

The second part of our analysis examines the home quarantine policy in Taiwan. Governments of SARS-affected areas adopted massive home quarantines to fight against the spread of the virus. For example, during the outbreak Taiwan put some 130,000 people in home quarantine, the single most pervasive home quarantine ever implemented within a national territory in modern times. The largest proportion of those affected were people who had traveled to Taiwan from areas that the WHO had designated as SARS-affected; some of the quarantined were confined in designated temporary homes such as hotels and establishments affiliated with the military.

Guarding Borders against Germs

Like other preventive measures, the key policies in reducing SARS risks were attempts to guard against the spread of viruses from person to person and from country to country. However, the unusual speed with which SARS spread globally increased pressure to implement quarantines and warn against travel. While the travel advisory was meant to place warning signs on national and regional borders, home quarantine was intended to place warning signs on people with high SARS risk and therefore drew borders between them and others. Ways to draw such borders ranged from the high-tech to lay person solutions. National borders at airports were equipped with high-tech temperature-taking machines to prevent people with fevers from entering without further health examination. In the case of home quarantine, borders were drawn around the home as a boundary, a practice especially tricky in apartments where people share the same building. In extreme cases, the border was drawn by means of only a few physical barriers, such as the logs used by villagers in the Chinese countryside.

The border consciousness in these efforts to prevent SARS is ironic, especially in light of the emphasis on borderless collaboration in fighting the disease. Ever since the outbreak of SARS, health authorities have stressed the borderless nature of SARS transmission and therefore called for collaboration across borders. For example, in June 2003, Taiwan's delegates to the WHO's Global Conference on SARS used the slogan "SARS: a borderless struggle." Nevertheless, SARS prevention measures also enhanced the salience of the "borders" of SARS risks.

To draw borders around risk-ridden people and places, both the quarantine measures and the travel advisory to SARS-affected areas involved risk classification. Since SARS symptoms are not easy to identify and the source of SARS—the virus—is not observable even with the help of the most advanced laboratory equipment, prevention measures perceived to be effective seemed inevitably to begin with designating and classifying danger zones in order to locate and contain the virus. These zones could be people or places in which there was believed to be a higher likelihood that the virus was present. If the zones were people, the answer was to quarantine them. If the zones were places, then people were banned from entering them, or people from them were banned from entering other places.

This process first involves classification. As Evitar Zerubavel has pointed out, while all classification aims to carve up reality and turn it into islands of meaning (such as high-risk people and affected areas), all classification works to make distinct clusters out of a reality that is continuous.[7] As a result, such classification efforts almost invariably involve an arbitrary cutoff point when dissecting this continuous reality. Arbitrary borders need to be established first to carve out classes from the continuous reality of dangers such as a virus. As Ruth Simpson suggested, discussing how people assign danger signs to certain objects—that is, classify risk groups—helps us to understand the tenuous connection between the objective world of danger and the corresponding perceptions of danger.[8]

The following example serves to illustrate this tenuous connection between objective dangers and subjective perceptions. During the SARS outbreak, Taiwanese health authorities decided to quarantine people coming back from a SARS-affected area, basing such decisions on the judgment that travelers with a history of travel to affected areas belonged to the high risk category. While governments of affected countries like Taiwan complained that the WHO was homogenizing places where SARS risks were diverse by designating the whole city or region as an affected area, these governments themselves treated travelers from other affected areas similarly, quarantining those coming from other homogenized affected areas. In a sense, the WHO and the governments of affected countries were all doing the same thing—that is, transferring borders from a political existence to a biomedical reality.

This example reveals the irony of treating national borders as meaningful lines for locating a virus. Taiwan placed people coming from other affected countries in home quarantine, but all of Taiwan was at that time designated a SARS-affected area by the WHO, and everybody residing in Taiwan was in effect classified as high risk and accordingly subject to being quarantined. As a matter of fact, when SARS was initially confined to the capital, Taipei, proposals were brought forth by municipal governments outside Taipei that people from the capital who entered their municipalities should be quarantined. Of course, that did not happen since such an act lacks political legitimacy. After all, it was assumed that the Taiwanese people should bear any risk caused by others if they were our fellow citizens. Yet it was also assumed that the Taiwanese people wanted to avoid the possible danger associated with travelers from outside, even though many of these were Taiwanese citizens traveling between Taiwan, Hong Kong, and China for business or tourism. The only fact that mattered for a person's classification, therefore, was whether he or she lived inside or outside the national border. At this point, dangers ceased to be objective facts and needed to be perceived within existing classification systems such as national territory.

Another example of arbitrary classification of risk is the WHO's decisions on issuing and the travel advisory for certain areas and later lifting it. To designate certain places as virus-ridden zones is a much more difficult classification than to designate certain people as dangerous. While it is sometimes possible to tell when a virus is present among people, it is almost impossible to detect when a virus is present in the environment of certain places. Therefore, the designation of areas of risk is inherently more arbitrary than the classification of people of risk. Arbitrary decisions are based more on subjective perceptions than on rigorous scientific reasoning. We argue that the adoption of SARS prevention measures stemmed from the health authorities' subjective interpretations and inferences about the objective dangers of SARS.

Global Governance

Constructing SARS as a Global Danger

The following quotes by the executive director of the WHO offer important insights into the way in which a public health authority such as the WHO defined and presented the threat of SARS to the general public.

> We've had killer outbreaks of new diseases before, like Ebola, but they have never spread internationally . . . We've never faced anything on this scale with such a global reach.

> .   .   .

> In the world today an infectious disease in one country is a threat to all: infectious diseases do not respect international borders.[9]

We found that the perceived danger of SARS to public health was not limited to its biomedical features. Compared to Ebola and other deadly epidemics, SARS was described as especially threatening because of the outbreak's "global reach." SARS, therefore, became the latest item to be listed among global dangers, like water and air pollution, that "do not respect international borders."

A significant number of SARS cases apparently originated in Guangdong, China, in mid-February 2003, and the disease spread outward rapidly from there.[10] During late February 2003, SARS moved beyond the Chinese mainland when a doctor from Guangdong who had treated SARS patients infected at least sixteen visitors to Hong Kong, who then spread the disease internationally. The threat of SARS hence came to be associated with the fact that it spread to a wide geographical area in a relatively short period of time. The global spread of SARS was mainly caused by increased international travel, linked to processes of globalization such as transnational investment, tourism, immigration, and transnational networking, all of them part and parcel of the globalization process. Therefore, SARS was highlighted as much more threatening to people in wider geographical areas than previous epidemics. While it took many months for the great flu epidemic to move around the world in 1918–19, the SARS virus was able to reach other countries within hours. Many official reports, including those released by national governments and the WHO, argue that the rapid global spread of infectious diseases such as SARS is a negative consequence of the globalization process.[11] This recognition of SARS as a global danger made both national governments and the WHO act promptly to introduce extreme measures to prevent the disease from leaping across national borders.

Governing International Health: SARS and the WHO

With its rapid international spread, SARS posed a special challenge in governing international health, especially to the WHO as a supranational health authority. An organization established to respond to the international spread of epidemics in the first part of twentieth century, the WHO has encountered more and more challenges when it comes to preventing epidemics from spreading in an era of hypermobility. According to the WHO, SARS was the first severe infectious disease to emerge in the globalized society of the twenty-first century.[12] However, the WHO's role in controlling SARS is part of a series of changes in global health governance that has lasted for more than a decade.[13] The emergence of new diseases like SARS has spurred extensive discourse on the globalization of public health threats, as Obijiofor Aginam notes: "Because communicable diseases do not respect the geopolitical boundaries of nation states, and state sovereignty is an alien concept in the microbial world, all of humanity is now vulnerable to the emerging and re-emerging threats of communicable diseases."[14]

In addition, SARS has had a profound impact on approaches to the control of infectious disease. First, the need to build knowledge about SARS prompted international collaboration in terms of sharing resources and information. Second, the outbreak of SARS empowered supranational organizations like the WHO to fight a microbial world that has no "respect" for national boundaries. As Ulrich Beck has pointed out: "The objectivity of global dangers is to further the construction of (centralized) transnational institutions. This point of view, often suspected of being naïve, thus involves—or even produces—a considerable impetus to power."[15]

Fidler has argued that the SARS outbreak represents "the coming of age of a governance strategy for infectious diseases more radical than any previous governance innovation in this area of international relations."[16] He stresses that among the innovations, the travel advisories were particularly radical for a number of reasons. First, in issuing travel advisories regarding SARS, the WHO acted without the consent of targeted countries. Second, in issuing such advisories, the WHO exercised its power of setting policy against the interests of the targeted countries. Third, through travel advisories, the WHO directed its recommendations directly to nonstate actors such as travelers, rather than communicating through state actors. Here we may consider that technological advances in communication such as the Internet have greatly enhanced the WHO's ability to disseminate information. Evidently, the availability of the Internet has helped to link the WHO directly to individuals and has therefore transformed its direct subjects of governance actions to include nonstate actors. People with access to the Internet could easily check on the status of the SARS outbreak and see warnings on the WHO Web site. As a matter of fact, during the SARS outbreak the WHO Web site updated its news and advisories on a daily basis. This kind of information dissemination would be simply unthinkable without the existence of the Internet.

Preventing the Global Spread of SARS

One of the WHO's most important roles in preventing the global spread of SARS was to designate affected areas. In this context, an affected area is defined as an area in which local chains of transmission of SARS are occurring, as reported by the national public health authorities. The WHO then gives advice to travelers who plan to travel to such affected areas. National governments also make use of such designations to identify people needing special screening when they cross national borders. By contrast, previous efforts to prevent infectious diseases from spreading transnationally were initiated mostly by national governments, guarding their borders by restricting tourists and immigrants infected with specific diseases from entering their territory. However, during the SARS outbreak, the WHO took a very active role in discouraging mobility across national boundaries. Prior to the outbreak, the WHO had only issued travel recommendations for international travelers to certain areas affected by communicable diseases. Such recommendations, however, were not intended to discourage trips to the affected areas, but only to highlight important guidelines for safeguarding against sources and transmission mechanisms of communicable diseases.

The prediction that SARS would rapidly spread around the world prompted the WHO to issue a rare worldwide emergency travel advisory on March 15, 2003, warning international travelers, healthcare workers, and airlines workers to be aware of SARS symptoms. Paul Farmer applauded that move:

> Disease surveillance and control must be as transnational as the epidemics themselves—not unilateral or bilateral. As SARS broke out, public-health specialists found themselves shouted down by mayors or ministers of trade and tourism, not only in authoritarian China but even in Canada. WHO correctly and courageously issued its travel advisory, despite being derided for triggering panic, fueling prejudices and damaging the global economy. The job of the WHO is to protect health rather than tourism or stock markets; thankfully, the international body proved itself able to resist national interests in its response.[17]

In response to the Amoy Gardens outbreak of SARS in Hong Kong, an event that pointed to the possibility of environmental contamination as a risk factor for transmission of the SARS virus, the WHO further issued a first travel warning to international travelers to some SARS-affected areas on April 2. This travel advisory stated: "As a measure of precaution, WHO is now recommending that persons traveling to Hong Kong and Guangdong Province of China consider postponing all but essential travel."[18] In the English media, this advisory was called a travel warning or travel ban. As the SARS crisis evolved, more cities and countries were named as regions to which people were warned against traveling. The effect of such travel warnings was tremendous. The advisories had a great negative economic impact in SARS-affected areas such as Guangdong, Hong Kong, and Toronto, some of the world's fastest-growing areas in international travel, trade, and tourism. For example, during the travel advisory periods, the number of inbound travelers to Taiwan decreased to only 10 percent of the ordinary volume.

This travel advisory was issued when the WHO took into consideration that more risk factors of SARS transmission patterns were present in certain SARS-affected areas such as Guangdong and Hong Kong. The travel advisory was issued in conjunction with the following statement of risk communication:

> The SARS situation in the Hong Kong Special Administrative Region has developed features of concern: a continuing and significant increase in cases with indications that SARS has spread beyond the initial focus in hospitals. These developments have suggested environmental routes of transmission from a SARS infected person which may be related to contamination of common systems that link rooms or flats together. Despite the implementation of strict measures to control the outbreak, there have continued to be a small number of visitors to Hong Kong who have been identified as SARS cases after their return from Hong Kong. The epidemic in Guangdong Province of China, situated adjacent to Hong Kong, is the largest outbreak of SARS reported and has also shown evidence of spread in the wider community.[19]

This statement offers a comprehensive explanation for the decision to issue a travel advisory to these areas. The WHO later established three factors to consider in decisions about issuing and lifting advisories against trips to certain SARS-affected areas: the number of probable SARS cases, community transmission, and the export of cases to other countries. During the SARS outbreak, a watch list of twenty-two countries was evaluated on a daily basis by the WHO to see if any of them should be put on the travel advisory list. Soon, such classification pressures pushed the WHO to release numerical and therefore seemingly more objective criteria: there should be no more than sixty hospitalized SARS patients in a region and the number of new cases of SARS patients there must not exceed five in three consecutive days for an advisory to be lifted. In regard to the basis for such a move toward numerical specifications, David Heymann, the executive director of communicable diseases at the WHO, pointed out that there was no scientific basis for choosing sixty hospitalized patients as a cutoff point for classifying certain regions as unsuitable for travel, because the WHO experts could not predict when the peak of SARS—a new disease—would be over. The number was chosen based on epidemiologists' intuition that sixty was an appropriate upper limit.[20]

The perception framework for danger adopted by the WHO should be further analyzed. Ruth Simpson has argued that by analyzing the perception framework for danger and safety, we no longer perceive danger only as an objective world but also as an intersubjective matter. She proposes that we perceive dangers within one of three larger frameworks: the cautious, the confident, or the neutral.[21] We found that the WHO, in its attempts to block the international spread of epidemics, had tended to adopt the neutral framework, according to Simpson's conceptualization, until the SARS outbreak. The neutral framework begins with the assumption that the environment is neutral, and marks certain entities as dangerous. Travel recommendations previously issued by the WHO to advise international travelers to epidemic-affected areas reflect such a neutral framework. These recommendations gave advice to individual travelers by marking specific sources and transmission routes of epidemics as dangerous, but assumed that other unmarked environments were neutral. In its attempts to block the spread of SARS, however, the WHO chose to adopt the cautious framework—which assumes things are dangerous until proven safe—as revealed by the travel advisories it issued. To list certain areas as SARS-affected and advise against nonessential trips to such areas was to treat these places as dangerous until proven safe.

Simpson did not systematically investigate what kinds of danger could compel us to adopt a cautious perception framework. We might infer that since the adoption of a cautious framework drastically raises the amount of physical as well as psychological resources invested in avoiding a danger, this framework is more likely to be adopted when aspects of a danger are uncertain.

When WHO officials shifted their position on SARS to embrace a cautious framework and consequently issued a very different kind of travel warning, the need arose to establish rigid and objective criteria on the basis of which to list danger zones. There was a great discrepancy between scientific evidence and decisions of prevention measures. It seems to be quite contradictory for the WHO to acknowledge its inability to know how SARS would develop, on the one hand, and to establish scientific criteria for listing danger zones, on the other hand. To establish objective criteria may have helped the WHO to fit into the conventional definition of a modern expert system—that is, a system generating more knowledge but not more uncertainties. The home quarantine that we will discuss in the next section can be understood similarly, as a policy response to both risks and uncertainties. Home quarantine was also implemented by means of objective criteria that involved the establishment of arbitrary cutoff points, on the basis of subjective perceptions of risk by health authorities.

Governance at Home

The Emergence of Home Quarantine in Taiwan

The Ministry of Health in Singapore issued a Home Quarantine Order (HQO) on March 24, 2003, which started the large scale of preventive measures focusing on healthy people. Under this HQO, persons who had had close contact with SARS patients had to stay at home for ten days and minimize their contact with other people. Before March 24, the major strategies to prevent the spread of SARS recommended by the WHO were the proper isolation of SARS cases and, for individuals who had been to affected areas or had had close contacts with SARS cases, and who then showed high fever or respiratory symptoms, the immediate seeking of medical attention. Even in Singapore, on March 23, 2003, the government still emphasized that "unless you have the symptoms AND a similar travel history or personal contact with infected persons, the Ministry urges the public to seek the advice of a GP first."[22] This meant that before the introduction of home quarantine measures, only ill persons became part of preventive measures for further transmission. The issuing of the HQO in Singapore signified a brave new measure that isolated people who did not show any symptoms. On the first day after the measure was instituted, around 300 people in Singapore were placed on the government's list of individuals requiring home quarantine.

Home quarantine was an additional precautionary measure, implemented after the government had already collected suspected and probable cases in a central place and added protection measures for hospital staff.[23] Based on the epidemiological theory of a transmission pyramid, the government believed that attention should be focused on preventing the increase of SARS cases from secondary and tertiary transmission. The fact that no further cases occurred among hospital staff meant that the secondary transmission in the medical setting had been effectively controlled. Efforts were made to contain the spread of the disease among the family and friends of SARS cases. Home quarantine allowed detection of infected cases in a shorter time period. Therefore, those who were subject to the HQO had to check regularly for fever; if they were ill, a specially equipped ambulance would transport them to a hospital.

The implementation of home quarantine policies in Singapore immediately became an exemplary case and spurred experts and local authorities in Taiwan to argue for more stringent measures. The first case of SARS in Taiwan, then known as atypical pneumonia, was publicized on March 14. One week later, when the patient's family and coworkers exhibited some symptoms, heated debates started among government officials and experts as to whether the government should add SARS to the official list of transmitted diseases and use that as legal justification to isolate suspected cases. Although the debate in Taiwan focused on how to manage suspected cases, several experts and the media used the establishment of home quarantine in Singapore to argue that stringent control measures were necessary.

Singapore was presented in Taiwan as a model of "stringency," in contrast to the image of Hong Kong's handling as "sloppy." This interpretation paved the way for a sudden implementation of home quarantine in Taiwan. Two days after Singapore issued the HQO, four engineers in Taiwan who had been to Beijing were identified as SARS cases, starting another wave of social upheaval. This event ended the controversy on the legal status of SARS; the Centers for Disease Control (CDC) in Taiwan immediately listed SARS as an official transmitted disease. At the same time, Taiwan issued its first home quarantine orders. Thus, while the WHO had been the major institution that the Department of Health in Taiwan followed closely, Singapore emerged as another significant model to learn from when policymakers in Taiwan needed to modify their measures of control.

More a Political Response than a Scientific Measure

We argue here that, different from the situation in Singapore, the introduction of home quarantine in Taiwan was more a response to a political crisis than a scientific, evidence-based control measure. The stage of the SARS outbreak in Taiwan differed from that in Singapore, and Taiwan did not follow all the control measures that Singapore took. While Singapore followed the epidemiological theory of the transmission pyramid in order to use home quarantine to prevent a further spread of SARS via secondary and tertiary transmission, the four SARS cases in Taiwan that triggered the new measures were index cases. One important lesson that both the WHO and the Singapore government learned was to protect healthcare workers, but Taiwan did not follow suit. On March 16, the WHO announced that 90 percent of SARS cases were healthcare workers, and when Singapore issued the HQO, half of the SARS cases in Singapore were doctors, nurses, and other hospital staff. When the Ministry of Health in Singapore announced ten measures to contain SARS, three of them concerned the infection control system in the hospital setting (enhanced infection control procedures in hospitals, enhanced protection procedures in emergency departments at hospitals, and additional isolation facilities in public hospitals).[24] Even though no new cases occurred among hospital staff, the enhancement of protective measures among healthcare workers was still one of the four precautionary measures that the Ministry of Health announced on March 22.[25] Nevertheless, the emphasis on control procedures in hospitals was not taken seriously enough in Taiwan, and this fact partly led to the most serious SARS outbreak in Taipei's Hoping Hospital, which began in early April.[26] As Charles Rosenberg has observed, quarantine has been considered by authorities as a politically feasible choice since the fourteenth century, even when such measures did not have scientific support.[27] Compared to the loose practices in hospital control procedures in late March in Taiwan, home quarantine seemed to be singled out as a dramatic ritual that could easily demonstrate state power during a social crisis that demanded more visible state intervention.

Until March 26, scientific evidence, although limited, suggested that only those who showed symptoms were infectious. Therefore the isolation of SARS cases was deemed one of the most effective strategies to prevent the spread of SARS. The WHO immediately supported Singapore's home quarantine system: "Several countries are introducing maximum measures, including quarantine, to prevent the further spread of SARS. New diseases such as SARS are poorly understood as they emerge. At the beginning of an outbreak, it is sound public health policy to institute maximum control measures needed to prevent further spread."[28]

That statement did not minimize past scientific reports regarding infectious patterns. Home quarantine was meant to help detect suspected cases more efficiently, rather than being offered on the basis of any new scientific finding on the nature of the virus or infectious channels. Still, such measures dramatically transformed the perception framework among laypeople.

Transformation of the Risk Perception Framework

From the very beginning of the implementation of home quarantine in Taiwan, serious discrimination existed. Some neighbors kept their distance from healthy quarantined people or rejected contact with their family members who did not have to follow the home quarantine procedures. Several cases were reported of healthy people who committed suicide not due to the severity of any illness but because of social discrimination. Obviously, the community viewed people under home quarantine procedures as infectious. By contrast, authorities and experts emphasized that people under home quarantine were not infectious. Vice Minister Lee Hsien Loong of Singapore directly stated: "People on HQOs are not dangerous, neither have they done anything wrong."[29] The U.S. Centers for Disease Control and Prevention, as well as the Singapore government, emphasized that as long as people did not have symptoms, "they are not infectious."[30] A huge gap in the perception of danger thus existed between the layperson and the expert.

We argue that it is not due to any lack of scientific knowledge that laypeople had such a wrong perception. Rather, we want to emphasize that the imposition of home quarantine itself helped create such a perception. First of all, the policy marked an easily visible group as posing a possible danger, which was much easier for the public to identify as a threat than the invisible virus itself. Before the implementation of home quarantine, health authorities in Singapore, Hong Kong, and Taiwan advocated that individuals should seek medical attention whenever they had suspected symptoms. Except for those who returned from affected areas, few among the masses were considered to have been exposed to danger. However, attention soon moved from symptoms to persons; home quarantine clearly identified specific subjects in the community who might have a higher possibility of infectiousness than others. Secondly, the content of these measures treated people in home quarantine as "sick persons" and "dangerous persons." For example, in Singapore the health authorities asked employers to treat the quarantine period as "paid hospitalization sick leave." Such a measure associated people under home quarantine with the ill. Electronic cameras and other surveillance measures were used to supervise their activities. Such stringent strategies created the image of danger. Thirdly, in Taiwan, the Chinese translation of quarantine means isolation. Although the U.S. CDC and the governments of Canada and Singapore emphasized the difference between quarantine and isolation, the Chinese translation used a single term, *geli*. This terminology blurred the boundary between the ill who needed hospital isolation and the healthy who only needed to observe their health more closely. Therefore, with the introduction of home quarantine during the SARS outbreak, a new type of danger was created, which led to further misunderstanding and social disruption in the community.

Conclusions

Paul Basch comments: "The essence of things international lies in the crossing of borders, those imaginary lines on which so much of the world's emotion, energy, and treasure are spent."[31] This chapter raises the question of whether emotion, energy, and treasure were well spent in preventing the SARS virus from spreading across nations. In general, we have learned three lessons from fighting the danger of SARS at the dawn of the twenty-first century.

First, good governance against germs cannot be built solely upon belief in scientific or technical models. As Dorothy Nelkin points out, "the fundamental uncertainties about the nature and extent of the risks inherent in many technological choices often defy systematic analysis and scientific consensus."[32] In the case of SARS, health authorities were unaware that risk communication cannot be confined to technical terms. Sometimes the effort to quantify risks and benefits actually masks real technical uncertainties. Establishing criteria for designating areas for travel advisories shows the problem of such masking of uncertainties.

In governing the SARS risk, we found that health authorities based the political legitimacy of their policies solely on the belief in scientific knowledge as a trustworthy source for communicating information about risk control to their constituents. As a result of this, limited space was left for people to view public health policies as the result of both risk selection and political responses. The present analysis of policy responses suggests that there is a fundamental contradiction between health authorities' acknowledging their inability to know how new epidemics such as SARS develop and the establishment of rigorous scientific criteria to list danger zones.

Second, by transcending technical models for analyzing health policies and introducing politics into the scene, we found that the interests of both the WHO and state governments in maintaining good governance over germs influenced their choice of a cautious framework of risk perception in fighting the SARS risk. A cautious risk framework is evident in the following statement offered by the executive director of communicable disease at the WHO, David Heymann: "In SARS there is no place for complacency. We cannot be wooed into false security over the successful containment efforts that have interrupted human transmission, as false security could become our worst enemy."[33]

To health authorities in the WHO and state governments, the selection of a cautious perception framework for fighting SARS was rooted in political considerations to respond to the emerging pressures on policymakers to guard people's right to be healthy.

Third, epidemics prevention policies increasingly involve more the proper balance between risk control and risk taking. For one thing, it is simply impossible to carry out germ governance to such an extent that every single danger related to epidemics is addressed. As Giddens argues, the advancement of technological innovation does not lead to increasing certainty and security in the world. He suggests that, in some ways, the opposite is true.[34]

In the quote above, Heymann fails to give us specifics about what kind of security should be regarded as false. As a result, we do not know what true security would be like in the case of SARS.

There is an inherent difficulty in establishing safety zones in dealing with all kinds of dangers. Ruth Simpson offers very good reasons for why this is the case:

> Because danger is often unobservable, it is impossible to determine for certain when we are safe. While it is sometimes possible to tell when danger is present, it is impossible to tell for certain that it is *completely* absent . . . In addition, safety does not manifest itself in any observable way. There are no "safety signs" to establish unequivocally when we are safe, as danger signs warn against harm. *Safety, ironically, may be a more uncertain and unstable state than danger*: in safety, there is always the possibility that danger lurks unseen.[35]

The difficulty of establishing safety zones under the cautious framework is especially true in the case of dealing with the dangers of SARS.

Since the microbial world is unobservable to the unaided human eye, there is probably no such thing as true security. This leads us to wonder whether true security is a feasible goal in fighting SARS. Viruses, like bacteria, have for a long time been part of our planet and, indeed, our bodies. This is the reason why Rosenberg wrote in *Explaining Epidemics* that "we have not, it seems, freed ourselves from the constraints and indeterminacy of living in a web of biological relationships—not all of which we can control or predict."[36] Taking this perspective, the true nightmare for human beings in fighting epidemics might not be that we are often wooed into false security, but that we choose to establish a belief that true security against epidemics is feasible and possible. This is probably the central fear of the modern age.

NOTES

The authors wish to thank the editors of this book, Angela K. C. Leung and Charlotte Furth, for suggesting ways to improve the arguments and focus of our writing. We also want to thank Judith Leavitt, Lewis Leavitt, Lü Tsung-Hsueh, and Fu Daiwei for reading the manuscript and providing helpful comments. This chapter especially benefits from key literature on the development of international health governance brought to our attention by Lü Tsung-Hsueh. All translations are ours, unless otherwise indicated.

1. World Health Organization, "Consensus Document on the Epidemiology of Severe Acute Respiratory Syndrome (SARS)."

2. N. King, "Security, Disease, Commerce."

3. See, for example, Irwin, *Risk and the Control of Technology*, and Jasanoff, *Risk Management and Political Culture*.

4. Giddens, "Risk Society," 25.

5. Fidler, "Germs, Governance, and Global Public Health in the Wake of SARS," 802.

6. Ibid.

7. Zerubavel, 1–2.

8. Ruth Simpson, "Neither Clear Nor Present," 553.

9. David Heymann, executive director of communicable diseases at the WHO: The first quote is from a news report on March 30, 2003, "World Health Officials Prepare for the 'Big One'" by Emma Ross. Available at http://www.resonant.org/newsarticles/2003/2003.03.30-world_health_officials_prepare_for_sars-seacoast online.com.html. The second quote is from his presentation at the WHO Global Con-

ference on SARS on June 17, 2003, published online on the WHO Web site: http://
www.who.int/csr/sars/conference/june_2003/materials/presentations/en/index
.html.

10. World Health Organization, "WHO Issues a Global Alert about Cases of Atypical Pneumonia."

11. Health Canada, "Learning from SARS."

12. World Health Assembly, "Severe Acute Respiratory Syndrome (SARS)," 4.

13. Fidler, "Germs, Governance, and Global Public Health in the Wake of SARS,"
801.

14. Obijiofor, "International Law and Communicable Diseases," 946.

15. Beck, "World Risk Society as Cosmopolitan Society?" 5.

16. Fidler, "Germs, Governance, and Global Public Health in the Wake of SARS,"
801.

17. Farmer, "SARS and Inequality," 6.

18. World Health Organization, "Update 17."

19. Ibid.

20. Lam, *SARS*, 103.

21. Simpson's three frameworks begin with default assumptions about safety and
danger. The confident framework assumes everything is safe until proven dangerous;
the cautious framework assumes everything is dangerous until proven safe; and the
neutral framework assumes the environment is neutral until marked as explicitly
safe or dangerous. See "Neither Clear nor Present," especially 553–57.

22. Singapore Ministry of Health, "Update (x) on SARS Cases in Singapore."

23. Singapore Ministry of Health, "Enhanced Precautionary Measures to Break
SARS Transmission."

24. Singapore Ministry of Health, "Measures Taken to Control the SARS Outbreak
in Singapore."

25. Singapore Ministry of Health, "Enhanced Precautionary Measures to Break
SARS Transmission."

26. Chen D. and Wu, "Dushi, chuanran jibing yu shehui zhengyi."

27. Rosenberg, *Explaining Epidemics*, 282.

28. World Health Organization, "Update 10."

29. H. Lee, "May Day Rally Speech."

30. Hsien Loong Lee. "CDC Telebriefing Transcript: CDC Update on Severe Acute
Respiratory Syndrome (SARS)." Available on the CDC Web site at www.cdc.gov/od/
oc/media/transcripts/+030508.htm.

31. Basch, *Textbook of International Health*, 42.

32. Nelkin, "Communicating Technological Risk," 100.

33. Heymann, Preface, ii.

34. Giddens, "Risk Society," 23.

35. R. Simpson, "Neither Clear nor Present," 551.

36. Rosenberg, "Explaining Epidemics," 287.

Afterword

Biomedicine in Chinese East Asia:
From Semicolonial to Postcolonial?

Warwick Anderson

In 1968, Owsei Temkin, the retiring director of the Institute of the History of Medicine at Johns Hopkins University, warned that "the tradition of the Western approach to the history of medicine is too narrow a basis for the historical comprehension of medicine as it is developing in our era." The "Western" or "scientific" medicine to which he had devoted so much study was changing rapidly into "global" medicine, about which he knew little. Already to a few younger, more anthropologically minded historians, he said, "scientific medicine appears as a system on a par with other, indigenous, systems, so that a kind of comparative history of medicine is cultivated." While the epistemological consequences of such equipoise gave Temkin pause, he recognized the need to broaden the scope of the history of medicine, to acknowledge the cosmopolitan reach of its subject matter. "If world health is a common concern," he concluded, "history focused upon global medicine is a legitimate aim."[1]

While historians proved dilatory in taking up their global burden, some anthropologists in the 1970s displayed considerable interest in comparing the elite or learned medical traditions of Asia with their Western counterpart.[2] Frequently these systemic comparisons turned out static and narrowly textual analyses, which obscured the dynamism and complexity of ordinary healthcare. Even so, hints of contact and exchange, eclecticism and hybridity, and stress and subjugation within and between the great traditions do sometimes emerge in these accounts. Charles Leslie avoided the terms "Western" and "scientific," preferring to use "cosmopolitan" to describe the elite system of medicine that had spread from Europe and superseded other traditions and practices.[3] Arthur Kleinman pointed out that anthropologists were comparing systems of personalized healthcare and disease prevention, and not the public health apparatus. Provocatively, he stated that the "comparative study of public health begins with its introduction as a system into other cultures." Comparative study of public health was thus inherently part of the genealogy of imperialism and globalization. In 1973, Kleinman sketched the history of public health in China, emphasizing the impact of missionaries and the development of rudiments of state action in the treaty ports. The young historian of medicine—who was soon diverted toward anthropology—noted the Manchurian plague prevention service constituted, in 1910, the first public health program of the national government. "Public health had finally become part of the construction of the modern Chinese nation," he wrote.[4]

As early as 1968, Ralph Croizier was urging further investigation of the "slow, painful, but irresistible introduction of modern medicine" into China.[5] Since then—mostly since the 1980s—historians have extensively charted the development of this "modern medicine" in Africa and South Asia, showing how European medical ideas and practices, now cosmopolitan, frequently traced the contours of empire and nation, commonly adding pathological depth to older categories of race and gender.[6] Critical studies of colonial hygiene and public health now jostle on the bookshelves with nuanced examinations of colonial clinical activities, especially psychiatry. More instrumentalist accounts of colonial medicine sit uneasily beside social and cultural histories. We find investigations of the impact of empire on disease patterns and social suffering as well as descriptions of the colonization of bodies and minds, of forced yet subtle alterations of sensibility and structure of feeling. Many of these African and South Asian case studies of the codependency of biomedicine and empire point assertively toward the more pervasive globalization of Western medicine in our own times, helping to explain how this particular tradition or system has become so pervasive. Yet until recently there were few such critical studies of colonial public health and medicine in East Asia—despite the distant pleas of Croizier, Kleinman, and John Bowers, among others.[7] Belatedly, this collection of essays begins to answer their calls.

Perhaps China's role in the colonial drama of the nineteenth and twentieth centuries is too ambiguous or marginal to insert it readily into the analysis of the medical dimensions of imperialism. It is not as though medicine in China has evaded scholarship altogether. Clearly delimited historical and anthropological studies of traditional Chinese medicine, in elite and vernacular forms, abound.[8] Some scholars still favor systemic comparisons with other bounded traditions.[9] Indeed, it is tempting to attribute the relative immunity to postcolonial critique of Chinese medicine to its apparent durability and continuing appeal—yet ayurveda proved similarly resilient and attractive in India, the *locus classicus* for studies of colonial impact. More likely, the conceptual challenge of an oddly variegated and elusive patterning of imperial formations in the region—Mao Zedong's semicolonial condition[10]—explains the late arrival of the critical study of colonial public health and hygiene in China. Bravely, many contributors to this collection are now prepared to engage with the multiple and various incarnations of colonialism in Northeast Asia, whether the mercantile, minimalist version present in the treaty ports; the scientific and disciplinary forms of Japanese occupation; or, perhaps more tangentially, the complex internal colonialisms rife in the region. Taken together, their essays complicate, or perhaps simply extend, the "colonial" of colonial medicine. The influence of the German notion of hygiene police on the practices of Japanese imperialism is especially interesting, suggesting yet another way to medicalize, and thereby empower, the late colonial state. In discovering this misplaced repertoire of twentieth-century imperialism, these essays reveal other late styles of colonialism, other ways to fashion colonial and protonational subjects, differing (at least in degree) from those familiar in African and South Asian histories.[11]

It may be worthwhile taking a moment to reflect on the late styles of medical colonialism. As elsewhere, the predominant modality of the late colonial state was disciplinary and benevolent, or progressive within limits, using reform of personal and domestic hygiene to produce certain sorts of self-governing individuals, actors in a humanitarian narrative. The colonial subject was registered, inspected, told what to eat, when to wash, and how to defecate responsibly. Such modern rituals of hygiene were linked intimately to the making of potential citizens and their surveillance. Self-government of body, involving proper conduct and comportment, became a necessary precondition for political self-government or national sovereignty. Disputes arose between colonizers and nationalists not so much over the character of the trajectory, but about the exact location reached on the imagined arc toward achievement of self-government of person and polity. The biopolitics of the late colonial state were therefore as much about deferral as discipline.[12] Yet as Sean Hsiang-lin Lei, Ruth Rogaski, and others demonstrate here, "benevolence" was not the only medical modality of late colonialism. At times of perceived crisis, coercive operations on "bare life"—manifested in segregation, quarantine, biological control, and vaccination—could take the place of the making of colonial subjects. Adroitly, the late colonial state thus alternated between the biopolitics of the clinic, or bureau of health, and the camp—or between the *bios* of conditional civic recognition and *zoë* of the state of exception.[13]

In making legible the markings of the state on the bodies of its subjects, historians of colonial medicine are often prone to teleological narratives focused on citizenship and nationality. Sometimes our ostensibly critical accounts come to appear just another way of telling the national story. Observing that global medicine was developing at a time of unprecedented "national consciousness" in non-Western countries, Temkin long ago cautioned against medical history's "threatening fragmentation into national histories."[14] That is, he worried that the future history of global medicine would fail its dispersive and inclusive aims and instead dwindle into serial nationalisms. Yet reading the essays in this volume, it is surprisingly difficult to detect any national grand narrative. Perhaps the location of many of the authors in a liminal and largely unrecognized state without a nation explains in part their reticence and reserve. They give us instead a variety of case studies of state medicine and public health, sensitive to social and epidemiological difference, to overlapping and contending sovereignties, offered up with transcolonial and transnational comparison in mind. Taiwan, Manchuria, and the lower Yangzi delta never quite congeal into "China"—rather, they link more closely to other places, other colonial sites.

These studies pose, but cannot answer, the question of what is comparable in the history of public health. Both Temkin and Kleinman have suggested that international public health is amenable to genealogical inquiry but relatively resistant to the systemic or typological comparisons that are applied to the great traditions of clinical medicine. We should, they suggest, follow ideas, practices, careers, and models from one site to the next, from Germany to Japan to China, for example—or track Patrick Manson from Amoy to London, and follow plague fighters from Malaya via Cambridge to Manchuria.[15] They recommend attention to local adaptations and transformations of public health action, as well as resistance or indifference to it. As many of the essays in this collection indicate, we need to be especially sensitive in such comparisons to the sensuous and emotional register of bodily reform and personal hygiene, to the affective elements of colonial medicalization, to the more intimate and private parts of public health.[16] Sometimes disease prevention and disinfection are indistinguishable from cultivation of a certain sensibility and the restructuring of feelings about body and self.[17] On other occasions, of course, they serve merely as herding or sorting mechanisms.

As Temkin predicted, through studies such as the ones collected here we will better understand what he called "global" medicine, and thus discern more clearly the modern relations of bodies to places, of bodies to other bodies, and of those same delicate, exposed bodies to the nation-state and international governance.

NOTES

I am grateful to Bridget Collins for research assistance on this essay. Many of these ideas arose from a collaborative residency in 2005 with Adele E. Clarke at the Bellagio Study Center, courtesy of the Rockefeller Foundation.

1. Temkin, "Comparative Study of the History of Medicine," 362, 365, 368.

2. Leslie, *Asian Medical Systems.* See also Kleinman, "Toward a Comparative Study of Medical Systems" and "Concepts and a Model for the Comparison of Medical Systems as Cultural Systems"; and Kleinman and Mendelsohn, "Systems of Medical Knowledge."

3. Leslie, "Introduction," 5.

4. Kleinman, "The Background and Development of Public Health in China," 6, 14. See also Bowers, "The History of Public Health in China to 1937."

5. Croizier, *Traditional Medicine in Modern China*, 56.

6. Some seminal works are Packard, *White Plague, Black Labor*; Vaughan, *Curing Their Ills*; Keller, *Colonial Madness*; Arnold, *Colonizing the Body*; and Harrison, *Public Health in British India.*

7. But see Rogaski, *Hygienic Modernity*; Benedict, *Bubonic Plague in Nineteenth-Century China*; and Lo, *Doctors within Borders*. For Southeast Asia, see Manderson, *Sickness and the State*; Monnais-Rousselot, *Médecine et Colonisation*; and Anderson, *Colonial Pathologies.*

8. For example, Sivin, *Chinese Science* and *Medicine, Philosophy and Religion in Ancient China*; and Unschuld, *Medicine in China.* For more recent interactive accounts, see Scheid, *Chinese Medicine in Contemporary China* and *Currents of Tradition in Chinese Medicine, 1626–2006*; and Taylor, *Chinese Medicine in Early Communist China, 1945–63.*

9. For example, Lloyd and Sivin, *The Way and the Word*; and Kuriyama, *Expressiveness of the Body and the Divergence of Greek and Chinese Medicine.*

10. Mao wrote around 1940: "China today is colonial in the Japanese-occupied

areas and basically semi-colonial in the Kuomintang areas, and it is predominantly feudal or semi-feudal in both" (*On New Democracy*, 4).

11. By "late style" I mean to refer to Said, *On Late Style*.

12. On the supposedly progressive or liberal late-colonial state, see J. Darwin, "What Was the Late Colonial State?" I elaborate on medical styles of late colonialism in Anderson, *Colonial Pathologies*. This characterization is indebted to Foucault, *Discipline and Punish* and *History of Sexuality*, Vol. 1; and Stoler, *Race and the Education of Desire*. On the colonial deferral of modernity, see Chakrabarty, *Provincializing Europe*.

13. The terminology draws on Agamben, *Homo Sacer*. L. Cohen ("Operability, Bioavailability, and Exception") argues that states of exception may also produce subjectivities—though not civic recognition.

14. Temkin, "Comparative Study of the History of Medicine," 367.

15. Haynes, *Imperial Medicine*; and Wu L., *Plague Fighter*. For a more extensive review of this approach, see Anderson, "Postcolonial Histories of Medicine." One might argue this is the "contamination," rather than "configuration," model of the comparative history of medicine (Rosenberg, "Explaining Epidemics," 295).

16. See Anderson, "States of Hygiene."

17. That is, one might do more to bring Clifford Geertz and Raymond Williams into conversation with the history of medicine. On moral sensibilities, see Geertz, "Found in Translation." On structures of feeling, see Williams, *Marxism and Literature*.

Timeline

1600–1046 BCE	Shang dynasty.
1122–256 BCE	Zhou dynasty (including the Western Zhou and the Spring and Autumn and Warring States Periods).
206 BCE–220 CE	Han dynasty.
618–907	Tang dynasty.
960–1279	Song dynasty.
1271–1368	Yuan (Mongol) dynasty.
1368–1644	Ming dynasty.
1644	Beginning of Qing (Manchu) dynasty.
1842	China defeated in the First Opium War. Signing of the Nanjing Treaty, ceding Hong Kong to the British and opening Guangzhou (Canton), Shanghai, Ningpo, Fuzhou, and Xianmen to foreign trade.
1851–64	Taiping rebellion.
1854	Japan forced to open up to foreign trade.
1856	China defeated in the Second Opium War.
1858	Signing of the Tianjin Treaty, opening up additional treaty ports and giving foreign missionaries the right to preach in China.
1860	Burning of the Yuanming Yuan (Summer Palace) by joint British-French forces and Signing of the Beijing Convention whereby Kowloon Peninsula was ceded to Great Britain.

1866   Arrival of Dr. Patrick Manson in China, as a medical official in the Maritime Customs office.

1867   German Staatemedizin adopted in Japan.

1868   Beginning of Meiji reforms in Japan. Medical Westernization is made official.

1872   Establishment of Donghua (Tung Wah) hospital of Chinese medicine in colonial Hong Kong.

1893   Administration of public health in Japan transferred to the Police Department.

1894–95   Bubonic plague in Yunnan, Guangdong, Hong Kong, and Taiwan.

1895   China defeated in the first Sino-Japanese War. The Treaty of Shimonoseki cedes the island of Formosa (Taiwan) to the Japanese.

1895   Japanese prohibition of the practice of traditional Chinese medicine.

1897   Discovery by the Japanese bacteriologist Shiga Kiyoshi of *Shigella dysenteriae.*

1898   Failure of political reforms by the Qing government.

1899   Sotokufu Medical School established in Taiwan.

1900   Boxer Uprising suppressed by allied forces.

1905   Russia defeated in the Russo-Japanese War. The Treaty of Portsmouth cedes southern Sakhalin Island and Russian territory in Manchuria to Japan.

1905   First population census in Taiwan.

1910   Japanese occupation of Korea.

1910–11   Pneumonic plague in northeastern China.

1911   End of Qing dynasty and establishment of the Republic of China (ROC).

1914   Japan officially joins the Central Powers. First World War extends to East Asia.

1918   End of First World War.

1918–20   Global Spanish flu epidemic.

1920   First population census in Japan.

1921   Establishment of the League of Nations.

1926–27   Northern expedition in China by Republican forces against local warlords.

1928   Establishment of the Nationalist-led ROC government in Nanjing.

1929   Beginning of campaign to suppress traditional medicine in China.

1930   Establishment of the Japan Society of Racial Hygiene.

1931   Japanese occupation of inner Manchuria; establishment of the puppet regime Manchukuo.

1932   Japanese invasion of Shanghai.

1933   Japanese withdrawal from the League of Nations.

1934   China and Japan both sign the International Health Regulations in Paris.

1937–45   Second Sino-Japanese War.
Japan establishes a medical school at Taihoku (Taipei) Imperial University.

1940   Japan issues the National Eugenics Law. The Institute of Public Health is established in Japan with funding from the Rockefeller Foundation.

1941   Japanese attack on Pearl Harbor.

1945   Defeat of Japan and return of Formosa (Taiwan) and Manchuria to China. Division of Korea into North and South Korea.

1945–49   Civil war in China between the Nationalists and the Communists.

1946   The Rockefeller Foundation helps establish a malaria research institute in Taiwan.

1947   Japan's Police Department abolishes the administration of public health.

1949   The ROC retreats to Taiwan; establishment of the communist People's Republic of China (PRC) on the mainland.

1950–53 PRC involvement in the Korean War.

1952   Beginning of the Patriotic Hygiene Movement in the PRC.

1958   Global antimalaria campaigns by the WHO. Great Leap Forward movement in the PRC.

1961   Beginning of family planning in Taiwan, in cooperation with the University of Michigan and the U.S. Population Council.

1965   The WHO announces the eradication of malaria in Taiwan.

1965   Beginning of the barefoot doctor program in the PRC.

1966–76 Cultural Revolution in the PRC.

1971   The ROC (Taiwan) withdraws from the UN, and the PRC takes China's seat on the Security Council.

1975   Death of Chiang Kai-shek in Taiwan.

1976   Death of Mao Zedong in China.

1980   Beginning of economic reforms in the PRC under Deng Xiaoping.

1987   End of martial law in Taiwan.

1994   National health insurance begins in Taiwan.

1997   Hong Kong becomes a Special Administrative Region (SAR) of the PRC.

1999   Macao becomes an SAR of the PRC.

2003   Global SARS epidemic.

Glossary

a-pô 阿婆

ba da chuanranbing 八大傳染病

Baihua 百花

baisituo 百斯脫

banlangen 板籃根

baojia (hokō) 保甲

Baoshan 寶山

baowei 保衛

bingqi 病氣

biyi 避疫

Buyun 步雲

Caopu 曹普

chaihu 柴胡

Changchun 長春

Changhua 昌化

Changling 長嶺

changshan 常山

Changshu 常熟

changzhi fusi 腸窒扶斯

Cheng Wuji 成無己

Chiang Kai-shek (Jiang Jieshi) 蔣介石

chili 赤痢

chong 蟲

chuanran xing 傳染性

chuanran xitong tu 傳染系統圖

chuanranbing 傳染病

chuanshi 傳屍

chuanzhu 傳注

dafeng lai 大風癩

Dagong Bao 大公報

Dai-tō-a Kyōeikenhe 大東亞共榮圈

Dalian/Dairen 大連

dao mazi 倒馬子

dayi 大疫

Deng Kunhe 鄧坤和

Denzenbyō Kenkyusho 傳染病研究所

difang zizhi 地方自治

diqi 地氣

Dongfang zazhi 東方雜誌

Dong Xiaoping 董小平

Dongzha 東柵

Duan Xianzeng 段獻增

duzhuo 度著

eisei (weisheng) 衛生

fangtu zhi qi 方土之氣

fangyi 防疫

fazhen zhifusi 發疹窒扶斯

feidianxing feiyan 非典型肺炎

feilao 肺癆

feiyong 肥壅

fenchang 糞廠

Feng Heling 馮鶴齡

fengshui 風水

fengtubing 風土病

fu xiang jianran 復相漸染

fulian 伏連

gan 疳

ganran 感染

geli 隔離

Gotō Kioshi 後藤清

gu 蠱

guaili 乖戾

guochan yaowu kexue yanjiu 國產
　藥物科學研究

guoquan 國權

guzhang 臌脹

Haining 海寧

Haining Ribao 海寧日報

Haiyan 海盐

Hang-Ki (Heng Qi) 恒祺

Hangzhou 杭州

haoqiao 毫竅

Harbin 哈爾濱

hokō 戶口

Hsinchu (Xinzhu) 新竹

huachong zhi duqi 化蟲之毒氣

huangbing 黃病

Huangpu 黃浦

Huangwan 黃灣

huanyi 換易

huasheng zhi wu 化生之物

huchou 狐臭

huliela 虎列剌

Hunan 湖南

Huo Yuanjia 霍元甲

huoxuelong 活血龍

huxiang chuanran 互相傳染

Huzhou 湖州

Ishii Shirō 石井四郎

Jia'nan 嘉南

Jiangnan 江南

Jiangxi 江西

jianran 漸染

jianyi 檢疫

Jiashan 嘉善

Jiaxing 嘉興

Jiedao Ting 街道廳

jiedu 解毒

Jilin 吉林

Jilong (Keelung) 基隆

Jin Yuehua 金月華

jing 經

Jingbao 警保

Jingwu Tiyu Hui 精武體育會

Jingxiang 淨湘

jingyan 鏡驗

jiu ran wu su 舊染汙俗

kaitogu igaku 開拓醫學

Kaohsiung (Gaoxiong) 高雄

ke 科

Kerqin 科爾沁

Kitasato Shibasaburo 北里柴三郎

lai 癩

Lai Guangxing 賴光興

lao 癆

li 里

li 裏

Liang Qichao 梁啟超

Lianhe Bao 聯合報

Liaodong 遼東

liqi 癘氣

li su 俚俗

Li Youping 李幼平

Longnan 龍南

mafeng 麻風

Magara Masanao 真柄正直

Manchukuo 滿洲國

Mantetsu 滿鐵

Manzhouli 滿洲里

masha 麻痧

mazi 馬子
miemen 滅門
nanho igaku 南方醫學
Nanjing 南京
Nong'an 農安
Pingfang 平房
Pinghu 平湖
potu 破土
qi 氣
qingdao 清道
qingre 清熱
qingre jiedu 清熱解毒
qiwei 氣味
ran 染
ranbing 染病
ranyi 染易
ranzhuo 染著
refeng yi 熱風疫
sán-pô 產婆
Sandai 三代
Shang (dynasty) 商
shang 傷
shanghan 傷寒
Shao Rong 邵榮
Shen Junru 沈鈞儒
Shen Qingfa 沈慶法
sheng zhu 生注
Shengjing Shibao 盛京時報
Shenshi nongshu 沈氏農書
Shenshu 沈墅
Shenyang 瀋陽
shi 時
Shi Youquan 施有銓
Shi Zhaoji 施肇基
Shidai 十代
shifu dili 實扶的里
shilao 尸癆
shiyi 時疫

Shuanglin 雙林
Shuangshan 雙山
shuitu bufu 水土不服
shuyi 鼠疫
sifen 四分
sishi liuyin 四時六淫
Sota Nagamune 曾田長宗
Su Delong 蘇德隆
Suzhou 蘇州
Tachikawa Yoshio 立川義男
Taichung (Taizhong) 台中
Taihu 太湖
Tianjin 天津
tianran dou 天然痘
tiansheng 天生
Tongliao 通遼
Tongxiang 桐鄉
wei 衛
wei ran wang hua 未染王化
weisheng (eisei) 衛生
weisheng du chong 微生毒蟲
weisheng wu 微生物
wenbing 溫病
Wenhui Bao 文匯報
wenyi 瘟疫
Wu Yi 吳儀
wugu 無辜
Wuhu 蕪湖
Wushantou 烏山頭
Xi Liang 錫良
xiangchuan 相傳
xiangran 相染
xiangran yi 相染易
xiangran zhuo 相染著
Xiashi 硤石
Xieqiao 斜橋
xinghongre 猩紅熱
Xincheng 新塍

Xinjing 新京
Xinmin 新民
Xu Bihui 徐碧輝
Xu Jianguo 徐建國
Xuancheng 宣城
xue 血
xuepai 學派
xulao 虛勞
yangmei chuang 楊梅瘡
Yao Hubao 姚胡寶
yi (eki) (epidemic) 疫
yi (exchange) 易
ying 營
yinyang yi 陰陽易
yiqi 疫氣
yong 壅
yousi 有司
Yu Yue 俞樾
zaqi 雜氣
zeifeng 賊風
zhai 瘵
zhang 丈

zhang 瘴
Zhang Ji 張機
Zhang Xiaorui 張曉瑞
zhangli 瘴癘
zhangqi 瘴氣
Zhejiang 浙江
zheng 癥
Zhili 直隸
Zhong xi yi hezuo 中西醫合作
Zhong xi yi jiehe 中西醫結合
Zhong xi yi tuanjie 中西醫團結
Zhongdai 鍾埭
Zhouzhen 周鎮
zhu (pouring) 注
zhu (stationing) 住
zhuan xiang wu ran 轉相污染
zhuan xiangran yi 轉相染易
zhuangre 壯熱
zhuanqu 專區
zhuo 著
zhuyi 注易

Bibliography

Abraham, Thomas. *Twenty-First Century Plague: The Story of SARS*. Baltimore: Johns Hopkins University Press, 2005.

Ackerknecht, Erwin Heinz. *A Short History of Medicine*. Rev. ed. Baltimore: Johns Hopkins University Press, 1982.

Agamben, Giorgio. *Homo Sacer: Sovereign Power and Bare Life*. Stanford, Calif.: Stanford University Press, 1998.

Anderson, Benedict. *Imagined Communities*. London: Verso, 1983.

Anderson, Warwick. *Colonial Pathologies: American Tropical Medicine, Race, and Hygiene in the Philippines*. Durham, N.C.: Duke University Press, 2006.

———. "Postcolonial Histories of Medicine." In *Medical History: The Stories and Their Meanings*, edited by John Harley Warner and Frank Huisman, 285–307. Baltimore: Johns Hopkins University Press, 2004.

———. "States of Hygiene: Race 'Improvement' and Biomedical Citizenship in Australia and the Colonial Philippines." In *Haunted by Empire: Geographies of Intimacy in North American History*, edited by Ann Laura Stoler, 94–115. Durham, N.C.: Duke University Press, 2006.

———. "Where Is the Postcolonial History of Medicine?" *Bulletin of the History of Medicine* 79, no. 3 (1998): 522–30.

Ando, K., K. Kurauchi, and H. Nishimura. "A New Plague Endemic Area in the Northeastern Part of Inner Mongolia." *Kitasato Archive for Experimental Medicine* 8, no. 1 (January 1932): 35–38.

Andrews, Bridie. "Tuberculosis and the Assimilation of Germ Theory in China, 1895–1937." *Journal of the History of Medicine and Allied Sciences* 52 (1997): 114–57.

Ang, Erik Sze-Wee, et al. "Evaluating the Role of Alternative Therapy in Burn Wound Management: Randomized Trial Comparing Moist Exposed Burn Ointment with Conventional Methods in the Management of Patients with Second-Degree Burns." *Medscape/General Medicine* 3 (2001): 3–18.

Anker, Peder. *Imperial Ecology: Environmental Order in the British Empire, 1895–1945*. Cambridge: Harvard University Press, 2002.

Anonymous. "Josanpu sotsugyo shiki 助產婦卒業式 [Graduation Ceremony of Midwives]. *Taiwan igakkai zasshi* 59 (1907): 376.

Apple, Rima. "Constructing Mothers: Scientific Motherhood in the Nineteenth and Twentieth Centuries." *Social History of Medicine* 8 (1995): 161–78.

———. *Mothers and Medicine: A Social History of Infant Feeding, 1890–1950*. Madison: University of Wisconsin Press, 1987.

Arnold, David. *Colonizing the Body: State Medicine and Epidemic Disease in Nineteenth-Century India*. Berkeley: University of California Press, 1993.

———. "Introduction: Tropical Medicine before Manson." In *Warm Climates and Western Medicine: The Emergence of Tropical Medicine, 1500–1900*, edited by David Arnold, 1–19. Amsterdam: Rodopi, 1996.

———. *Science, Technology, and Medicine in Colonial India*. Vol. 3, part 5, *The New Cambridge History of India*, edited by Gordon Johnson. Cambridge: Cambridge University Press, 2000.

Aronowitz, Robert. "Lyme Disease: The Social Construction of a New Disease and Its Social Consequences." *Milbank Quarterly* 69, no. 1 (1991): 79–112.

Atkinson, J. M. *A Historical Survey of Plague in Hong Kong since Its Outbreak in 1894*. Hong Kong: n.p., 1907.

Bao Shichen 包世臣. *Qimin sishu* 齊民四術 [Four ways to govern the people]. Beijing: Zhonghua shuju, 2001 [1851].

Barclay, G. W. *From Far Formosa: The Island, Its People and Missions*. New York: F. H. Revell, 1896.

Barenblatt, Daniel. *A Plague upon Humanity: The Secret Genocide of Axis Japan's Germ Warfare Operation*. New York: Harper Collins, 2004.

Bartholomew, James R. "Japanese Nobel Candidates in the First Half of the Twentieth Century." *Osiris* 13 (1998): 238–84.

Basch, Paul. *Textbook of International Health*. New York: Oxford University Press, 1993.

Beck, Ulrich. "World Risk Society as Cosmopolitan Society?" *Theory, Culture and Society* 12, no. 4 (1996): 1–32.

Benedict, Carol. *Bubonic Plague in Nineteenth-Century China*. Stanford, Calif.: Stanford University Press, 1996.

———. "But What was the Disease? Framing Epidemics in China's Past." Unpublished paper presented at workshop, "Epidemics in China," Fairbank Center for East Asian Research, Harvard University, April 16–17, 2005.

Berdmore, Sept. "The Principles of Cooking." In *Health Exhibition Literature*, vol. 4: *Health in Diet*, ed. Anonymous, 163–250. London: William Clowes and Sons, 1884.

Bijker, Wiebe E. *Of Bicycles, Bakelites and Bulbs: Toward a Theory of Sociotechnical Change*. Cambridge: MIT Press, 1995.

Birn, Anne-Emanuelle, and Armando Solorzano. "Public Health Policy Paradoxes: Science and Politics in the Rockefeller Foundation's Hookworm Campaign in Mexico in the 1920s." *Social Science and Medicine* 49 (1999): 1197–213.

Blake, Henry. *Bubonic Plague in Hong Kong: Memorandum; On the Result of the*

Treatment of Patients in Their Own Houses and in Local Hospitals, During the Epidemic of 1903. Hong Kong: Noronha, 1903.

Blyth, Alexander Wynter. "Diet in Relation to Health and Work." In *Health Exhibition Literature*, vol. 4: *Health in Diet*, edited by Anonymous, 251–354. London: William Clowes and Sons, 1884.

Bowers, John Z. "The History of Public Health in China to 1937." In *Public Health in the People's Republic of China*, edited by Myron E. Wegman, Tsung-Yi Lin, and Elizabeth F. Purcell, 26–46. New York: Josiah Macy Jr. Foundation, 1973.

———. *Western Medicine in a Chinese Palace: Peking Union Medical College, 1917–1951.* New York: Josiah Macy Jr. Foundation, 1972.

Brown, Peter J. "Culture and the Global Resurgence of Malaria." In *The Anthropology of Infectious Disease: International Health Perspectives*, edited by M. C. Inhorn and Peter J. Brown, 119–41. Amsterdam: Gordon and Breach, 1997.

Cain, P. J., and A. G. Hopkins. *British Imperialism: Innovation and Expansion, 1688–1914.* London: Longman, 1993.

Cao Dongyi 曹東義, ed. *Zhongyi qun yingzhan SARS: SARS yu zhongyi waigan rebing zhenzhi guifan yanjiu* 中醫群英戰 SARS: SARS 與中醫外感熱病診治規藩研究 [Chinese medicine completely fights SARS: SARS and Chinese medicine externally afflicted heat diseases, research on the outlines of diagnosis and treatment]. Beijing: Zhongyi guji chubanshe, 2006.

Cao Hongqin 曹洪欣 and Weng Weiliang 翁維良, eds. *SARS wenyi yanjiu* 瘟疫研究 [SARS: Research on Epidemics]. Beijing: Zhongyi guji chubanshe, 2005.

Cao Jinqing 曹錦清, Zhang Letian 張樂天, and Chen Zhongya 陳中亞. *Dangdai Zhebei xiangcun de shehui wenhua bianqian* 當代浙北鄉村的社會文化變遷 [Cultural changes in rural villages of modern northern Zhejiang]. Shanghai: Shanghai yuandong chubanshe, 2001.

Cao Shuji 曹樹基 and Li Yushang 李玉尚. *Shuyi: Zhangzhen yu heping* 鼠疫：戰爭與和平 [Plague: War and peace]. Jinan, China: Shangdong huabao chubanshe, 2006.

Castiglioni, Arturo. *A History of Medicine.* Translated by E. B. Krumbhaar. New York: Knopf, 1941.

Chakrabarty, Dipesh. "Postcoloniality and the Artifice of History: Who Speaks for 'Indian' Pasts?" In *A Subaltern Studies Reader 1986–1995*, edited by Ranajit Guha, 263–93. Minneapolis: University of Minnesota Press, 1997.

———. *Provincializing Europe: Postcolonial Thought and Historical Difference.* Princeton, N.J.: Princeton University Press, 2000.

Chambers, David Wade, and Richard Gillespie. "Locality in the History of Science: Colonial Science, Technoscience, and Indigenous Knowledge." In *Nature and Empire: Science and the Colonial Enterprise*, edited by Roy MacLeod (Osiris, second series, vol. 15), 221–40. Chicago: University of Chicago Press, 2000.

Chang, Chia-feng 張嘉鳳. "Dispersing the Foetal Toxin of the Body: Conceptions of Smallpox Aetiology in Pre-Modern China." In *Contagion: Perspectives from Pre-*

modern Societies, edited by Lawrence I. Conrad and Dominik Wujastyk, 23–38. Aldershot, England: Ashgate, 2000.

———. "Yiji yu xiangran—yi 'Zhubing Yuanhou Lun' wei zhongxin shilun Wei-Jin zhi Sui-Tang zhijian yiji de jibing guan 疫疾與相染 — 以諸病源候論為中心試論魏晉至隋唐之間醫籍的疾病觀 [Disease, epidemics and mutual contamination—the concept of illness between the Wei-Jin and Sui-Tang Periods]." *Taida lishi xuebao* 台大歷史學報 27 (2001): 37–82.

Chao En-xiang 晁恩祥. "Guanyu zhongyiyao fang zhi Feidian gongzuo de sikao 觀于中醫藥防治非典工作的思考 [Analysis of work on the prevention and treatment of SARS with TCM]." *Tianjin zhongyiyao* 20, no. 4 (August 2003): 5–7.

Chao Yuanfang 巢元方. *Zhubing yuanhou lun* 諸病源候論 [On the origins and symptoms of all diseases]. Annotated ed. *Zhubing yuanhou zong lun jiao zhu* 諸病源候總論集注 [On the origins and symptoms of all diseases, annotated]. Beijing: Renmin weisheng chubanshe, 1996 [610].

Chatterjee, Partha. *Nationalist Thought and the Colonial World: A Derivative Discourse?* London: Zed Books for the United Nations University, 1986.

Chen, C. C. [Chen Zhiqian]. *Medicine in Rural China: A Personal Account*. Berkeley: University of California Press, 1989.

Chen, C. T., Y. T. Wu, and H. C. Hsieh. "Differences in Detectability of Minor Splenomegaly through Variation in the Recumbent Position of the Patient." *Journal of the Formosan Medical Association* 53, no. 9 (1954): 561–67.

Chen Chaochang 陳超常, Yuan Qilong 袁啓龍, and Ye Zhen 葉蓁. "Yinian lai Jiaxing dingluoshi tianran ganran zhuxuexichongbing weiyou zhi diaocha 一年來嘉興釘螺蛳天然感染住血吸蟲病尾蚴之調查 [A one-year study on schistosomiasis in snails in Jiaxing]." *Kexue* 32, no. 8 (1950): 242–44.

Chen Dongsheng 陳東升 and Wu Jialing 吳嘉苓. "Dushi, chuanran jibing yu shehui zhengyi 都市、傳染疾病與社會正義 [Cities, infectious disease, and social justice]." *Qingnian yanjiu xuebao* 7, no. 1 (January 2004): 83–96.

Chen Fu 陳敷. *Nong shu* 農書 [Book on agriculture]. *Siku quanshu* edition, vol. 730. Taibei, China: Shangwu yinshuguan, 1983 [1149].

Chen, J. W. H. "Pneumonic Plague in Harbin (Manchurian Epidemic, 1921)." *China Medical Journal* 1923: 7–17.

Chen, M. S., and C. L. Huang. "Industrial Workers' Health and Environmental Pollution under the New International Division of Labor: The Taiwan Experience." *American Journal of Public Health* 87, no. 7 (1997): 1223–31.

Chen Shaoxin 陳紹馨. *Taiwan de renkou bianqian yu shehui bianqian* 臺灣的人口變遷與社會變遷 [Population changes and social changes in Taiwan]. Taipei: Lianjin, 1979.

Chen Shou 陳壽. "Wu shu 吳書 [Book on the kingdom of Wu]." In *San guo zhi* 三國志 [History of the three kingdoms], *juan* 46–65:1093–1470. Beijing: Zhonghua shuju, 1982 [late 3rd century].

Chen Sicheng 陳司成. *Meichuang milu* 霉瘡秘錄 [Secret record of rotten sores]. Edition based on the 1885 edition. Beijing: Xueyuan chubanshe, 1994 [1632].

Chen Wanli 陳萬裏 and Pu Nangu 蒲南穀. "Zhejiangsheng fangzhi jiangpianchong-bing chubu gongzuo baogao 浙江省防治薑片蟲病初步工作報告 [Preliminary report on the prevention of fasciolopsiasis in Zhejiang Province]." *Zhonghua yixue zazhi* 23, no. 8 (1937): 1105–11.

Chen Yan 陳言. *Chen Wuze san yin fang* 陳無擇三因方 [Chen Yan on the three causes of diseases]. 1927. Reprint, Taipei: Tailian guofeng chubanshe, 1991 [1174].

Cheng Jiong 程迥. *Yijing zhengben shu* 醫經正本書 [Orthodox book on medical classics]. *Congshu jicheng* edition, 44:3–5. Taipei: Xinwenfeng chubanshe, 1985 [1176].

Cheyne, George. *The English Malady*. Edited with an introduction by Roy Porter. London: Routledge, 1991.

Christie, Dugald. *Thirty Years in Moukden, 1883–1913: Being the Experiences and Recollections of Dugald Christie*. London: Constable, 1914.

"Chuanranbing 傳染病 [Infectious disease]." *Yixue shijie* 醫學世界 6 (1908): 66–74.

Cohen, Lawrence. "Operability, Bioavailability, and Exception." In *Global Assemblages: Technology, Politics, and Ethics as Anthropological Problems*, edited by Aihwa Ong and Stephen J. Collier, 79–90. Oxford: Blackwell, 2005.

Cohen, Paul A. *China and Christianity: The Missionary Movement and the Growth of Chinese Antiforeignism, 1860–1870*. Cambridge: Harvard University Press, 1963.

Collingham, E. M. *Imperial Bodies: The Physical Experience of the Raj, c. 1800–1947*. Cambridge: Polity, 2001.

Conrad, Lawrence I. "A 9th-Century Muslim Scholar's Discussion of Contagion." In *Contagion: Perspectives from Pre-modern Societies*, edited by Lawrence I. Conrad and Dominik Wujastyk, 163–78. Aldershot, England: Ashgate, 2000.

Croizier, Ralph C. *Traditional Medicine in Modern China: Science, Nationalism, and the Tensions of Cultural Change*. Cambridge: Harvard University Press, 1968.

Cunningham, Andrew. "Transforming Plague: The Laboratory and the Identity of Infectious Disease." In *The Laboratory Revolution in Medicine*, edited by Andrew Cunningham and Perry Williams, 209–44. Cambridge: Cambridge University Press, 1992.

Cunningham, Andrew, and Perry Williams, eds. *The Laboratory Revolution in Medicine*. Cambridge: Cambridge University Press, 1992.

Darwin, Charles. *The Descent of Man, and Selection in Relation to Sex*. With an introduction by John Tyler Bonner and Robert M. May. Princeton, N.J.: Princeton University Press, 1981.

Darwin, John. "What Was the Late Colonial State?" *Itinerario* 23 (1999): 73–82.

Davis-Floyd, Robbie, and Carolyn F. Sargent, eds. *Childbirth and Authoritative Knowledge: Cross-Cultural Perspectives*. Berkeley: University of California Press, 1997.

De Chaumont, Francis, and Stephen Bennett Francois. "Practical Dietetics Especially in Relation to Preserved and Condensed Foods." In *Health Exhibition Literature*, vol. 6: *Health in Diet*, edited by Anonymous, 59–82. London: William Clowes and Sons, 1884.

Delaporte, François. *Disease and Civilization: The Cholera in Paris, 1832*. Translated by Arthur Goldhammer. Cambridge: MIT Press, 1986.

Dickersin, Kay, and Eric Manheimer. "The Cochrane Collaboration: Evaluation of Health Care and Services Using Systematic Reviews of the Results of Randomized Controlled Trials." *Clinical Obstetrics Gynecology* 41, no. 2 (June 1998): 315–31.

Dikotter, Frank. *Narcotic Culture: A History of Drugs in China*. Chicago: University of Chicago Press, 2004.

Ding Fubao 丁福保. *Zhong xi yifang huitong* 中西醫方彙編 [An integrated compilation of Chinese and Western medical formulas]. Shanghai: Wenming shuju, 1909.

Duara, Prasenjit. *The Global and Regional in China's Nation-Formation*. London: Routledge, 2009.

———. *Sovereignty and Authenticity: Manchukuo and the East Asian Modern*. Lanham, Md.: Rowman and Littlefield, 2003.

Dudgeon, John H. "Diet, Dress, and Dwellings of the Chinese in Relation to Health." In *Health Exhibition Literature*, vol. 19: *Miscellaneous Including Papers on China*, 253–486. London: William Clowes and Sons, 1884.

———. *The Diseases of China: Their Causes, Conditions, and Prevalence, Contrasted with Those of Europe*. Glasgow: Dunn and Wright, 1877.

———. "Dr. John Dudgeon's Report on the Health of Peking for the Half Year Ended 30th September, 1872." *Half-Yearly Medical Reports of the Chinese Maritime Customs* 6 (1874): 7–10.

———. "Dr. John Dudgeon's Report on the Physical Conditions of Peking, and the Habits of the Pekingese as Bearing upon Health (First Part)." *Half-Yearly Medical Reports of the Chinese Maritime Customs* 2 (1871): 73–82.

———. "Dr. John Dudgeon's Report on the Physical Conditions of Peking, and the Habits of the Pekingese as Bearing upon Health (Second Part)." *Half-Yearly Medical Reports of the Chinese Maritime Customs* 4 (1873): 29–42.

Dunell, G. R. "Great Britain. Food." In *Health Exhibition Literature*, vol. 18: *Miscellaneous Including Jury Awards and Official Catalogue*, edited by Anonymous, 189–92. London: William Clowes and Sons, 1884.

Echenberg, Myron. *Plague Ports: The Global Urban Impact of Bubonic Plague, 1894–1901*. New York: New York University Press, 2007.

Elman, Benjamin A. *A Cultural History of Modern Science in China*. New Histories of Science, Technology and Medicine. Cambridge: Harvard University Press, 2006.

———. *On Their Own Terms: Science in China 1550–1900*. Cambridge: Harvard University Press, 2005.

Evans, Charles W. DeLacy. *How to Prolong Life: An Inquiry into the Cause of Old Age and Natural Death; Showing the Diet and Agents Best Adapted for a Lengthened Prolongation of Existence*. London: Baillière, Tindall, and Cox, 1885.

Faber, Ernst. *Zixi cudong* 自西徂東 [From West to East]. Originally published as *Civilization, Chinese and Christian*. Shanghai: Shanghai shudian, 2002 [1884].

Fairbank, John King. "The Creation of the Treaty System." In *The Cambridge History of China*, vol. 10: *Late Ch'ing, 1800–1910*, edited by Denis Twitchett and John King Fairbank, part 1, 213–63. Cambridge: Cambridge University Press, 1978.

Fan Yen-choiu [Fan Yanqiu] 范燕秋. "Nüeji fangzhisuo 瘧疾防治所 [Malarial prevention station]." In *Taiwan lishi cidian* 臺灣歷史辭典 [Dictionary of Taiwan history], edited by Xu Xueji 許雪姬, 1032. Taipei: Xingzhengyuan wenhua jianshe weiyuanhui, 2004.

———. "Riben diguo fazhan xia zhimin Taiwan de renzhong weisheng (1895–1945) 日本帝國發展下殖民台灣的人種衛生(1895–1945) [Racial hygiene in colonial Taiwan under the development of Japanese imperialism]." Ph.D. diss., National Chengchi University, 2001.

———. "Yixue yu zhiming kuozhang: Yi rizhi shiqi Taiwan nüeji yanjiu weili 醫學與殖民擴張—以日治時期臺灣瘧疾研究為例 [Medicine and the colonial expansion: Taiwanese malaria research in the Japanese colonial period as an example]." *Xinshixue* 新史學 7, no. 3 (1996): 133–73.

Fan Ye 范曄. *Hou Han shu* 後漢書 [Book on the Later Han dynasty]. Beijing: Zhonghua shuju, 1966 [5th century].

Fan Zhenglun 樊正倫 and Zhang Xiaotong 張曉彤. "Zhongyi bu pa Feidian 中醫不怕非典 [Chinese medicine does not fear SARS]." Pamphlet distributed by the Cui Yueli Center of Research on Traditional Chinese Medicine in Beijing 北京 崔月犁傳統醫學研究中心, April 20, 2003.

Fang Bao 方苞. "Chen Yuxu muzhiming 陳馭虛墓誌銘 [Epitaph of Chen Yuxu]." In *Fang Bao ji* 方苞集 [Collection of Fang Bao], edited by Liu Jigao 劉季高, 295–96. Shanghai: Shanghai guji chubanshe, 1983 [1851].

Fang Xingzhun 范行准. *Zhonguo yufang yixue sixiang shi* 中國預防醫學思想史 [A history of Chinese preventive medical thought]. Shanghai: Hudong yiwu shenghuo chubanshe, 1953.

Farid, M. A. "Views and Reflections on Anti-Malaria Programs in the World." *Kaohsiung Journal of Medical Science* 7 (1991): 243–55.

Farmer, Paul, "SARS and Inequality." *Nation*, May 26, 2003, 6.

Fayrer, Joseph. *Tropical Dysentery and Chronic Diarrhoea*. London: J. and A. Churchill, 1880.

Fellman, Anita Clair, and Michael Fellman. *Making Sense of Self: Medical Advice Literature in Late Nineteenth-Century America*. Philadelphia: University of Pennsylvania Press, 1981.

Feng Huiling 馮惠玲, ed. *Gonggong weiji qishi lu dui SARS de duo wei shen shi* 公共危機啟示錄-對SARS 的多維審視 [Record of enlightening remarks on public crisis: Several remarkable and careful observations about SARS]. Beijing: Zhongguo renmin daxue chubanshe, 2003.

Fiddes, Nick. *Meat: A Natural Symbol*. London: Routledge, 1991.

Fidler, David P. "Germs, Governance, and Global Public Health in the Wake of SARS." *Journal of Clinical Investigation* 113, no. 6 (2004): 799–804.

———. *International Law and Infectious Diseases*. Oxford: Oxford University Press, 1999.

Finlay, Mark R. "Early Marketing of the Theory of Nutrition: The Science and Culture of Liebig's Extract of Meat." In *The Science and Culture of Nutrition, 1840-1940*, edited by Harmke Kamminga and Andrew Cunningham, 48–74. Amsterdam: Rodopi, 1995.

Fisher, Carney T. "Zhongguo lishi shang de shuyi 中國歷史上的鼠疫 [The plague in Chinese history]." Trans. Lin Yumei and Liu Cuirong. In *Jijian suo zhi: Zhongguo huanjing shi lunwen ji* 積漸所至: 中國環境史論文集 [Sediments of time: Environment and society in Chinese history], edited by Liu Cuirong (Liu T'sui-jung) 劉翠溶 and Mark Elvin, 673–747. Taipei: Zhongyang yanjiuyuan jingji yanjiusuo, 1995.

Fisher, Claude S. *America Calling: A Social History of the Telephone to 1940*. Berkeley: University of California Press, 1992.

Flohr, Carsten. "The Plague Fighter: Wu Lien-Teh and the Beginning of the Chinese Public Health System." *Annals of Science* 53 (1996): 360–81.

Fou Shanyong, ed. 缶善永, *Hainingshi weisheng zhi* 海甯市衛生志 [Public health history of Haining]. Unpublished manuscript. 1995.

Foucault, Michel. *Discipline and Punish: The Birth of the Prison*. Translated by Alan Sheridan. New York: Pantheon, 1977.

———. *The History of Sexuality*. Vol.1. Translated by Robert Hurley. New York: Pantheon, 1978.

Fu Daiwei 傅大為. *Yaxiya de xin shenti: Xingbie, yiliao, yu jindai Taiwan* 亞細亞的新身體: 性別、醫療、與近代台灣 [Assembling the new body: Gender/sexuality, medicine, and modern Taiwan]. Taipei: Qunxue, 2005.

Fu, Xiaobing, Hengguo Wang, and Zhiyong Sheng. "Advances in Wound Healing Research in China: From Antiquity to the Present." *Wound Repair and Regeneration* 9, no. 1 (2001): 2–10.

Gamsa, Mark. "The Epidemic of Pneumonic Plague in Manchuria 1910–1911." *Past & Present* 190 (February 2006): 147–84.

Ge Hong 葛洪. *Zhouhou beiji fang* 肘後備急方 [Handy recipes for urgent uses]. Beijing: Renmin weisheng chubanshe, 1983 [4th century].

Geertz, Clifford. "Found in Translation: On the Social History of the Moral Imagination." In *Local Knowledge: Further Essays in Interpretive Anthropology*, 36–54. New York: Basic, 1983.

Gesuidō Tokyo hyakunenshi hensan iinkai 下水道東京100年史編纂委員會, eds. (Editorial committee of the Hundred Year History of Tokyo sewer system). *Gesuidō Tokyo hyakunenshi* 下水道東京100年史 [Hundred-year history of the sewer system in Tokyo]. Tokyo: Tokyoto gesuidōkyoku, 1989.

Giddens, Anthony. "Risk Society." In *The Politics of Risk Society*, edited by Jane Franklin, 23–34. Oxford: Blackwell, 1998.

Ginzburg, Carlo. "Clues: Roots of an Evidential Paradigm." In *Clues, Myths, and the Historical Method*, edited by Carlo Ginzburg, 96–125. Baltimore: Johns Hopkins University Press, 1988.

Gong Tingxian 龔廷賢. *Jishi quanshu* 濟世全書 [Complete book to save the world]. In *Gong Tingxian yixue quanshu* 龔廷賢醫學全書 [Complete medical works by Gong Tingxian], edited by Li Shihua 李世華, 845–1088. Beijing: Zhongguo zhongyiyao chubanshe, 1999 [1636].

Gordon, Charles Alexander. *China from a Medical Point of View in 1860 and 1861: To Which Is Added a Chapter on Nagasaki as a Sanitarium*. London: John Churchill, 1863.

————. *An Epitome of the Reports of the Medical Officers to the Chinese Imperial Maritime Customs Service, from 1871 to 1882. With Chapters on the History of Medicine in China; Materia Medica; Epidemics; Famine; Ethnology; and Chronology in Relation to Medicine and Public Health*. London: Ballière, Tindall, and Cox, 1884.

Grant, Mark. *Galen on Food and Diet*. London: Routledge, 2000.

Greenfeld, Karl Taro. *China Syndrome: The True Story of the 21st Century's First Great Epidemic*. New York: Harper Collins Publishers, 2006.

Guo Liping 郭利平, Ma Rong 馬融, et al., eds. *SARS huanzhe huifu qi de zhongyiyao liaoxiao fenxi* SARS 患者恢复期的中醫藥療效分析 [Analysis of the curative effect of SARS patients treated by TCM during the recovery stage]. *Tianjin zhongyiyao* 20, no. 4 (August 2003): 12–13.

Guoshiguan 國史館 (Academia Historica), ed. *Taiwan zhuquan yu yige zhongkuo lunshu dashiji* 臺灣主權與一個中國論述大事紀 [A chronology of relevant events of Taiwan sovereignty and one-China discourse, 1943–2001]. Taipei: Guoshiguan, 2002.

Habib, S. Irfan, and Dhruv Raina, eds. *Situating the History of Science: Dialogues with Joseph Needham*. New Delhi: Oxford University Press, 1999.

————, eds. *The Social History of Science in Colonial India*. New Delhi: Oxford University Press, 2007.

Haebara Chōhō 南風朝原保. "Taiwan ni okeru nyūyōji shibō ni tsuite 台灣に於ける乳幼児死亡に就て [Infant and child death in Taiwan]." Privately published manuscript, Taipei: Haebara in 南風原醫院 [Haebara Hospital], 1938.

————. "Taiwan ni okeru nyūji hashōfū ni tsuite 台灣に於ける乳兒破傷風に就て [Tetanus among infants and children in Taiwan]." *Nihon kōshū hoken kyōkai zasshi* 14 (1938): 1–11.

Hai Xia 海霞. 2003. "Guangdong sheng zhongyiyuan zhiliao Feidianxing feiyan linchuang jingyan 廣東省中醫院治療非典型肺炎臨床經驗 [Clinical experiences of treating SARS lung inflammation in Guangdong Hospital of TCM]." *Tianjin zhongyiyao: Feidian zhuanti* [Tianjin journal of traditional Chinese medicine: Special papers on SARS] 20, no. 3 (June 2003): 24–25.

Hangzhoushi zhi. Weisheng pian 杭州市志衛生篇 [Gazetteer of Hangzhou City. Public health section]. Mimeograph in Hangzhoushi weishengju tushushi 杭州市衛生局圖書室 [Library of Hangzhou Municipal Health Bureau].

Hanson, Marta. "Inventing a Tradition in Chinese Medicine: From Universal Canon to Local Medical Knowledge in South China, the 17th to the 19th Century." Ph.D. diss., University of Pennsylvania, 1997.

———. "Robust Northerners and Delicate Southerners: The Nineteenth-Century Invention of a Southern Medical Tradition." In *Innovation in Chinese Medicine*, edited by Elizabeth Hsu, 262–91. Cambridge: Cambridge University Press, 2001.

———. Review of *At the Epicentre: Hong Kong and the SARS Outbreak*, by Christine Loh and Civic Exchange, eds. *China Review International* 13, no. 1 (2006): 218–24.

Harris, Sheldon. *Factories of Death: Japanese Biological Warfare 1932–45 and the American Coverup*. London: Routledge, 1994.

Harrison, Mark. *Climates and Constitutions: Health, Race, Environment and British Imperialism in India, 1600–1800*. New Delhi: Oxford University Press, 1999.

———. *Public Health in British India: Anglo-Indian Preventive Medicine, 1859–1914*. Cambridge: Cambridge University Press, 1994.

———. "Science and the British Empire." *Isis* 96 (2005): 56–63.

———. "'The Tender Frame of Man': Disease, Climate, and Racial Difference in India and West Indies, 1760–1860." *Bulletin of the History of Medicine* 70, no. 1 (spring 1996): 68–93.

Hatori Shigeo 羽鳥重郎. "Taiwan oyobi nanpō shokuminchi hikaku eisei tōkei 台灣及南方殖民地比較衛生統計 [Comparative health statistics in Taiwan and the colonies in the south]." *Taiwan igakkai zasshi* 173 (1917): 163–83.

Hayashizawa Eijirō 林澤榮次郎. "Shoseiji hashōfū no jikken 初生兒破傷風の實驗 [Experiment of tetanus treatment for the newborn]." *Taiwan igakkai zasshi* 52 (1907): 63–67.

Haynes, Douglas M. *Imperial Medicine: Patrick Manson and the Conquest of Tropical Disease*. Philadelphia: University of Pennsylvania Press, 2001.

He Gangde 何剛德 ed. "Fujun nongchan kaolüe 撫郡農產考略 [A brief survey of agriculture in Fuzhou]." In *Zhongguo jindai nongye shi ziliao* 中國近代農業史資料 [Notes on Chinese agricultural history], edited by Li Wenzhi 李文治, 1:593–94. Beijing: Sanlian shudian, 1957.

He Lianchen 何廉臣. *Quanguo mingyi yan'an leibian* 全國名醫驗案類編 [A compilation of cases from the experience of nationally renowned doctors]. Shanghai: Dadong shuju, 1929.

———. "Yi yu guojia guanxi lun 醫與國家關係論 [On the relationship between medicine and the state]." *Yixue zazhi* 醫學雜誌 [Magazine of medicine], no. 59 (1930): 15–18.

Health Canada. "Learning from SARS: Renewal of Public Health in Canada." A report of the National Advisory Committee on SARS and Public Health, October 2003. Publication number 1210. http://www.phac-aspc.gc.ca/publicat/sars-sras/naylor/index.html.

Heaton, Charles. *Medical Hints for Hot Climates and for Those out of Reach of Professional Aid*. London: W. Thacker, 1897.

Henderson, James. *Shanghai Hygiene or Hints for Preservation of Health in China*. Shanghai: Presbyterian Mission Press, 1863.

Henry, Todd. "Sanitizing Empire: Japanese Articulations of Korean Otherness and the Construction of Early Colonial Seoul, 1905–1919." *Journal of Asian Studies* 64, no. 3 (August 2005): 639–75.

Hevia, James. *English Lessons: The Pedagogy of Imperialism in Nineteenth-century China*. Durham, N.C.: Duke University Press 2003.

Heymann, David. Preface. In *SARS: The Truth behind the WHO*, by Esther Lam, ii–iv. Hong Kong: Infowide Publication, 2003.

Hirst, L. Fabian. *The Conquest of Plague: A Study of the Evolution of Epidemiology*. Oxford: Clarendon Press of Oxford University Press, 1953.

Hitōgawa Hachigorō 下村八五郎. "Tainanshōshita niokeru mararia bōatsusagyō no jisai to sono seiseki" 臺南州下ニ於ケルマラリア防遏作業ノ實際ト其成績 [The situation and the achievement of malaria prevention in Tainan]." *Taiwan igakkai zasshi* 臺灣醫學會雜誌 34 (1935): 56–76.

Hong Kong Baptist University. School of Chinese Medicine. *Xianggang jinhui daxue Zhongyi xueyuan kang yanxing dong shilu* 香港浸會大學中醫學院抗炎行動實錄 [Hong Kong Baptist University School of Chinese Medicine records of infection-fighting activities]. Hong Kong: Jinhui daxue zhongyiyao xueyuan mishu chu, 2003.

Hong Kong Government Logistics Department. *SARS in Hong Kong: From Experience to Action: A Summary Report of the SARS Expert Committee*. Hong Kong: Government Logistics Department, 2003.

Hong Kong Hospital Authority. *Report of the Hospital Authority Review Panel on the SARS Outbreak*. Hong Kong: Hospital Authority, 2003.

Hong Kong Museum of Medical Sciences Society. *Plague, SARS and the Story of Medicine in Hong Kong*. Hong Kong: Hong Kong University Press, 2006.

Hong Mai 洪邁. *Yijian zhi* 夷堅志 [Record of Yijian]. *Siku quanshu* edition, *juan* 1047. Taibei, China: Shangwu yinshuguan, 1983 [Southern Song].

Hong Youxi 洪有錫 and Chen Lixin 陳麗新. *Xianshengma, chanpo, yu fuchanke yishi* 先生媽、產婆、與婦產科醫師 [Lay midwives, certified midwives, and obstetricians]. Taipei: Qianwei, 2002.

Hoong, Chua Mui, Maria Almenoar, and Teh Joo Lin, eds. *A Defining Moment: How Singapore Beat SARS*. Singapore: Institute of Policy Studies, 2004.

Horiuchi Tsuguo 崛內次雄. "Taiwan nyūyōji shibō no bōshisaku 台灣乳幼兒死亡の防止策 [Policies for reducing infant and child death in Taiwan]." *Taiwan shakai-jigyō no tomo* 18 (1930): 190–95.

House, Edward H. *Japanese Expedition to Formosa*. Tokyo, 1875.

Howard-Jones, Norman. *The Scientific Background of the International Sanitary Conferences 1851–1938*. Geneva: World Health Organization, 1975.

Hsiung Ping-chen 熊秉真. *Youyou: Chuantong Zhongguo de qiangbao zhi dao* 幼幼：傳統中國的襁褓之道 [Infant care in traditional China]. Taipei: Lianjing, 1995.

Hsu, Hong-Yen, and Su-Yen Wang. 1985. *The Theory of Feverish Diseases and Its Clinical Applications*. Long Beach, Calif.: Oriental Healing Arts Institute, 1985.

Huang Pi-Sung 黃碧松 et al., eds. *2004 nian wenbing guoji xueshu yantaohui* 2004 年溫病國際學術研討會 [2004 international academic research on *wenbing*]. Taibei, Taiwan: Cheng Sui-Tsung, 2004.

Huang Shaohong 黃紹竑. *Wushi huiyi* 五十回憶 [Memories at fifty]. Changsha, China: Yuelu shushe, 1999.

Huang Yulan 黃玉蘭. *Shiyong linchuang chuanranbing xue* 實用臨床傳染病學 [Practical and clinical epidemiology of infectious disease]. Beijing: Renmin junyi chubanshe, 1990.

Huangdi neijing suwen 黃帝內經素問 [The Yellow Emperor's inner canon: Plain questions]. Beijing: Renmin weisheng chubanshe, 1994 [1st century].

Huazhong shifan daxue lishi yanjiusuo, Suzhou shi dang'an'guan (Institute of History of Huazhong Normal University, and Suzhou Municipal Archives) 華中師範大學歷史研究所、蘇州市檔案館, ed. *Suzhou shanghui dang'an congbian* 蘇州商會檔案叢編 [A collection of archival texts of commercial associations in Suzhou]. Vol. 1: *1905–1911*. Wuhan, China: Huazhong shifan daxue chubanshe, 1991.

Hunt, Nancy Rose. *A Colonial Lexicon: Of Birth Ritual, Medicalization, and Mobility in the Congo*. Durham, N.C.: Duke University Press, 1999.

Iijima Wataru 飯島涉. "Infectious and Parasitic Disease Studies in Taiwan, Manchuria, and Korea under the Japanese Empire: Brief History of Japanese Colonial Medicine." Paper presented at the International Conference on the Ideas, Organization, and Practice of Hygiene in Han Society from the Traditional to the Modern Periods, Research Center for Humanities and Social Sciences, Academia Sinica, Taipei, November 22–23, 2004.

———. *Pesuto to kindai Chūgoku: Eisei no "seidoka" to shakai henyō* ペストと近代中國：衞生の「制度化」と社會変容 [Plague and modern China: The institutionalization of public health and social change]. Tokyo: Kenbun shuppan, 2000.

International Plague Conference. Report of the International Plague Conference held at Mukden, April 1911. Manila: Bureau of Printing, 1912.

Irwin, Alan. *Risk and the Control of Technology: Public Policies for Road Traffic Safety in Britain and the United States*. Dover, N.H.: Manchester University Press, 1985.

Jamieson, Robert Alexander. "Dr. Alexander Jamieson's Report on the Health of Shanghai for the Half Year Ended 30th September, 1871." *Half-Yearly Medical Reports of the Chinese Maritime Customs* 2 (1871): 33–43.

———. "Dr. Alexander Jamieson's Report on the Health of Shanghai for the Half Year Ended 30th September, 1873." *Half-Yearly Medical Reports of the Chinese Maritime Customs* 6 (1874): 54–69.

Jarcho, Saul. "Galen's Six Non-naturals: A Bibliographic Note and Translation." *Bulletin of the History of Medicine* 44, no. 4 (July–August 1970): 372–77.

Jasanoff, Sheila. *Risk Management and Political Culture: A Comparative Analysis of Science.* New York: Russell Sage Foundation, 1986.

Jiang Zhichai 蔣芷儕. "Dumen shi xiaolu 都門識小錄 [Brief record of the capital]." In *Qing dai yeshi* 清代野史 [Unofficial history of the Qing dynasty], 4:243–86. Chengdu, China: Bashu shushe, 1987 [1920].

Jiaxing difang jianshe xiehui xianzheng jianshe kaochatuan baogaoshu ji fulu 嘉興地方建設協會縣政建設考察團報告書及附錄 [County constructions survey report of the Jiaxing government]. Special issue of *Jiaxing minguo shibao* 嘉興民國時報, 1937.

Jiaxingshi zhengxie wenshi ziliao weiyuanhui (Committee of the Compilation of Cultural Materials of Jiaxing Municipality) 嘉興市政協文史資料委員會. *Song wenshen: Jiaxing diqu xuefang gongzuo jishi* 送瘟神:嘉興地區血防工作紀實 [Farewell to the plague god: Prevention of schistosomiasis in Jiaxing]. Beijing: Zhongguo kexue jishu chubanshe, 1995.

Jiaxingshi zhi bianzuan weiyuanhui (Editorial Committee of the Jiaxing Muncipal Gazetteer) 嘉興市志編纂委員會. *Jiaxingshi zhi* 嘉興市志 [Gazetteer of Jiaxing City]. Beijing: Zhongguo shuji chubanshe, 1997.

Jones, Alfred G. *North China English Baptist Mission: Hints about Climate, Living and Outfit, &C., Intended for the General Information of Missionaries Proceeding Thither.* London: Alexander and Shepheard, 1884.

Jones, Margaret. "Infant and Maternal Health Services in Ceylon, 1900–1948." *Social History of Medicine* 15 (2002): 263–89.

Kamminga, Harmke. "Nutrition for the People, or the Fate of Jacob Moleschott's Contests for a Humanist Science." In *The Science and Culture of Nutrition, 1840–1940*, edited by Harmke Kamminga and Andrew Cunningham, 15–47. Amsterdam: Rodopi, 1995.

Kamminga, Harmke, and Andrew Cunningham. Introduction. In *The Science and Culture of Nutrition, 1840–1940*, edited by Harmke Kamminga and Andrew Cunningham, 1–14. Amsterdam: Rodopi, 1995.

Kantō Totokufu Rinji Bōkibu (Plague Prevention Department of the Kanto Government) 關東都督府臨時防疫部. *Meiji yonjūsan-yonen Minami Manshū "pesuto" ryūkōshi. Furoku, shashinchō* 明治四十三、四年南滿洲「ペスト」流行誌.附錄・寫眞帖 [The plague in south Manchuria, 1910–11. Appendix, illustrated with photographs taken on the spot]. Port Arthur, Manchuria: Kantō Totokufu Rinji Bōekibu, 1912.

Keller, Richard C. *Colonial Madness: Psychiatry in French North Africa.* Chicago: University of Chicago Press, 2007.

King, F. H. *Farmers of Forty Centuries or Permanent Agriculture in China, Korea, and Japan.* 1911. Reprinted as *Farmers of Forty Centuries: Organic Farming in China, Korea, and Japan.* Mineola, N.Y.: Dover Publications, 2004.

King, Nicholas B. "Security, Disease, Commerce: Ideologies of Postcolonial Global Health." *Social Studies of Science* 32 (2002): 763–89.

Klein, Susan. *A Book for Midwives: A Manual for Traditional Birth Attendants and Community Midwives*. Palo Alto, Calif.: Hesperian Foundation, 1995.

Kleinman, Arthur. "The Background and Development of Public Health in China: An Exploratory Essay." In *Public Health in the People's Republic of China*, edited by Myron E. Wegman, Tsung-Yi Lin, and Elizabeth F. Purcell, 5–25. New York: Josiah Macy Jr. Foundation, 1973.

———. "Concepts and a Model for the Comparison of Medical Systems as Cultural Systems." *Social Science and Medicine* 12 (1978): 85–93.

———. "Toward a Comparative Study of Medical Systems." *Science, Medicine and Man* 1 (1973): 55–65.

Kleinman, Arthur, and Everett Mendelsohn. "Systems of Medical Knowledge: A Comparative Approach." *Journal of Medicine and Philosophy* 3 (1978): 314–30.

Kleinman, Arthur, and James Watson, eds. *SARS in China: Prelude to Pandemic?* Stanford: Stanford University Press, 2006.

Kline, Ronald, and Trevor Pinch. "Users as Agents of Technological Change: The Social Construction of the Automobile in the Rural United States." *Technology and Culture* 37 (1996): 763–95.

Kobayashi Hiroshi 小林博, ed. *Hikone shi no mararia taisaku* 彦根市ノマラリア對策 [Malaria strategies in Hikone City]. Hikone, Japan: Hikone shi eiseika, 1951.

Kobayashi Shigeru 小林茂. *Nihon shinyō mondai genryū kō* 日本屎尿問題源流考 [The origin of the question of excrement treatment in Japan]. Tokyo: Akashi shoten, 1983.

Kobayashi Takehiro 小林丈広. *Kindai nihon to kōshū eisei: Toshishakaishi no kokoromi* 近代日本と公衆衛生：都市社會史の試み [Modern Japan and public health: An attempt at urban social history]. Tokyo: Yuzankaku shuppan, 2001.

Koh, Tommy, Aileen Plant, and Eng Hin Lee, eds. *The New Global Threat: Severe Acute Respiratory Syndrome and Its Impacts*. Singapore: World Scientific, 2003.

Koseishō Imukyoku 厚生省醫務局. *Isei hachijūnen shi* 醫制八十年史 [Eighty years of history of medical institutions]. Tokyo: Koseishō imukyoku, 1955.

Kumar, Deepak. *Science and the Raj: A Study of British India*. Oxford: Oxford University Press, 2006.

Kuriyama, Shigehisa. *The Expressiveness of the Body and the Divergence of Greek and Chinese Medicine*. New York: Zone, 1999.

Laderman, Carol. *Wives and Midwives: Childbirth and Nutrition in Rural Malaysia*. Berkeley: University of California Press, 1983.

Lam, Esther. *SARS: The Truth behind the WHO*. Hong Kong: Infowide Publication, 2003.

Leavitt, Judith Walzer. *Brought to Bed: Child-Bearing in America 1750–1950*. New York: Oxford University Press, 1986.

Lee, Chor Lin, and Bryan van der Beek. *38°C: Remembering SARS*. Singapore: Singapore History Museum, 2004.

Lee, Hsien Long. "DPM Lee's May Day Rally Speech." Ministry of Foreign Affairs

press release. May 1, 2003. http://www.moh.gov.sg/mohcorp/speeches.aspx
?id=1710.

Lei, Sean Hsiang-lin. "From *Changshan* to a New Anti-malarial Drug: Re-networking
Chinese Drugs and Excluding Chinese Doctors." *Social Studies of Science* 29,
no. 3 (June 1999): 323–58.

———. "Habituate Individuality: Framing of Tuberculosis and Its Material Solutions in Republican China." Paper presented at the annual meeting of the Association for Asian Studies, Chicago, March 31 to April 3, 2005.

———. "When Chinese Medicine Encountered the State: 1910–1949." Ph.D. diss.,
University of Chicago, 1999.

———. "Why *Weisheng* Is Not about Guarding Life: Alternative Conceptions of
Hygiene, Self, and Illness in Republican China." Translated by Sabine Wilms.
Forthcoming in *East Asian Science, Technology and Society*.

Leslie, Charles, ed. *Asian Medical Systems: A Comparative Study*. Berkeley: University of California Press, 1976.

———. Introduction. In *Asian Medical Systems: A Comparative Study*, edited by
Charles Leslie, 1–17. Berkeley: University of California Press, 1976.

Leung, Angela K. C. 梁其姿. "Jibing yu fangtu zhi guanxi: Yuan zhi Qing jian yijie de
kanfa 疾病與方土之關係：元至清間醫界的看法 [Disorders and locality: Views of
doctors from the Yuan to the Qing]." In *Xingbie yu yiliao* 性別與醫療 [Gender and
medicine], edited by Huang Kewu 黃克武, 162–212. Taipei: Zhongyang yanjiuyuan jindai yanjiusuo, 2002.

———. *Shishan yu jiaohua* 施善與教化 [Charity and moral transformation]. Taipei:
Lianjing chubanshe, 1997.

Leung, Ping Chung, and Eng Eong Ooi, eds. *SARS War: Combating the Disease*. River
Edge, N.J.; Hong Kong: World Scientific, 2003.

Li Bozhong 李伯重. "Ming-Qing Jiangnan feiliao xuqiu de shuliang fenxi 明清江南
肥料需求的數量分析 [Quantitative analysis of night soil fertilizer in Jiangnan
during the Ming and Qing dynasties]." *Qingshi yanjiu* 清史研究 1 (1999): 30–38.

Li Guoqi 李國祁. *Zhongguo xiandaihua de quyu yanjiu: Min Zhe Tai diqu, 1860–1916*
中國現代化的區域研究：閩浙臺地區，1860–1916 [Regional study of Chinese
modernization in Fujan, Zhejiang, and Taiwan, 1860–1916]. Taipei: Institute of
Modern History, Academia Sinica, 1982.

Li Jianmin 李建民. "Contagion and Its Consequences: The Problem of Death Pollution in Ancient China." In *Medicine and the History of the Body: Proceedings of the
20th, 21st, and 22nd International Symposium on the Comparative History of Medicine*, edited by Shigehisa Kuriyama et al., 201–22. Ishiyaku EuroAmerica, 1999.

———. "Xian Qin liang Han bingyin guan ji qi bianqian—yi xin chutu wenwu wei
zhongxin 先秦兩漢病因觀及其變遷—以新出土文物為中心 [Etiological concepts
and their changes in the Qin and Han dynasties, based on recent archaeological
findings]." Unpublished manuscript. September 2006.

Li Shang-Jen (Shang-Jen Li). "Moral Economy and Health: John Dudgeon on Hygiene in China." *Bulletin of the Institute of History and Philology* 76, no. 3 (2005): 467–509.

Li Shizhen 李時珍. *Bencao gangmu* 本草綱目 [Compendium of *materia medica*]. Facsimile of the 1885 edition. Taipei: Wenguang tushu gongsi, 1955 [1579–93].

Li Shunbao 李順保, ed. *Wenbingxue quanshu* 溫病學全書 [Complete collection of warm disease studies]. Beijing: Xueyuan chubanshe, 2002.

Li Wei 李偉, Chen Xiumin 陳秀敏, and Guo Hongjie 郭宏杰. "Shirun shaoshanggao zhiliao ruchuang 33 li liaoxiao guancha 濕潤燒傷膏治療褥瘡33例療效觀察 [Clinical efficacy of MEBO in treating bedsores in thirty-three cases]." *Guoyi luntan* 國醫論壇 18 (2003): 31.

Li Weipu 李蔚普. "Lei xuexicongbing de zhongyi wenxian ziliao 類血吸蟲病的中醫文獻資料 [Sources from Chinese medicine on quasi-schistosomiasis]." *Jiangxi zhongyiyao* 10 (October 1955): 22–33.

Li Yushang 李玉尚. "Huanjing yu ren: Jiangnan chuanranbingshi yanjiu (1820–1953) 環境與人：江南傳染病史研究 (1820–1953) [Environment and man: A study on the history of Jiangnan infectious diseases (1820–1953)]." Ph.D. diss., Fudan University, 2003.

———. "Jindai Zhongguo shuyi duiying jizhi 近代中國鼠疫對應機制 [Coping mechanisms for the plague in modern China]." *Lishi yanjiu* 歷史研究 1 (2002): 114–27.

Liang Gengyao 梁庚堯. "Nan Song chengshi de gonggong weisheng wenti 南宋城市的公共衛生問題 [Public health problems of Southern Song cities]." *Zhongyang yanjiuyuan lishi yuyan yanjiusuo jikan* 中央研究院歷史語言研究所集刊 70, no. 1 (1999): 119–63.

Liang Peiji 梁培基. "Shang fangbian yiyuan lun zhiyi fangyi shu 上方便醫院論治疫防疫書 [Letter on treating and preventing the plague submitted to the hospital]." *Zhongxi yixue bao* 中西醫學報 [Journal of Chinese and Western medicine] (1911): 1–6.

Liang Qingyin 梁慶寅, ed. *Feidian: Fansi yu duice* 非典:反思與對策 [SARS: Retrospection and countermeasures]. Guangzhou: Zhongshan daxue chubanshe, 2003.

Liang Qizi. See Leung, Angela K. C.

Lin Chin-ju. "Transforming Patriarchal Kinship Relations: Four Generations of 'Modern Women' in Taiwan, 1900–1999." Ph.D. diss., University of Essex, 2003.

Litt, Jacquelyn. *Medicalized Motherhood: Perspectives from the Lives of African-American and Jewish Women*. New Brunswick, N.J.: Rutgers University Press, 2000.

Liu Baoyan 劉保延 et al. "Zhong xi yi jiehe zaoqi ganyu dui SARS feibu yanzheng de yingxiang 中西醫結合早期干預對SARS肺部炎症的影響 [Effect of early intervention with integrated Chinese and Western medicine on pulmonary inflammation in SARS]." *Tianjin zhongyiyao* 21, no. 4 (August 2004): 268–71.

Liu Chun 劉純. *Liu Chun yixue quanshu* 劉純醫學全書 [Complete medical works of Liu Chun]. Beijing: Zhongguo zhongyiyao chubanshe, 1999 [late 14th–early 15th centuries].

Liu Cuirong 劉翠溶 and Liu Shiyong 劉士永. "Taiwan lishishang de jibing yu siwang 臺灣歷史上的疾病與死亡 [Disease and mortality in the history of Taiwan]." *Taiwan shi yanjiu* 臺灣史研究 4, no. 2 (1998): 90–132.

Liu Guohui. *Warm Diseases: A Clinical Guide*. Seattle: Eastland, 2001.

Liu Jinzao 劉錦藻. *Qingchao xu wenxian tongkao* 清朝續文獻通考 [General compilation of Qing institutions]. Hangzhou, China: Zhejiang guji chubanshe, 1988 [1912].

Liu, Lydia H. *The Clash of Empires: The Invention of China in Modern World Making*. Cambridge: Harvard University Press, 2004.

Liu Mei 劉梅. "Tian Fenlan jiaoshou tan zhongyi zhiliao 'Feidian' 田芬蘭教授談中醫治療非典 [Professor Tian Fenlan's discussion on using Chinese medicine to treat SARS]." *Tianjin zhongyiyao* 20, no. 4 (August 2003): 17–18.

Liu Shiyung 劉士永. "Differential Mortality in Colonial Taiwan (1895–1945)." *Annales de Démographie Historique* 1 (2004): 229–47.

———. "'Qingjie,' 'weisheng,' yu 'baojian': Rizhi shidai Taiwan shehui gonggong weishengnian de gaibian 「清潔」,「衛生」, 與「保健」：日治時代台灣社會公共衛生念的改變 ['Sanitation,' 'hygiene,' and 'public health': Changing thoughts on public health in colonial Taiwan]." *Taiwanshi yanjiu* 台灣史研究 8, no. 1 (2001): 41–88.

Liu Tingchun 劉庭春. *Riben ge zhengzhi jigou canguan xiangji* 日本各政治機構參觀詳記 [Detailed account of various Japanese political institutions visited]. 1907. Reprinted in *Riben zhengfa kaocha ji* 日本政法考察記 [Account of the visit to Japan's political and legal institutions], edited by Liu Xuemei 劉雪梅 and Liu Yuzhen 劉雨珍, 293–348. Shanghai: Shanghai guji chubanshe, 2002.

Liu, X., et al. "Chinese Herbs Combined with Western Medicine for Severe Acute Respiratory Syndrome (SARS)." *Cochrane Database of Systematic Reviews* 2 (January 2006): 1–68.

Liu Xuemei 劉雪梅 and Liu Yuzhen 劉雨珍, eds. *Riben zhengfa kaocha ji* 日本政法考察記 [Account of the visit to Japan's political and legal institutions]. Shanghai: Shanghai guji chubanshe, 2002.

Livingstone, David N. "Tropical Climate and Moral Hygiene: The Anatomy of a Victorian Debate." *British Journal for the History of Science* 32, part 1 (March 1999): 93–110.

Livingstone, Frank B. "Anthropological Implications of Sickle Cell Gene Distribution in West Africa." *American Anthropologist* 60 (1958): 533–62.

Lloyd, G. E. R., edited with an introduction. *Hippocratic Writings*, New York: Penguin Books, 1978.

Lloyd, G. E. R., and Nathan Sivin. *The Way and the Word: Science and Medicine in Early China and Greece*. New Haven, Conn.: Yale University Press, 2002.

Lo, Ming-cheng. *Doctors within Borders: Profession, Ethnicity, and Modernity in Colonial Taiwan*. Berkeley: University of California Press, 2002.

Lu Shizhong 路時中. *Wushang xuanyuan santian yutang dafa* 无上玄元三天玉堂大法 [Great method of the Jade Hall of the Three Heavens, of the supreme mysterious origin]. In *Zhonghua Daozang* 中華道藏 [Chinese Daoist canon], edited by Zhang Jiyu 張繼禹, *juan* 30. Beijing: Huaxia chubanshe, 2004 [ca. 12th century].

Lu Yunchang 陸允昌, ed. *Suzhou yangguan shiliao* 蘇州洋關史料 [Historical sources on foreign customs in Suzhou]. Nanjing: Nanjing daxue chubanshe, 1991.

Lusby, P. E., A. B. Coombes, and J. M. Wilkinson. "Honey: A Potent Agent for Wound Healing?" *Journal of Wound, Ostomy and Continence Nursing* 29, no. 6 (2002): 295–300.

Ma Xiaonan 馬筱楠. "Zhongyi zhuanjia: Linchuang jingyan zhengming zhongyao fangzhi feidian queshi you xiao 中醫專家:臨床經驗證明中藥防治非典確實有效 [Chinese medicine specialist: Clinical experience proves that treating SARS with Chinese herbs is truly effective]." *Shanghai qingnian bao* [Shanghai youth journal], April 24, 2003, pp. 1–2.

MacLeod, Roy. Introduction. In *Nature and Empire: Science and the Colonial Enterprise*, edited by Roy MacLeod (Osiris, second series, vol. 15), 1–13. Chicago: University of Chicago Press, 2000.

MacPherson, Kerrie L. *A Wilderness of Marshes: The Origins of Public Health in Shanghai, 1843–1893*. Hong Kong: Oxford University Press, 1987.

Manderson, Lenore. *Sickness and the State: Health and Illness in Colonial Malaya, 1870–1940*. Cambridge: Cambridge University Press, 1996.

Manheimer, Eric, and Brian Berman. "The Cochrane Column: Exploring, Evaluating, and Applying the Results of Systematic Reviews of CAM Therapies." *Explore* 1, no. 3 (May 2005): 210–15.

Manshū Ika daigaku; Minami Manshū Tetsudō Kabushiki Kaisha. Eiseika (Manchuria Medical School, and Public Health Section of the South Manchurian Railroad Co. Ltd) 滿洲醫科大學; 南滿洲鐵道株式會社. 衛生課. *Manshū Ika Daigaku daiikkai Tōmōjunkai shinryōhokoku: Taishō12 nen natsu* 滿洲醫科大學第一回東蒙巡廻診療報告: 大正十二年夏 [Report of the Manchuria Medical School First Mobile Clinic to East Mongolia]. Dairen, Manchuria: Mantetsu Eiseika, 1923.

Manshū Kekkaku Yobō Kyōkai (Manchurian TB Prevention Society) 滿洲結核豫防協會. *Manshū eisei no jittai chōsa* 滿洲衛生の實態調查 [On-the-Ground Survey of the Hygiene of Manchuria]. Hsinkyo: Manshū Kekkaku Yobō Kyōkai, 1939.

Manson, Patrick. "Dr. P. Manson's Report on the Health of Amoy for the Half Year Ended 30th September 1881." *Half-Yearly Medical Reports of the Chinese Maritime Customs* 22 (1882): 1–3.

Manson, Patrick, and David Manson. "The Drs. Mansons' Report on the Health of Amoy for the Half Year Ended 30th September 1873." *Half-Yearly Medical Reports of the Chinese Maritime Customs* 6 (1874): 20–32.

Mao Zedong 毛澤東. *Jianguo yilai Mao Zedong wengao* 建國以來毛澤東文稿 [Selected writings of Mao Zedong since 1949]. Vol. 8. Beijing: Zhongyang wenxian chubanshe, 1992 [1958].

———. *Mao Zedong shuxin ji* 毛澤東書信集 [Collection of Mao Zedong's letters]. Beijing: Renmin chubanshe, 1983.

———. *On New Democracy*. Peking: Foreign Languages Press, 1964 [1940].

Martin, Emily. *The Woman in the Body: A Cultural Analysis of Reproduction.* Boston: Beacon Press, 1987.

Martin, James Ronald. *The Influence of Tropical Climates on European Constitutions.* London: John Churchill, 1856.

McGaw, Judith A. "No Passive Victims, No Separate Spheres: A Feminist Perspective on Technology's History." In *In Context: History and the History of Technology; Essays in Honor of Melvin Kranzberg,* edited by Stephen H. Cutcliffe and Robert C. Post, 172–91. Bethlehem, Pa.: Lehigh University Press, 1989.

McKeown, Thomas. *The Role of Medicine: Dream, Mirage, or Nemesis.* Princeton, N.J.: Princeton University Press, 1979.

Meleney, Henry Edmund, and Ernest Carroll Faust. "The Intermediate Host of Schistosome Japonicum in China." *China Medical Journal* 37, no. 7 (July 1923): 547.

Mendelsohn, J. Andrews. "From Eradication to Equilibrium: How Epidemics Became Complex after World War I." In *Greater Than the Parts: Holism in Biomedicine, 1920–1950,* edited by Christopher Lawrence and George Weisz, 303–31. New York: Oxford University Press, 1998.

Meng Shujiang 孟澍江, ed. *Wenbing xue* 溫病學 [Warm disease studies]. Shanghai: Shanghai kexue jishu chubanshe, 1985.

Milles, Dietrich. "Working Capacity and Calorie Consumption: The History of Rational Political Economy." In *The Science and Culture of Nutrition, 1840–1940,* edited by Harmke Kamminga and Andrew Cunningham, 75–96. Amsterdam: Rodopi, 1995.

Minami Manshū Tetsudō Kabushiki Kaisha; Eiseika (Public Health Section of the South Manchurian Railroad Co. Ltd) 南滿洲鐵道株式會社. 衛生課. *Kōtoku ninendo pesuto bōeki gaikyō* 康德二年度ペスト防疫概況 [General report on epidemic prevention work in the Kangde 2 plague]. Hōten (Fengtian), Manchukuo: Minami Manshū Tetsudō Kabushiki Kaisha, 1936.

———. *Manshū fūdo eisei kenkyū gaiyō* 滿洲風土衞生研究概要 [Outline of research on the hygiene of Manchurian natural conditions and social customs]. Dairen (Dalian), Manchuria: Minami Manshū Tetsudō Kabushiki Kaisha Chihōbu Eiseika, 1936.

———. *Minami Manshū Tetsudō fuzokuchi eisei gaikyō: Shōwa 3 nendo* 南滿洲鐵道附屬地衞生概況: 昭和3年度 [Sanitary conditions of the lands administered by the South Manchurian Railway: Report for 1928]. Dairen (Dalian), Manchuria: Minami Manshū Tetsudō Kabushiki Kaisha Chihōbu Eiseika, 1930.

———. *Minami Manshū Tetsudō fuzokuchi eisei gaikyō: Taishō 10 nendo* 南滿洲鐵道附屬地衞生概況: 大正十年度 [Sanitary conditions of the lands administered by the South Manchurian Railway: Report for 1921]. Dairen, Manchuria: Minami Manshū Tetsudō Kabushiki Kaisha Chihōbu Eiseika, 1923.

Mirzaee, Mohammad. "Trends and Determinants of Mortality in Taiwan, 1895–1975." Ph.D. diss., University of Pennsylvania, 1979.

Mitchell, Timothy. *Rule of Experts: Egypt, Techno-Politics, Modernity.* Berkeley: University of California Press, 2002.

Mitter, Rana. *The Manchurian Myth*. Berkeley: University of California Press, 2000.

Miyauchi Isaburō 宮内豬三郎. "Shinkoku jijō tankenroku: Seishi oyobi hiryo 清国事情探検録 [Adventures in the empire of the great Qing]." In *Bakumatsu Meiji Chūgoku kenbunroku shūsei* 幕末明治中國見聞録集成 [A collection of writings on the sights and sounds in China in the Bakumatsu and Meiji Periods], edited by Kojima Shinji 小島晉治, 11:508–54. Tokyo: Yumani shobō, 1997 [1895].

Monnais-Rousselot, Laurence. *Médecine et Colonisation: L'Aventure Indochinoise, 1860–1939*. Paris: CNRS Editions, 1999.

Moore, W. J. *Health in the Tropics*. London: John Churchill, 1862.

Morel, Marie-France. "The Care of Children: The Influence of Medical Innovation and Medical Institutions on Infant Mortality 1750–1914." In *The Decline of Mortality in Europe*, edited by R. Schofield, D. Reher, and A. Bideau, 196–219. Oxford: Clarendon Press of Oxford University Press, 1991.

Morishita Kaoru 森下薫 and Nabika Hiroshi 並河汪. "Mararia chiryō kansuru kenkyū 5: Jōzan no mararia kansenni obosu eikyo マラリア治療關スル研究第5報常山ノマラリア感染ニ及ボス影響 [Researches on the treatment of malaria no. 5: The impact of dichroa Febrifuga on malaria infection]." *Taiwan igakkai zasshi* 臺灣醫學會雜誌 vol. 30, nos. 310–21 (1933): 741–46.

Morishita Kaoru 森下薫 and Ōda Junro 小田俊郎, producers, *Mararia* マラリア (Malaria) (film). Taihoku (Taipei): Taiwan Sōtokufu, 1939.

Morishita Kaoru 森下薫, Sugida Nobusuke 杉田慶介, and Hitōgawa Hachigorō 下村八五郎. "Shinchikushōshita shisaichihō ni botsuhatsu seru ryukosei mararia ni tsuite 新竹州下震災地方ニ勃發セル流行性マラリア」ニ就テ [The outbreak of epidemic malaria at the earthquake areas in Hsinchu]." *Taiwan igakkai zasshi* 臺灣醫學會雜誌 36 (1937): 1151–66 and 1666–1746.

Morishita Kaoru 森下薫 et al. "Wusandōni okeru mararia ryukō kyūsono bōatsuni All Quinization no kōkoni tsuite 烏山頭ニ於ケル「マラリア流行及其ノ防辺特ニ All Quinization ノ效果ニ就テ [About the "All Quinization" method of malaria prevention in Wushantou]." *Taiwan igakkai zasshi* 臺灣醫學會雜誌 30, nos. 310–21 (1933): 711–35.

Mozi 墨子 [Mozi]. *Mozi xian gu* 墨子閒詁 [Exegetical studies of Mozi], annotated by Sun Yirang 孫詒讓. Taipei: Huazheng shuju, 1987 [1893 Warring States Period].

Müller, Augustus, and Patrick Manson. "Drs. Müller and Manson's Report on the Health of Amoy for the Half Year Ended 30th September, 1871." *Half-Yearly Medical Reports of the Chinese Maritime Customs* 2 (1871): 10–23.

———. "Drs. Müller and Manson's Report on the Health of Amoy for the Half Year Ended 31st March, 1872." *Half-Yearly Medical Reports of the Chinese Maritime Customs* 3 (1872): 22–33.

Myers, Ramon H. "Japanese Imperialism in Manchuria: The South Manchuria Railway Company, 1906–1933." In *The Japanese Informal Empire in China, 1895–1937*, edited by Peter Duus, Ramon H. Myers, and Mark R. Peattie, 101–32. Princeton, N.J.: Princeton University Press, 1989.

Nagayo Sensai 長與專斎. "Shōkō shishi 松香私志 [A private account of Shōkō]." In

Matsumoto Jun jiden; Nagayo Sensai jiden 松本順自伝・長與専斎自伝 [Autobiography of Matsumoto Jun; autobiography of Nagayo Sensai], edited by Ogawa Teizō 小船鼎三 and Sakai Shizu 酒井シヅ, 101–214. Tokyo: Heibonsha, 1980 [1902].

Naimushō eiseikyoku (Public Health Bureau of the Ministry of Internal Affairs) 内務省衛生局, *Shanhai eisei jōkyō* 上海衛生状況 [Shanghai public health record]. Tokyo: Naimushō Eiseikyoku, 1916.

Nakayama Makiko 中山まき子. "Nihon no boshiseisaku no rekishi 日本の母子政策の歴 [The history of maternal and child health policy in Japan]." *Naruto kyōikudaigaku kenkyūkiyō* 15 (2000): 41–55.

Nathan, Carl F. *Plague Prevention and Politics in Manchuria, 1910–1931.* Cambridge: Harvard University Press, 1967.

Nelkin, Dorothy. "Communicating Technological Risk: The Social Construction of Risk Perception." *Annual Review of Public Health* 10 (1989): 100.

Nelson, T. "Medical Results of Recent Chinese Wars." *British and Foreign Medico-Chirurgical Review* 32 (1863): 203–19.

Ng, W. C. *The Silent War: 1 March–31 May 2003.* Singapore: Tan Tock Seng Hospital, 2004.

Noguchi Kinjirō 野口謹次郎, and Watanabe Yoshio 渡邊義雄. *Shanhai kyōdōsokai to kōbukyoku* 上海共同租界と工部局 [Shanghai concessions and municipal council]. Tokyo: Nikko Shoin, 1939.

Notomi Kaijirō 納富介次郎. "Shanghai zaji 上海雜記 [Miscellanea of Shanghai]." In *"Qiansuiwan" de Shanghai xing—Riben 1862 nian de Zhongguo guancha* 千歲丸″的上海行—日本1862年的中國觀察 [The *Chitosei Maru* in Shanghai: Observation of Japanese visitors on China in 1862], edited by Feng Tianyu 馮天瑜 and translated by Liu Bolin 劉柏林, 306–28. Beijing: Shangwu yinshuguan, 2001.

Notter, J. Lane. "The Hygiene of the Tropics." In *Hygiene and Diseases in the Warm Climates*, edited by Andrew Davidson, 25–80. Edinburgh: Young J. Pentland, 1893.

Nutton, Vivian. "The Seeds of Disease: An Explanation of Contagion and Infection from the Greeks to the Renaissance." Chapter 11 in *From Democedes to Harvey: Studies in the History of Medicine.* London: Variorum reprints, 1988.

Obijiofor Aginam. "International Law and Communicable Diseases." *Bulletin of the World Health Organization* 80, no. 12 (2002): 946.

Ōda Taibfumi 小田定文, Morishita Kaoru 森下薫, and Nabika Hiroshi 並河汪. "Mararia chiryo kansuru kenkyu 3: Saiko no mararia chiryo teki kōka マラリア治療ニ關スル研究 Ⅲ.柴胡ノ「マラリア治療的効果 [Research on malaria treatment no. 3: The effects of Bupleurum on malaria treatment]." *Taiwan igakkai zasshi* 臺灣醫學會雜誌 30, nos. 310–21 (1933): 99–109.

Omori Nanzaburo 大森南三郎. "Kotoshu no anofielishu ni tsuite 紅頭嶼ノ「アノフエレス」ニ就テ [On the anopheline mosquitoes of Kotoshu]." *Taiwan igakkai zasshi* 臺灣醫學會雜誌 36 (1937): 2800–01.

Omori Nanzaburo and Noda Hyowazo. "On an Anopheline Mosquito, *Anopheles Arbumbrosus*, Newly Found in Taiwan." *Studia Medica Tropicalis (Formosa)* 1 (1943): 919–20.

Ono Yoshirō 小野芳朗. *Seiketsu no kindai "eiseishōka" kara "kōkinguzzu"* 清潔の近代「衛生唱歌」から「抗菌グッズ」 [The modernization of hygiene: From "the songs of hygiene" to "antibiotic substances"]. Tokyo: Kodansha, 1997.

Oudshoorn, Nelly, and Trevor Pinch, eds. *How Users Matter: The Co-Construction of Users and Technology*. Cambridge: MIT Press, 2003.

Oxford American Dictionary and Thesaurus. 2nd ed. New York: Oxford University Press, 2003.

Packard, Randall M. *White Plague, Black Labor: Tuberculosis and the Political Economy of Disease in South Africa*. Berkeley: University of California Press, 1989.

Pelling, Margaret. *Cholera, Fever and English Medicine 1825–1865*. Oxford: Oxford University Press, 1978.

———. "Contagion/Germ Theory/Specificity." In *Companion Encyclopedia of the History of Medicine*, edited by W. F. Bynum and Roy Porter, 316–18. London: Routledge, 1993.

———. "The Meaning of Contagion: Reproduction, Medicine and Metaphor." In *Contagion: Historical and Cultural Studies*, edited by Alison Bashford and Claire Hooker, 15–38. London: Routledge, 2001.

Peng Shengquan 彭勝權 et al., eds. *Wenbingxue* 溫病學 [Warm diseases studies]. Beijing: Renmin weisheng chubanshe, 2000.

———. *Lingnan wenbing yanjiu yu linchuang* 嶺南溫病驗究與臨床 [Research and clinical experience of Lingnan's warm diseases]. First published in 1991 in China as part of a series on Chinese medicine and pharmacy in the Guangdong and Guangxi region titled *Lingnan zhongyiyao congshu* 嶺南中醫藥叢書 [Collectanea of Chinese medicine and pharmaceutics in Lingnan]. Taipei: Zhiyuan shuju, 2002.

———. "Lingnan wenbing xueshuo jianjie 嶺南溫病学说简介 [Analysis of the doctrines about Lingnan's warm diseases]." In *Lingnan wenbing yanjiu yu linchuang* 嶺南溫病驗究與臨床, edited by Peng Shengquan 彭勝權 et al., 1–22. Taipei: Zhiyuan shuju, 2002.

Peng Weihao 彭偉皓. "Qingdai Xuantong nianjian Dongsanshen shuyi fangzhi yanjiu 清代宣統年間東三省鼠疫防治研究 [A study of plague control during the Qing Xuantong period]." Master's thesis, Donghai University, Taichung, 2007.

Perrins, Robert. "Doctors, Disease and Development: Engineering Colonial Public Health in Southern Manchuria, 1905–1931." In *Building a Modern Japan: Science, Technology and Medicine in the Meiji Era and Beyond*, edited by Morris Low, 103–132. London: Palgrave MacMillan, 2005.

Porter, A. N., ed. *Atlas of British Overseas Expansion*. London: Routledge, 1991.

Porter, Roy. "Diseases of Civilization." In *The Companion Encyclopedia of the History of Medicine*, edited by W. F. Bynum and Roy Porter, 585–600. London: Routledge, 1993.

Prothero, R. M. "Foreword: Population Movement and Malaria Persistence in Rameswaram Island." *Social Science and Medicine* 22, no. 8 (1986): 879–80.

Qian Xinzhong 錢信忠. *Zhonghua Renmin Gongheguo xuexichong dituji* 中華人民共和國血吸蟲病地圖集 [Maps of schistosomiasis in the People's Republic of China]. Shanghai: Zhonghua ditu xueshe, 1987.

Qiu Jinzhang 丘瑾璋, and Xu Gongsu 徐公肅. "Shanghai gonggong zujie zhidu 上海公共租界制度 [Systems in Shanghai concessions]." In *Shanghai gonggong zujie shigao* 上海公共租界史稿 [History of the Shanghai concessions], 1–297. Shanghai: Shanghai renmin chubanshe, 1980.

Qiu Zhonglin 邱仲麟. "Mingdai Beijing de wenyi yu diguo yiliao tixi de yingbian 明代北京的瘟疫與帝國醫療體系的應變 [Plagues in Beijing in the Ming dynasty and occasional changes in the imperial healthcare system]." *Zhongyang yanjiuyuan lishi yuyan suo jikan* 中央研究院歷史語言所集刊 75, no. 2 (2004): 331–87.

Raina, Dhruv. *Images and Contexts: The Historiography of Science and Modernity in India*. New Delhi: Oxford University Press, 2003.

Rather, Lelland J. "The 'Six Things Non-Natural': A Note on the Origins and Fate of a Doctrine and a Phrase." *Clio Medica* 3 (1968): 337–47.

Reid, A. G. "Dr. A. G. Reid's Report on the Health of Hankow for the Half Year Ended 30th September, 1871." *Half-Yearly Medical Reports of the Chinese Maritime Customs* 2 (1871): 44–60.

Rennie, David Field. *Peking and the Pekingese: During the First Year of the British Embassy at Peking*. Vol. 1. London: John Murray, 1865.

Republic of China (Taiwan). Executive Yuan. Council for Economic Planning and Development. *Taiwan Statistical Data Book*. Taipei: Council for Economic Planning and Development, 2006.

Republic of China (Taiwan). Executive Yuan. Department of Health. *Health Statistics in Taiwan*. Taipei: Department of Health, 2005.

———. *Malaria Eradication in Taiwan*. Taipei: Department of Health, 1993.

Ri Tōgaku [Li Tengyue] 李騰嶽. "Taiwan ni okeru shōni shibōritsu oyobi nisan shōni sibōgen-in no tōkeikansatsu 台灣に於ける小兒死亡率及二三小兒死亡原因の統計觀察 [Statistical observations on mortality rates and some causes of death among the children in Formosa]." *Taiwan igakkai zasshi* 402 (1938): 1425–50.

Richardson, Ruth. *Death, Dissection, and the Destitute*. Chicago: University of Chicago Press, 2001.

Riley, James C. *The Eighteenth-Century Campaign to Avoid Disease*. Basingstoke, England: Macmillan, 1987.

Roberts, J. A. G. *China to Chinatown: Chinese Food in the West*. London: Reaktion, 2002.

Rogaski, Ruth. *Hygienic Modernity: Meanings of Health and Disease in Treaty-Port China*. Berkeley: University of California Press, 2004.

———. "Nature, Annihilation, and Modernity: China's Korean War Germ Warfare Experience Revisited." *Journal of Asian Studies* 61, no. 2 (May 2002): 381–416.

Rosen, George. *A History of Public Health*. Expanded ed. Baltimore: Johns Hopkins University Press, 1993.

Rosenberg, Charles E. "Explaining Epidemics." In *Explaining Epidemics and Other Studies in the History of Medicine*, 193–304. Cambridge: Cambridge University Press, 1992.

———. "Framing Disease: Illness, Society, and History." Introduction to *Framing Disease: Studies in Cultural History*, edited by Charles E. Rosenberg and Janet Golden, xiii–xxvi. New Brunswick, N.J.: Rutgers University Press, 1992.

Rothman, Barbara Katz. *In Labor: Women and Power in the Birthplace*. New York: Norton, 1982.

Said, Edward W. *On Late Style: Music and Literature against the Grain*. New York: Pantheon, 2006.

Sakaue Hirozō 坂上弘藏. "Shoseiji hashōfū ni tsuite oyobi sono nirei 初生兒破傷風 に就て及其二例 [Tetanus among newborns and a report of two cases]." *Taiwan igakkai zasshi* 99 (1911): 37–45.

Scheid, Volker. *Chinese Medicine in Contemporary China: Plurality and Synthesis*. Durham, N.C.: Duke University Press, 2002.

———. *Currents of Tradition in Chinese Medicine, 1626–2006*. Seattle: Eastland, 2007.

———. Foreword to *Warm Diseases: A Clinical Guide*, by Liu Guohui. Seattle: Eastland, 2001.

Schipper, Kristofer, and Franciscus Verellen, eds. *The Taoist Canon: A Historical Companion to the Daozang*. Chicago: University of Chicago Press, 2004.

Sen, S. N. "The Character of the Introduction of Western Science in India during the Eighteenth and the Nineteenth Centuries." In *The Social History of Science in Colonial India*, edited by S. Irfan Habib and Dhruv Raina, 69–82. New Delhi: Oxford University Press, 2007.

Seow, Doris. *SARS: Better Understanding & Prevention*. Singapore: Unlimited Graphic Pte., 2003.

Shah, Nayan. *Contagious Divides: Epidemics and Race in San Francisco's Chinatown*. Berkeley: University of California Press, 2001.

Shang shu 尚書 [Book of history]. Annotated ed. *Shang shu zhengyi* 尚書正義 [Correct interpretations of the book of history], annotated by Kong Yingda 孔穎達 *Sibu beiyao* edition. Taipei: Zhonghua shuju, 1972 [Spring and Autumn Period].

Shao Yuanping 邵遠平. *Jieshan shiwen cun* 戒山詩文存 [Writings and poems of Shao Yuanping]. 1684 edition.

Shen Bao 申報 [Shen Daily]. Publication in book form of all issues from 1872 to 1949. Shanghai: Shanghai shudian, 1983.

Shen Defu 沈德符. *Wanli yehuo bian* 萬曆野獲編 [Wild tales of the Wanli era]. Beijing: Zhonghua shuju, 1997 [1619].

Shen Zhiwen 沈之問. *Jiewei yuansou* 解圍元藪 [Sources of relief]. Modern edition based on the first published edition from 1816. Shanghai: Shanghai guji chubanshe, 1997.

Shengji zonglu 聖濟總錄 [Sages' salvation records]. Beijing: Renmin weisheng chu-banshe, 1992 [1111–17].

Shi Meiding 史梅定, ed. *Shanghai zujie zhi* 上海租界志 [History of the Shanghai concessions]. Shanghai: Shanghai shehui kexueyuan chubanshe, 2001.

Shi Runzhang 施閏章. *Shi Yushan ji* 施愚山集 [The works of Shi Yushan]. Hefei, China: Huangshan shushe, 1992 [1708].

Shikoku chūtongun shileibu (Headquarters of the [Japanese] Army in Qing China) 清國駐屯軍司令部, ed. *Qingmo Beijing zhi ziliao* 清末北京志資料 [On the history of Beijing in the late Qing]. Translated by Lü Yonghe 呂永和 and Zhang Zong-ping 張宗平. Beijing: Yanshan chubanshe, 1994. Originally published as *Pekinshi* 北京誌 [Gazetteer of Beijing] (Tokyo: Hakubunkan, 1908).

———. *Tenshinshi* 天津誌 [Gazetteer of Tianjin]. Tokyo: Hakubunkan,1909.

Shimizu Hideo 清水秀夫. *Jiyō eiseikowa* 實用衛生講話 [Practical hygiene prin-ciples]. Tokyo: Tomikura shoten, 1925.

Shoushi tongkao 授時通考 [A general investigation into agricultural time]. Re-printed as *Shoushi tongkao jiaozhu* 授時通考校注 [Collation and annotation and the general investigation into agricultural time], edited by Ma Zongsheng 馬宗勝. Beijing: Nongye chubanshe, 1992 [1737].

Simpson, Ruth. "Neither Clear nor Present: The Social Construction of Safety and Danger." *Sociological Forum* 11, no. 3 (1996): 549–62.

Simpson, W. J. *Report on the Causes and Continuance of Plague in Hong Kong and Suggestions as to Remedial Measures*. London: Waterlow and Sons, 1903.

Singapore Ministry of Health. "Enhanced Precautionary Measures to Break SARS Transmission." Press release. March 22, 2003. http://www.moh.gov.sg/mohcorp/pressreleases.aspx?id=1112.

———. "Measures Taken to Control the SARS Outbreak in Singapore." Press re-leases. March 17, 2003. http://www.moh.gov.sg/mohcorp/pressreleases.aspx?id=1100.

———. "Update (x) on SARS Cases in Singapore." Singapore Ministry of Health. April 23, 2003. http://www.moh.gov.sg/mohcorp/pressreleases.aspx?id=1114.

Singapore Ministry of Information, Communications, and the Arts. *Fighting SARS Together*. Singapore: Ministry of Information, Communications, and the Arts, 2003.

Sinn, Elizabeth. *Power and Charity: The Early History of Tung Wah Hospital*. Hong Kong: Oxford University Press, 1989.

Sivin, Nathan, ed. *Chinese Science*. Cambridge: MIT Press, 1972.

———. *Medicine, Philosophy and Religion in Ancient China: Researches and Reflec-tions*. Aldershot, England: Variorum, 1995.

Somerville, J. R. "Dr. J. R. Somerville's Report on the Health of Foochow (Pagoda Anchorage) for the Half Year Ended 30th September, 1871." *Half-Yearly Medical Reports of the Chinese Maritime Customs* 2 (1871): 24–32.

Spence, Jonathan. *To Change China: Western Advisers in China 1620–1960*. Boston: Little, Brown, 1969.

Spielman, Andrew, and Michael D'Antonio. *Mosquito: A Natural History of Our Most Persistent and Deadly Foe*. New York: Hyperion, 2001.

Stewart, J. A. "Dr. J. A. Stewart's Report on Health Conditions in Foochow." *Half-Yearly Medical Reports of the Chinese Maritime Customs* 18 (1880): 65–70.

Stocking, George W. *Victorian Anthropology*. New York: Free Press, 1987.

Stoler, Ann Laura. *Carnal Knowledge and Imperial Power: Race and the Intimate in Colonial Rule*. Berkeley: University of California Press, 2002.

———. *Race and the Education of Desire: Foucault's "History of Sexuality" and the Colonial Order of Things*. Durham: Duke University Press, 1995.

Strickmann, Michel. *Chinese Magical Medicine*. Edited by Bernard Faure. Stanford: Stanford University Press, 2002.

Suenaga Keiko 末永恵子. *Senji igaku no jittai: Kyū Manshū Ika Daigaku no kenkyū* 戦時医学の実態: 旧満州医科大学の研究 [The true nature of wartime medicine: Research on the former Manchuria Medical School]. Tokyo: Kinohanasha, 2005.

Sun Chengdai 孙承岱 et al., eds. *Diquo zhuyi qinlue Dalianshi congshu: Weisheng juan* 帝国主义侵略大连市丛书: 卫生卷 [Series on imperialism's invasion of Dalian: Medicine and public health]. Dalian: Dalian chuban she, 1999.

Sun Simiao 孫思邈. *Beiji qianjin yaofang* 備急千金要方 [Essential recipes for urgent uses worth a thousand gold pieces]. Beijing: Renmin weisheng chubanshe, 1995 [652].

Sutphen, Mary P. "Not What, but Where: Bubonic Plague and the Reception of Germ Theories in Hong Kong and Calcutta, 1894–1897." *Journal of the History of Medicine* 52 (1997): 81–113.

Suzhou bowuguan (Suzhou Museum) 蘇州博物館, ed. *Ming Qing Suzhou gong-shangye beike ji* 明清蘇州工商業碑刻集 [Collection of stele inscriptions for commerce and industries in Suzhou during the Ming and Qing dynasties]. Nanjing: Jiangsu renmin chubanshe, 1981.

Taipeishū keimubu 台北州警務部. *Taipeisyū keisatsu eisei tenrankai shashinchō* 台北州警察衛生展覽會寫真帖 [Picture book of the police and health exhibition in Taipei]. Taipei: Taiwan nichinichi shinpō, 1926.

Taiwan Executive Yuan, I. J. Su, et al., eds. *Memoir of Severe Acute Respiratory Syndrome Control in Taiwan*. Taipei: Department of Health, Center for Disease Control, 2003.

———. *SARS and Flu Prevention: Taiwan Experience*. Taipei: Department of Health, Center for Disease Control, 2004.

———. *SARS in Taiwan: One Year after the Outbreak*. Taipei: Department of Health, Center for Disease Control, 2004.

Taiwan Malaria Research Institute. *Annexes to the Plan of Operations for Malaria Eradication in China (Taiwan)*. Taipei; Taiwan Malaria Research Institute, 1963.

Taiwan nichinichi shinpōsha 台灣日日新報社 [Taiwan nichinichi Daily], ed. *Naichi-jin kenkōhō* 內地人健康法 [Health practices in Taiwan]. Taipei: Taiwan nichinichi shinpōsha, 1906.

Taiwan shakai jigyōsha 台灣社會事業社 [Taiwan Social Welfare Society]. "Jinteki shigen jūjitsu to jidōhogo 人的資源充實と兒童保護 [Human resources and child protection]." *Shakai jigyō no tomo* 139 (1940): 58–92.

Taiwan Sōtokufu eiseika (Taiwan Public Health Section under the Sotokufu [or Governor's Office]) 臺灣總督府衛生課. *Taiwan mararia gaikyō* 臺灣マラリア概要 [Summary of Taiwanese malaria]. Taipei: Taiwan Sōtokufu keimukyoku, 1935.

Taiwan Sōtokufu keimukyoku 台灣總督府警務局 [Taiwan Department of Police under the Sōtokufu]. *Taiwan keisatsu oyobi eisei tōkeisho* 台灣警察及衛生統計書 [Police and health statistics in Taiwan].Taipei: Taiwan sōtokufu keimukyoku, 1933.

Taiwansheng fuyou weisheng yanjiusuo (Taiwan Research Institute of Maternal and Child's Health) 台灣省婦幼衛生研究所. *Fuyou weisheng zhuyao tongji* 婦幼衛生主要統計 [Maternal and child health statistics]. Taichung: Taiwansheng fuyou weisheng yanjiusuo, 1992.

Taiwansheng jiaotongbu (Taiwan Ministry of Transportation) 臺灣省交通部. *Taiwansheng jiaotong jianshe* 臺灣省交通建設 [Transportation in Taiwan]. Taizhong: Taiwansheng zhengfu, 1987.

Taiwansheng wenxian weiyuanhui (Taiwan Provincial Archives) 臺灣省文獻委員會. *Taiwansheng tongzhi gao* 臺灣省通志稿 [A draft general history of Taiwan]. Taipei: Taiwansheng wenxian weiyuanhui, 1953.

Taiwansheng zhengfu (Taiwan Provincial Government) 台灣省政府. *Taiwan guangfu sanshi nian* 臺灣光復三十年 [The thirty-year restoration of Taiwan]. Taichung: Taiwansheng zhengfu, 1975.

Takagi Tomoe 高木友枝. *Taiwanjin no eisei jōtai* 台灣人の衛生狀態 [The health of the Taiwanese people]. Taipei: Taiwan kōikai, 1910.

Takigawa Tsutomu 滝川勉. "Higashi Azia nōgyō ni okeru chiryoku saiseisan wo kangaeru—Funnyō riyō no rekishiteki kōsatsu 東アジア農業における地力再生産を考える—糞尿利用の歴史的考察 [A reflection on the replenishment of agricultural soil in East Asia: A survey of the history of the use of excrement]." *Azia Keizai* アジア経済 45, no. 3 (2004): 59–76.

Tamanoi, Mariko. "Knowledge, Power, and Racial Classifications: The 'Japanese' in Manchuria." *Journal of Asian Studies* 59, no. 2 (May 2000): 248–76.

Tanaka Jirō 田中次郎. *Santō gaikan* 山東概觀 [Introduction to Shandong Province]. Tokyo: Teishindaijin kanbokeirika, 1915.

Tang Dalie 唐大烈. *Wuyi huijiang* 吳醫彙講 [Collected discussions of Wu medicine]. Shanghai: Kexue jishu chubanshe, 1983 [1814].

Taylor, Kim. *Chinese Medicine in Early Communist China, 1945–63: Medicine of Revolution*. London: RoutledgeCurzon, 2004.

Temkin, Owsei. "Comparative Study of the History of Medicine." *Bulletin of the History of Medicine* 42 (1968): 362–71.

Ter Haar, Barend. *Telling Stories: Witchcraft and Scapegoating in Chinese History*. Leiden, the Netherlands: Brill, 2006.

Thomas, Nicholas. *Entangled Objects: Exchange, Material Culture, and Colonialism in the Pacific*. Cambridge: Harvard University Press, 1991.

Tian Xiangyang 田向陽, ed. *Liugan yu qinliugan: Fangkong zhishi duben* 流感與禽流感：防控知試讀本 [Transmission and poultry transmission: Reader on prevention and knowledge]. Beijing: Zhongguo zhongyiyao chubanshe, 2006.

Tianjin zhongyiyao: Feidian zhuanti 天津中醫藥：非典專題 [Tianjin journal of Chinese medicine: Special papers on SARS] 20, no. 3 (June 2003).

Tissot, Samuel August David. *An Essay of Diseases Incidental to Literary and Sedentary Persons.* London: E. and C. Dilly, 1768.

Tokuhashi Yō 德橋曜, ed. *Kankyō to keikan no shikaishi* 環境と景観の社会史 [Social history of environment and scenery]. Tokyo: Bunkashobo hakubunsha, 2004.

Touati, François-Olivier. "Contagion and Leprosy: Myth, Idea and Evolution in Medieval Minds and Societies." In *Contagion: Perspectives from Pre-modern Societies*, edited by Lawrence I. Conrad and Dominik Wujastyk, 179–201. Aldershot, England: Ashgate, 2000.

Toyoda Hidezō 豐田秀造. *Toman to eisei* 渡滿と衞生 [Immigration to Manchuria and hygiene]. Tokyo: Sanseido, 1933.

Toyoda Tarō 豐田太郎. *Manshū no iji eisei kotoni densenbyō* 滿洲の醫事衞生殊に傳染病 [Medicine and hygiene in Manchuria, with particular reference to contagious disease]. Fukuoka, Japan: Kyushu Teikoku Daigaku Igakubu Gakuyūkai Shuppanbu, 1935.

Tran, Thi Trung Chien. *Hoat dong phong chong SARS tai Viet Nam = SARS Containment Activities in Vietnam.* Hanoi: National Government, 2003.

Trotter, Thomas. *An Essay Medical, Philosophical and Chemical on Drunkenness and Its Effects on the Human Body.* Edited with an introduction by Roy Porter. London: Routledge, 1988.

———. *A View of the Nervous Temperament.* London: Longman, Hurst, Ress, and Orme, 1807.

Tsukiyama Kiichi 築山揆一. "Mararia yobōhō 麻剌里亞豫防法 [Malaria preventive methods]." *Taiwan igakkai zasshi* 臺灣醫學會雜誌 29 (1905): 89–101.

Turner, Bryan S. *Regulating Bodies: Essays in Medical Sociology.* London: Routledge, 1992.

Underwood, G. R. "Dr. G. R. Underwood's Report on the Health of Kiukiang, for the Year Ended 31st March 1887." *Half-Yearly Medical Reports of the Chinese Maritime Customs* 33 (1887): 19–24.

Unschuld, Paul U. *Medicine in China: A History of Ideas.* Berkeley: University of California Press, 1985.

Uruno Katsuya 宇留野勝彌. *Manshū no chihōbyō to densenbyō* 滿洲の地方病と傳染病 [Endemic and contagious diseases of Manchuria]. Tokyo: Kainan Shobō, 1943.

Vaughan, Megan. *Curing Their Ills: Colonial Power and African Illness.* Stanford, Calif.: Stanford University Press, 1991.

Volkmar, Barbara. "The Concept of Contagion in Chinese Medical Thought: Empirical Knowledge versus Cosmological Order." *History and Philosophy of Life Sciences* 22 (2000): 147–65.

Wada Toyotane 和田豐種. "Mahisei chihō no mararia ryohō 麻痺性痴呆ノ「マラリア

療法 [Malariotherapy for paralysis dementia]." *Taiwan igakkai zasshi* 臺灣醫學會雜誌 36 (1939): 203–9.

Wagner, Wilhelm. *Chūgoku Nōsho* 中国農書. Translated by Takahashi Yōkichi 高山洋吉. Tokyo: Tokoshoin, 1972. Originally published as *Die Chinesische Landwirtschaft* (Berlin: P. Parey, 1926).

Wailoo, Keith. *Drawing Blood: Technology and Disease Identity in Twentieth-Century America*. Baltimore: Johns Hopkins University Press, 1997.

Wajcman, Judy. "Reflection on Gender and Technology Studies: In What State Is the Art?" *Social Studies of Science* 30, no. 3 (2000): 447–64.

Wang Ang 汪昂, *Bencao beiyao* 本草備要 [Complete Essentials of Materia Medica]. Taipei: Hualien publisher, 1973 [1683].

Wang Qiao 王樵. *Fang Lu ji* 方麓集 [The works of Fang Lu]. *Siku quanshu* edition, 1285:97–476. Taibei, China: Shangwu yinshuguan, 1986 [16th century].

Wang Tao 王燾. *Waitai miyao* 外臺秘要 [Arcane essentials from the imperial library]. Taipei: Zhongguo yiyao yanjiusuo, 1985 [752].

Wang Ximeng 王希孟. *Shanghai xiaomie xuexichongbing de huigu* 上海消滅血吸蟲病的回顧 [A look back at the elimination of schistosomiasis in Shanghai]. Shanghai: Shanghai kexue jishu chubanshe, 1985.

Wang Yaoguang 王耀光, Ma Rong 馬融, et al. "Zhongyi bianzheng shi zhi peihe xiyao zhiliao shenchu qi he xishou qi chuanranxing Feidianxing feiyan 10 li linchuang baogao 中醫辨證施治配合西藥治療滲出期和吸收期傳染性非典型肺炎10例臨床報告 [Clinical report of 10 cases with SARS at exudative and absorbent phases treated by integrated traditional Chinese and western medicine]." *Tianjin zhongyiyao* 20, no. 4 (August, 2003): 14–16.

Wang Zuorong 王作榮. *Women ruhe chuangzaole jingji qiji* 我們如何創造了經濟奇蹟 [How we created the economic miracle]. Taipei: Shibao, 1987.

Warren, Kenneth S. "Farewell to the Plague Spirit: Chairman Mao's Crusade against Schistosomiasis." In *Science and Medicine in Twentieth-century China: Research and Education*, edited by John Z. Bowers, J. William Hess, and Nathan Sivin, 123–40. Ann Arbor: Center for Chinese Studies, the University of Michigan, 1988.

Watson, James. "Dr. James Watson's Report on the Health of Newchwang for the Half Year Ended 30th September, 1871." *Half-Yearly Medical Reports of the Chinese Maritime Customs* 3 (1872): 10–15.

Watson, R. B., and K. C. Liang. "Seasonal Prevalence of Malaria in Southern Formosa." *Indian Journal of Malariology* 4 (1950): 471–86.

Watson, R. B., J. H. Paul, and K. C. Liang. "A Report on One Year's Field Trial of Chlorguanide (Paludrine) as a Suppressive and as a Therapeutic Agent in Southern Taiwan (Formosa)." *Journal of the National Malaria Society* 9, no. 1 (1950): 25–43.

Wei Baolin 魏葆琳, Sun Zengtao 孫增濤, and Lian Fu 廉富. "Yiqi huoxue fa wei zhu zhiliao SARS huifu qi 15 li liaoxiao fenxi 益氣活血法為主治療SARS恢复期15例理療效分析 [Analysis of curative effect in 15 SARS patients in convalescence mainly treated by supplementing qi and promoting blood circulation]." *Tianjin zhongyi-yao* 21, no. 2 (April 2004): 116–17.

Wei Jian 魏健. *Gaibian renlei shehui de ershi zhong wenyi* 改變人類社會的二十種瘟疫 [The twenty epidemics that changed human society]. Beijing: Jingji ribao chubanshe, 2003.

Weishengshu (Public Health Bureau) 衛生署. *Taiwan diqu gonggong weisheng fazhanshi* 臺灣地區公共衛生發展史 [A history of the development of public health in the Taiwan area]. Taipei: Weishengshu, 1995.

White, Luise. *Speaking with Vampires: Rumor and History in Colonial Africa.* Berkeley: University of California Press, 2000.

Williams, Raymond. *Marxism and Literature.* Oxford: Oxford University Press, 1977.

Wong, K. Chimin, and Wu Lien-teh. *History of Chinese Medicine: Being a Chronicle of Medical Happenings in China from Ancient Times to the Present Period.* 1936. Reprint, Taipei: Southern Materials Center, 1977.

Worboys, Michael. *Spreading Germs: Diseases, Theories, and Medical Practice in Britain, 1865–1900.* Cambridge: Cambridge University Press, 2000.

World Health Assembly. "Severe Acute Respiratory Syndrome (SARS)." Resolution of the Fifty-Sixth World Health Assembly, Geneva, May 28, 2003. http://apps.who.int/gb/archive/pdf_files/EB112/eeb1122.pdf.

World Health Organization. "Consensus Document on the Epidemiology of Severe Acute Respiratory Syndrome (SARS)." Produced by the Severe Acute Respiratory Syndrome (SARS) Epidemiology Working Group and the participants at the Global Meeting on the Epidemiology of SARS, May 16–17, 2003. Department of Communicable Disease Surveillance and Response. 2003, http://www.who.int/entity/csr/sars/WHOconsensus.pdf.

———. *Epidemiology and Control of Schistosomiasis.* Geneva: World Health Organization, 1980.

———. "Malaria." Fact sheet no. 94, updated January 2009. http://www.who.int/mediacentre/factsheets/fs094/.

———. *SARS: Clinical Trials on Treatment Using a Combination of Traditional Chinese Medicine and Western Medicine.* Geneva: World Health Organization, 2004.

———. "SARS: Status of the Outbreak and Lessons for the Immediate Future." Department of Communicable Disease Surveillance and Response, May 20, 2003. http://www.who.int/csr/media/sars_wha.pdf.

———. "Update 10: Data from China, Countries Introduce Stringent Control Measures." Department for Epidemic and Pandemic Alert and Response (EPR), March 2003. http://www.who.int/entity/csr/sars/archive/2003_03_26a/en/.

———. "Update 17: Travel Advice; Hong Kong Special Administrative Region of China, and Guangdong Province, China." Department for Epidemic and Pandemic Alert and Response (EPR). April 2003. http://www.who.int/csr/sars/archive/2003_04_02/en/.

———. "WHO Issues a Global Alert about Cases of Atypical Pneumonia." Press release, March 12, 2003. http://www.who.int/csr/sars/archive/2003_03_12/en/.

Wu Baodian 吳寶鈿. "Tao dafen de 掏大糞的 [Those who clean chamber pots]." In *Beijing wangshi tan* 北京往事談 [Old stories of Beijing], edited by Zhengxie Beijing shi weiyuanhui wenshi ziliao yanjiu weiyuanhui (Beijing Municipal Cultural Archival Committee) 政協北京市委員會文史資料研究委員會, 279–82. Beijing: Beijing chubanshe, 1988.

Wu Chia-Ling 吳嘉苓. "Yiliao zhuanye, xingbie, yu guojia: Taiwan zhuchanshi xingshuai de shehuixue fenxi 醫療專業、性別、與國家：台灣助產士興衰的社會學分析 [The medical profession, gender, and the state: A sociological analysis of the rise and decline of midwives in Taiwan]." *Taiwan shehuixue yanjiu* 台灣社會學研究 4 (2000): 191–268.

Wu Chia-Ling, and Fu Daiwei. "Research Agenda, Public Policy, and the Social Construction of Cesarean Sections in Taiwan." Paper presented at the Fourth International Conference of Bioethics, National Taiwan University, June 25–27, 2004.

Wu Lien-teh 伍連德. *Dongsansheng fangyi shiwu zongchu daquanshu* 東三省防疫事務總處大全書 [Complete report of the General Office for the Prevention of Plague in the Three Eastern Provinces] Vols. 3 and 4, 1922 and 1924. Dongsansheng fangyi shiwu zongchu.

———. "Plague." In *North Manchurian Plague Prevention Service: Reports 1914–1917*, 45–50. Peking: Peking Gazette Press, 1917.

———. *Plague Fighter: The Autobiography of a Modern Chinese Physician.* Cambridge: W. Heffer and Sons, 1959.

———. "The Second Pneumonic Plague Epidemic in Manchuria, 1920–21." *The Journal of Hygiene* 21, no. 3 (May 1923): 262–88.

———. *A Treatise on Pneumonic Plague.* Paris: Berger-Levrault, 1926.

Wu Qian 吳謙, ed. *Yizong jinjian* 醫宗金鑒 [Golden mirror of the medical tradition]. Beijing: Renmin weisheng chubanshe, 1990 [1742].

Wu Yingen 吳銀根 and Shen Qingfa 沈慶法. *Zhongyi waigan rebingxue* 中醫外感熱病學 [Externally inflicted heat disease studies in Chinese medicine]. Shanghai: Shanghai kexue jishu chubanshe, 1991.

Wu Youxing 吳有性. *Wenyi lun* 溫疫論 [On epidemics due to the warm factor]. Reprinted as *Wenyi lun buzheng* 溫疫論補正 [On epidemics due to the warm factor, with appendices]. Taipei: Xinwenfeng, 1985 [1642].

Wu Yu-lin. *Memories of Dr. Wu Lien-Teh: Plague Fighter.* Singapore: World Scientific Publishing Company, 1995.

Wu Zhuoliu 吳濁流. *Yaxiya de guer* 亞細亞的孤兒 [The orphan in Asia]. Translated from the Japanese by Wu Zhuoliu 吳濁流 and Huang Yuyan 黃玉燕. Hsinchu, Taiwan: Xinzhuxian wenhuaju, 2005.

Wyatt, Sally. "Non-Users Also Matter: The Construction of Users and Non-Users of the Internet." In *How Users Matter: The Co-Construction of Users and Technology*, edited by Nelly Oudshoorn and Trevor Pinch, 67–80. Cambridge: MIT Press, 2003.

Xi Liang 錫良 et al. "Xuyan 緒言 [Preface]." In *Dongsansheng yishi baogaoshu* 東三省疫事報告書 [Report on the epidemic in the three eastern provinces], edited by Zhang Yuanqi 張元奇 et al., 1–8. Fengtian, China: Fengtian fangyi zhongju, 1911.

Xia Renhu 夏仁虎. *Jiu jing suoji* 舊京瑣記 [Miscellaneous records of the old capital]. Beijing: Guji chubanshe, 1986 [1912–49].

Xiao Rongwei 蕭榮煒 and Ye Jiafu 葉嘉馥. *Xuexichongbing* 血吸蟲病 [Schistosomiasis]. Beijing: Renmin weisheng chubanshe, 1959.

Xiao Xiaoting 蕭曉亭. *Fengmen quanshu* 瘋門全書 [A complete book on leprosy]. Guangdong: Jingyetang, 1854 [late 18th century].

Xie Xialing 謝遐齡, Yu Hai 于海, and Fan Lizhu 藩麗珠, eds. *SARS, quanqiuhua yu Zhongguo* 全球化與中國 [SARS, globalization, and China]. Shanghai: Shanghai renmin chubanshe, 2004.

Xie Xueshi 解學詩. "'Xinjing' shuyi moulue—1940 nian" 新京鼠疫謀略—1940年 [The 1940 Xinjing plague strategy]. In *Zhanzheng yu eyi* 戰 爭与惡疫 [War and plague], edited by Xie Xueshi and Matsumura Takao 松村高夫, 58–122. Beijing: Renmin chubanshe, 1998.

Xie Yongguang 謝永光. *Xianggang zhongyiyao shihua* 香港中醫藥史話 [A history of Chinese medicine in Hong Kong]. Hong Kong: Sanlian shudian, 1998.

Xie Zhaozhe 謝肇淛. *Wu za zu* 五雜俎 [Five miscellaneous groupings]. Beijing: Zhonghua shuju, 1959 [1616].

Xinshengzhen zhi bianzuan weiyuanhui 新塍鎮志編纂委員會. *Xinshengzhen zhi* 新塍鎮志 [Gazetteer of Xinsheng Town]. Shanghai: Shanghai shehui kexueyuan chubanshe, 1998.

Xu Xuan 徐鉉. *Ji shen lu* 稽神錄 [Records of the deities]. *Siku quanshu* edition, vol. 1042. Taipei: Shangwu yinshuguan, 1983 [10th century].

Xu Yaoqin 許堯欽 and Chen Rongzhou 陳榮洲. "Pifu chuangyang zhengzhi sixiang yu shengji lei fangji de yanjiu 皮膚瘡瘍證治思想與生肌類方劑的研究 [Promoting the granulation of sores.]" *Zhongyiyao zazhi* 中醫藥雜誌 11, no. 4 (2000): 173–88.

Xue Yong. "Treasure Nightsoil as if It Were Gold: Economic and Ecological Links between Urban and Rural Areas in Late Imperial Jiangnan." *Late Imperial China* 26, no. 1 (2005): 41–71.

Yang Cui 楊翠. *Riju shiqi Taiwan funü jiefang yundong* 日據時期台灣婦女解放運動 [Women's liberation in Taiwan during the Japanese occupation]. Taipei: Shibao wenhua, 1993.

Yang Lien-sheng. "The Concept of 'Pao' as a Basis for Social Relations in China." In *Chinese Thought and Institutions*, edited by John King Fairbank, 291–309. Chicago: University of Chicago Press, 1957.

Yang Wen Shan, and Ying-hui Hsieh. "Infant Mortality in Colonial Taiwan 1905–1945: Evidence of the Historical Household Registration Data of Taiwan." Paper presented at the International Conference on the Ideas, Organization, and

Practice of Hygiene in Han Society from the Traditional to the Modern Periods, Research Center for Humanities and Social Sciences, Academia Sinica, Taipei, November 22–23, 2004.

Yanjing zaji 燕京雜記 [Miscellanea of the capital]. Beijing: Beijing guji chubanshe, 1986 [1878].

Yasui Keinosuke 安井慧之助 and Sakai Kiyoshi 酒井潔. *Taiwan ni okeru ikuji sōdan* 台灣に於ける育兒相談 [Consultation on child care in Taiwan]. Taipei: Taipei shinpō shuppansha, 1934.

Yin Haiguang 殷海光. "Fangong dalu wenti 反攻大陸問題 [The problem of re-conquest of China]." *Ziyou zhongguo* 自由中國 17 (1957): 3.

Yip, Ka-che. *Health and National Reconstruction in Nationalist China: The Development of Modern Health Services, 1928–1937*. Ann Arbor, Mich.: Association for Asian Studies, 1995.

Yoshitaka Komiya 小宮義孝. "Guanyu xuexichongbing fangzhi gongzuo de yijian-shu 關於血吸蟲病防治工作的意見書 [Comments on the prevention of schistosomiasis]." *Zhonghua yixue zazhi* 4 (1957): 297–302.

You Jianming 游鑑明. "Riju shiqi Taiwan de zhiye funü 日據時期台灣的職業婦女 [The career woman in Japanese colonized Taiwan]." Ph.D. diss., National Taiwan Normal University, 1995.

Young, Louise. *Japan's Total Empire: Manchuria and the Culture of Wartime Imperialism*. Berkeley: University of California Press, 1998.

Yu Botao 余伯陶. *Shuyi juewei* 鼠疫抉微 [Nuances of the bubonic plague]. Shanghai: Shanghai guji chubanshe, 1910.

Yu Fenggao 余風高. "SARS: Lishishang cong weiyouguode chuanranbing 歷史上從未有過的傳染病 [SARS: A newly emergent contagious disease]." In *Liuxingbing: Cong changjue dao tuibai* 流性病從猖獗到頹敗, edited by Yu Fenggao 余風高, 282–94. Jinan: Shandong huabao chubanshe, 2003.

Yu Shunzhang 俞順章. "Yi Su Delong jiaoshou 憶蘇德隆教授 [In memory of professor Su De-long]." *Wenhui bao* 文汇报, August 14, 2004.

Yu Xinzhong 余新忠. "Public Health in Qing Dynasty Jiangnan: Focusing on Environment and Water Supply." *Frontiers of History in China* 2, no. 3 (2007): 379–415.

———. "Shinmatsu ni okeru 'eisei' kainen no tenkai 清末における「衛生」概念の展開 [On the evolution of the concept of "weisheng" in late Qing China]." Translated by Ishino Kazuharu 石野一晴. *Tōyōshi kenkyū* 東洋史研究 64, no. 3 (2005): 104–40.

———. *Qingdai Jiangnan de wenyi yu shehui—yi xiang yi liao shehuishi de yanjiu* 清代江南的瘟疫與社會——一項醫療社會史的研究 [Epidemics and society in the Jiangnan region in the Qing dynasty: A study of the social history of medicine]. Beijing: Zhongguo renmin daxue chubanshe, 2003.

Yuan Hongchang 袁鴻昌, Zhang Shaoji 張绍基, and Jiang Qingwu 姜慶五. *Xuexichongbing fangzhi lilun yu shijian* 血吸蟲病防治理論與實踐 [Theory and practice of schistosomiasis control]. Shanghai: Fudan daxue chubanshe, 2003.

Zeigler, J. L. "Editorial: Tropical splenomegaly syndrome." *Lancet* 15, no. 1 (1976): 1058–59.

Zeng Zhikang. *Uniting in Combating* SARS. Hong Kong: Hong Kong Council of Social Service, 2003.

Zerubavel, Evitar. *The Fine Line: Making Distinctions in Everyday Life*. New York: Free Press, 1991.

Zhang Boli 張伯禮 and Zhang Junping 張軍平. "Zhong xi yi jiehe zhiliao SARS ruogan wenti tantao 中西醫結合治療SARS 若干問題探討 [Discussion of some problems in SARS treated by integrated Chinese and Western medicine]." *Tianjin zhongyiyao* 20, no. 4 (August 2003): 8–11.

Zhang Deyi 張德彝. *Xingmu qingxin lu* 醒目清心錄 [Record to clarify the view and purify the heart]. Beijing: Quanguo tushuguan suowei wenxian zhongxin, 2004 [1911].

Zhang Gao 張杲. *Yishuo* 醫說 [On medicine]. *Siku quanshu* edition, *juan* 742. Taipei: Shangwu yinshuguan, 1983 [1189].

Zhang Ji 張機. *Shanghan lun* 傷寒論 [Treatise on cold-damage disorders]. Commentary by Cheng Wuji 成無己. Taipei: Zhonghua shuju, 1966 [Eastern Han; commentary 1156].

Zhang Jinsheng 張晉生 et al., eds. *Yongzheng Sichuan tongzhi* 雍正四川通志 [General gazetteer of Sichuan province, Yongzheng period]. *Siku quanshu* edition, vols. 559–61. Taibei, China: Shangwu yinshuguan, 1986 [1781].

Zhang Lu 張璐. *Zhangshi yitong* 張氏醫通 [A general medical treatise by Zhang Lu]. Shanghai: Shanghai kexue jishu chubanshe, 1990 [1695].

Zhang Lüxiang 張履祥. *Bu Nongshu jiaoshi* 補農書校釋 [Annotated version of the supplemented book of agriculture]. Beijing: Nongye chubanshe, 1983 [1658].

Zhang Weixiong 張偉雄 and Zheng Hailin 鄭海麟, eds. *Huang Zunxian wenji* 黃遵憲文集 [Collection of essays by Huang Zunxian]. Kyoto: Zhongwen chubanshe, 1991.

Zhang Yuanqi 張元奇, et al., eds. *Dongsansheng yishi baogaoshu* 東三省疫事報告書 [Report on the epidemic in the three eastern provinces]. Fengtian, China: Fengtian fangyi zhongju, 1911.

Zhang Zaitong 張在同, Xian Rijin 咸日金 eds., *Minguo yiyao fagui xuanbian 1912–1948* (民國醫藥衛生法規選編 1912–1948). Tai'an (Shandong): Shandong daxue chubanshe, 1990.

Zhejiangsheng xuexichongbing fangzhi bianweihui (Editorial committee of the History of Prevention and Control of Schistosomiasis in Zhejiang Province) 浙江省血吸蟲病防治史編委. *Zhejiang xuexichongbing fangzhi shi* 浙江省血吸蟲病防治史 [The history of schistosomiasis prevention in Zhejiang]. Shanghai: Shanghai kexue jishu chubanshe, 1991.

Zheng Guanying 鄭觀應. "Sheng shi wei yan 盛世危言 [Words of warning in an age of prosperity]." In *Zheng Guanying ji* 鄭觀應集 [Collection of Zheng Guanying], edited by Xia Dongyuan 夏東元, 1:255–940. Shanghai: Shanghai renmin chubanshe, 1982 [1894].

Zheng Weiru 鄭偉如, Lin Zhaoqi 林兆耆, and Zhong Xueli 鐘學禮. "Riben zhuxue-xichongbing zhi linchuangguan: 355 li bing'an zhi fenxi 日本住血吸蟲病之臨床觀:三五五例病案之分析 [An analysis of 355 cases of schistosomiasis in Japan]." *Zhonghua yixue zazhi* 37, no. 10 (1951): 829–47.

Zhonggong Zhejiang shengwei chusihai jiang weisheng bangongshi (Office for the Elimination of the Four Pestilences and Promotion of Hygiene under the Communist Party of the Zhejiang Province) 中共浙江省委除四害講衛生辦公室. *Zhejiangsheng Hainingxian fangzhi xuexichongbing de zhongda shengli* 浙江省海寧縣防治血吸蟲病的重大勝利 [Victory over schistosomiasis in Haining County, Zhejiang Province]. Shanghai: Shanghai weisheng chubanshe, 1958.

Zhongguo zhongyi yanjiuyuan 中國中醫驗究院, ed. *Zhongyiyao fang zhi Feidian-xing feiyan (SARS) yanjiu* 中醫藥防治非典型肺炎 (SARS) 驗究 [Research on the prevention and treatment of SARS with TCM]. 2 volumes. Beijing: Zhongyi guji chubanshe, 2003.

Zhou li 周禮 [The rites of Zhou]. Taipei: Kaiming shudian, 1984 [Spring and Autumn Period].

Zhou Pingan 周平安 et al. "SARS hebing guzhi sunhai zhiliao chutan SARS合並骨質損害治療初探 [Primary consideration of the treatment of SARS complicated with osseous damage]. *Tianjin zhongyiyao* 21, no. 2 (April 2004): 132–34.

Zhou Yangjun 周揚俊. *Wenre shuyi quanshu* 溫熱暑疫全書 [A complete book on summer epidemics caused by warm and hot factors]. *Zhongguo Yixue Dacheng* 中國醫學大成 edition, vol. 3. Changsha, China: Yuelu shushe, 1990 [1679].

Zhu Mei 朱梅. "Guangzhou zhongyiyao daxue yifuyuan jizhen ke shou zhi Feidian 37 li linchuang zongjie 廣州中醫藥大學一附院急診科收之非典37例臨床總結 [Clinical summary of treating thirty-seven cases of SARS in the emergency room of the First Hospital affiliated with the Guangzhou University of Traditional Chinese Medicine]." *Tianjin zhongyiyao: Feidian zhuanti* [Tianjin journal of traditional Chinese medicine: Special issue on SARS] 20, no. 3 (June 2003): 15–16.

Zhu Xi 朱熹. *Huian xiansheng Zhu Wengong wenji* 晦菴先生朱文公文集 [Writings by Zhu Xi]. Taipei: Zhongwen chubanshe, 1972 [mid-13th century].

Zhuang Yongming 莊永明 *Taiwan geyao zhuixiangqu* 臺灣歌謠追想曲 (Nostalgic melody of Taiwanese folk song). Taipei: Qianwei, 1995.

Contributors

Warwick ANDERSON is a research professor in the Department of History and the Centre for Values, Ethics and the Law in Medicine at the University of Sydney. His books include *The Collectors of Lost Souls: Turning Kuru Scientists into Whitemen* (2008), *Colonial Pathologies: American Tropical Medicine, Race, and Hygiene in the Philippines* (2006), and *The Cultivation of Whiteness: Science, Health and Racial Destiny in Australia* (2003). In 2009 he co-edited a special issue of the journal *East Asia Science, Technology and Medicine* titled "Emergent Studies of Science and Technology in Southeast Asia."

Charlotte FURTH is a professor of history emerita at the University of Southern California. She is the author of *A Flourishing Yin: Gender in China's Medical History, 960–1665* (1999), and a co-editor of *Thinking with Cases: Specialist Knowledge in Chinese Cultural History* (2007).

Marta E. HANSON is an assistant professor of the history of medicine at Johns Hopkins University. She has published on the history of disease, regionalism, medical conceptions of geography and human variation, the politics of medicine in the Qing court, and the art of memory in the history of medicine in China. She is the author of a forthcoming book in the Needham Research Institute Series, Asian Studies, Routledge Press, *Speaking of Epidemics in Chinese Medicine: Disease and the Geographic Imagination in Late Imperial China.*

Sean Hsiang-lin LEI is an associate research fellow at the Institute of Modern History of the Academia Sinica. He co-edited *Techno-science Aspires for Society: Taiwan STS Reader I* (2005) and *Techno-science Aspires for Gender: Taiwan STS Reader II* (2005).

Angela Ki Che LEUNG is a research fellow at the Institute of History and Philology of the Academia Sinica, and a professor of history at the Chinese University of Hong Kong. She is the author of *Leprosy in China: A History* (2009) and *Charity and Moral Transformation: Philanthropic Organizations of the Ming and Qing Periods* (in Chinese, 1997), and the editor of *Medicine for Women in Imperial China* (2006).

Shang-Jen LI is an associate research fellow at the Institute of History and Philology of the Academia Sinica. He works on the history of British imperial medicine and has published articles in *Isis, Journal of the History of Biology*, and *Bulletin of the Institute of History and Philology*.

LI Yushang is a research fellow in history at Shanghai Jiao Tong University. He is a coauthor of *The Plague: War and Peace—Environment and Social Change in China, 1230–1960* (in Chinese, 2006).

LIN Yi-ping is an assistant professor at the Institute of Science, Technology, and Society at the National Yang-Ming University, in Taipei. Her specialty is public health. She has also edited books on science, technology, and society in Chinese.

LIU Shiyung is an associate research fellow at both the Institute of Taiwan History and the Academia Sinica's Research Center for the Humanities and Social Science. He is the author of *Prescribing Colonization: the Role of Medical Practice and Policy in Japan-Ruled Taiwan, 1895–1945* (2009) and "Malariology in colonial Taiwan," in *Disease, Colonialism, and the State: Malaria in Modern East Asian History*, edited by Ka-che Yip (2008). He and Stephan Morgan are the authors of "Was Japanese Colonialism Good for the Welfare of Taiwanese?" *China Quarterly* (December 2007).

Ruth ROGASKI is an associate professor of history at Vanderbilt University. The author of *Hygienic Modernity: Meanings of Health and Disease in Treaty-Port China* (2004), she is working on a book about the history of science in Manchuria.

TSENG Yen-fen is a professor of sociology at National Taiwan University. She is the co-author, with Wu Chia-Ling, of "Beyond Technical Models: Governing SARS Risk in Taiwan, 2003" (*Taiwanese Sociology*, 2006), and the author of "Governing Migrant Workers at a Distance" (*International Migration*, forthcoming).

WU Chia-Ling is an associate professor of sociology at the National Taiwan University. She has recently published on the risk governance of SARS, new reproductive technologies and gender politics in Taiwan, and public participation methods in newly democratic societies. Her current research focuses on the processes of framing risk in reproductive medicine in Taiwan, examining the high rate of cesarean section, multiple embryo implantation in IVF, and the bankruptcy of sperm banks.

YU Xinzhong is a professor of history at Nankai University, in Tianjin, China. He is the author of *Epidemics and Society in Jiangnan during the Qing Dynasty: A Study of the Social History of Medicine* (in Chinese, 2003) and *The History of the Family in the Ming and Qing Dynasties*, volume 4 of *A General History of the Chinese* (in Chinese, 2007). He is also the editor of *Disease, Medical Treatment and Hygiene Since the Qing Dynasty from the Perspective of Social and Cultural History* (in Chinese, 2009).

Index

Academia Sinica, 2–3
aesthetics of public health, 61, 63, 65
Africa, colonial, 140–41, 147, 154
Aginam Obijiofor, 261
agricultural resettlement, hygienic challenges, 135–36
agriculture: malaria and, 185; night soil use in, 51, 54, 206–8, 220; schistosomiasis and, 207–8
alcohol consumption in a hot climate, 114–15, 119–20
Altman, Lawrence K., 229
Anatomy Act, 153
Anderson, Benedict, 114
anemia, 118
Anglo-Indian bodily perceptions, 124
Anglo-Indian medicine, 123
antiplague measures, bubonic plague: Chinese medicine, challenges from, 85–87; Chinese perspective on, 139; effectiveness of, 139; quarantine, 83, 139; resistance to, 83; sanitary police, 139; stories of vampires, 141; vaccination, 138–39, 148–49
antiplague measures, enforcing, 78–80, 84, 102n28, 139
antiplague measures, pneumonic plague: autopsies, 144–45, 154–55; blocking the network of infection, 92–93; cremation, 83, 145–46; detention and quarantine, 81–82; draconian, 82–84, 144; gauze masks, 79–81; inspections and vaccinations, 151; police actions enforcing, 84; railway traffic restrictions,

81, 145; resistance to, 79–80, 87; rumors, stories, and fears, 139, 145, 147–52
Arnold, David, 4, 111

bacteriology, contagion theories, 27
Bao Shichen, 56
Basch, Paul, 269
bayberry sores (*yangmei chuang*), 39–40
bazimamoto (men who steal blood), 140, 147, 154
Beard, George, 121
Beck, Ulrich, 261
Beijing Convention, 110, 127n6
Bencao gangmu (Li Shizhen), 39
Benedict, Carol, 82
biological warfare, 14; Unit 731 and, 14, 133, 141–43, 155
biomedicine: Chinese medicine vs., 234–35; midwives incorporation of, 170; modern beliefs about, duality in, 155. *See also* Western medicine
Blake, Henry, 86
bodily fluids, disease transmission through, 33–34, 42–43
bodily perception and borders, 124
body of the nabob, 124
Book on agriculture (*Nong shu*) (Chen), 35, 37
borders: bodily perception, 124; colonizer-colonized, blurring of, 133, 140; crossing, 269; guarding against germs, 256–59; isolation vs. quarantine, 269; racial, policing of, 125

Boxer Uprising, 77–78
Brown, Peter, 185
bubonic plague (*shuyi*), Unit 731 caused, 142
bubonic plague, Hong Kong (1894): anti-plague measures, 83, 85–87; corpse dumping statistics from, 103n42; death statistics from, 86; migration statistics from, 92; pneumonic plague compared to, 78, 80, 85–87
bubonic plague, Manchuria (1940): anti-plague measures, 138–39, 148–49; death statistics from, 139; vampires, stories of, 141
Buckle, Henry Thomas, 117
bug toxin (*gu*), 32, 35
burial practices, 44

Chakrabarty, Dipesh, 155
chamber pot cleaner (*dao mazi*), 53
Chao Yuanfang, 30–35, 36
Chen Chaochang, 211
Chen Fu, 35, 37
Cheng Jiong, 37
Cheng Wuji, 36
Chen Shaoxin, 199
Chen Sicheng, 39
Chen Yan, 36, 38
Cheyne, George, 126
Chiang Kai-Shek, 196–97
Childbirth: infant mortality, Taiwan, 166–69; social networks in traditions of, 15, 172–75; women's narratives of, 163–66, 168–69, 172–74. *See also* midwives
children: disease transmission in, 32–34; East Indies dietary practices of, 124
China: colonial identity in, crisis of, 5; modern identity of, 4–5, 135; modernity and, path to, 11; opening of, 110; public health policy and infrastructure in, catalyst for, 97, 99, 274; rural hygiene in, 12, 149–51, 210–12. *See also* People's Republic of China (PRC)
Chinese, stereotypes of, 25, 51, 118

Chinese agriculture (*Die Chinesiche Land-wirtschaft*) (Wagner), 56
Chinese civil war, 232
Chinese herbs for SARS prevention and treatment, 9, 230, 243–44, 248, 253n41
Chinese medicine, classical: biomedicine vs., 234–35, 241–43; climates and constitutions in, 242, 244–46, 249–50; cutting the umbilical cord procedures in, 168; education programs of, 232, 234; inner-outer dyad of, 241–42, 245; integrated form of, 8–10, 231–32, 244, 246–48, 250; plague treatment in, challenges to, 84–88; scholarship on history of, 3–4; transformation of, 7–8
Chinese medicine, traditional (TCM): disease nomenclature in, 239; education and, 232–33, 240, 244; infectious disease treatment in, 241–42; integrated form of, 8–10, 231–32, 244, 246–48, 250; organ-based-environmental dyad, 242; SARS treatment using, 9–10, 243–44, 246; schistosomiasis treatment using, 212–13; the state in moderniz-ing, 100–101
Chinese medicine–Western medicine integration, 8–10, 231–32, 244, 246–48, 250
Chinese nationalism, 155
Chinese pharmaceutical industry, 230
Chinese pharmaceuticals, 232. *See also* Chinese herbs for SARS prevention and treatment
Chinese State Administration of Tradi-tional Chinese Medicine, 235, 246
cholera, 135, 137, 143, 159n51
Christie, Dugald, 87
chuanran: complexity of, 44; contagion vs., 27–28, 45, 90; dichotomy of mean-ings of, 89, 249; emergence and use of, as term, 35–37, 43, 88, 239; germ theory and, 45, 99, 239; late Imperial period understanding of, 37–45; mod-ern idea of, 45–46; overview of, 8–9; *ran*, early connotations of, 28–30; root

word of, 26; *wenyi* (epidemics) via, beliefs about, 25–26, 40–42, 45, 88–89. *See also* contagion

chuanranbing (infectious disease): disorders of, 96–97; eight classes of, 99–100; legal institution of, 97, 99–100; modern category of, Manchurian plague in creating, 9, 74–75, 93–94, 99, 249; modern international surveillance system over, 95; notifiable, 94–97, 99; notifiable infectious disease vs., 106n100

chuanshi (corpse transmission), 32–33, 38

chuan transmission of disease, 32–33

chuanzhu (outpour transmission), 32–34

Civilization, Chinese and Christian (Faber), 63

class structure: elites within the empire, 155; in modern midwifery, 172–73, 176

climate: in classical Chinese medicine, 8, 242, 244–46, 249–50; determining otherness with, 111–13; epidemics (*wenyi*) and, 238, 240–41, 242; identity and, 115; racial determinism and, 249; SARS outbreak and, 242; SARS treatment and, 244–46; tropical, and effect on health, 110–16, 125, 136. *See also* environment

Cochrane Center, 247

Cold Damage (*shanghan*), 8, 31, 36, 42, 240

Cold Damage (*shanghan*) doctrine, 9, 25

Collingham, E. M., 124

A Colonial Lexicon (Hunt), 140

colonial medical research, 140. *See also* Unit 731

colonial public health and hygiene: benevolent vs. coercive, 275–76; evil associated with, 139, 140; historians approaches to, 132; introduction overview, 11–15; volume conclusion, 274–77. *See also* Japan, colonial project of hygienic modernity

colonizer-colonized relation: boundaries of, blurring of and crossing, 133, 140;

introduction overview, 14; medical atrocities in, 140, 141–42, 155; midwifery education, 179n57; public health policy, exclusivity in, 137, 188–89

Complete Essentials of Materia Medica (*Bencao beiyao*) (Wang), 168

consumption (*lao* or *zhai*), 32, 35

contagion: *chuanran* vs., 27–28, 45, 90; environment and, 27, 29; germ theory integration, 249; historical understanding of, 26–27; modern understandings of, 27; overview of, 8–9; rituals to prevent, 35; root meaning, 28

contamination (*ran*), 28–31, 33, 36

corpses: desecration of, 139, 144–45, 153; polluting effect of, 32, 35, 38, 41, 44

cosmopolitan medicine, 161, 177n2, 273

cosmopolitan midwifery, 161

cosmopolitan science, 4, 161

cremation, 83, 145–46

Crozier, Ralph, 274

Cui Yueli Center for Traditional Medicine Research, 244

Cultural Revolution, 205

Cunningham, Andrew, 75

Dagong Bao, 25, 44

Dalian, public health protections in, 136–37

danger of bad milk, 33–34

danger-safety framework, 258, 264, 270, 272n21

D'Antonio, Michael, 194

Daoism, disease-transmission beliefs, 35–36

Darwin, Charles, 117

Delaporte, François, 27

Deng Kunhe, 60

Diamond, Jared, 249

diet: of British poor and laboring class, 126; Chinese, 109, 112–16, 119–27; European's health in China and, 109, 112–16, 119–22; identity and, 110; racial character and, 116–19, 122–26; SARS

diet (*cont'd*)
outbreak and, 242; social status and, 114
dietary studies, 125–26
Dikotter, Frank, 148
Ding Fubao, 93–94
discrimination: Japanese colonial public health policy, 137, 188–89; in midwifery education, 179n54, 179n57; students from SARS regions and, 229–30
disease, social characteristics of, 75, 97–98
disease transmission: by contamination and switching (7th-12th century) beliefs, 30–37; introduction overview, 8–9; Ming-Qing period (14th-19th centuries) beliefs, 37–43. *See also chuanran*
Dongfang Zazhi, 64
Donghua (Tung Wah) Hospital, 83, 85–86, 234
Dong Xiaoping, 236
Duan Xianzeng, 65
Dudgeon, John, 111, 119–21
dye by immersion (*jianran*), 29–30
dyeing, 28

Eastern Mongolia, 149–50
Eastern Railway, 77, 82
East Indies, childhood dietary practices, 124
economics: of Chinese diet, 121–22, 125; in malaria control, 198–200; of media coverage of SARS epidemic, 229–30; night soil trade, 10, 54–56, 60, 220; of schistosomiasis treatment, 219
education: classical Chinese medicine, 232, 234; midwifery programs, 172, 179n54, 179nn56–57; traditional Chinese medicine, 232–33, 240, 244
Egypt, malaria in, 185
eisei (modern sanitary movement, Japan), 7, 133–37, 148–51. *See also weisheng*
England: British medical professionals, qualifications for, 127n2; cholera con-

trol and, 153; diet of poor and laboring classes in, 126
Enlightenment scholarship, 3, 5
environment: contagion and, 27, 29; Japanese perception and adaptation to, 12; malaria and, 184–85, 198–99; provoking epidemic *qi*, 8, 29, 41–42; schistosomiasis and, 206–10. *See also* climate; pathogenic *qi*
epidemic control (*fangyi*), 17–20, 136–39
Epidemic Prevention and Water Purification Department. *See* Unit 731
epidemic *qi*, 8, 25, 29, 41–42
European imperialism, 115, 117, 124–25, 154, 249
European racial identity, 117
European's health: climate affecting, 110–16, 125; diet affecting, 109, 112–16, 119–22, 126; malaria control, 185
evil Japanese physician, 139, 142–43, 147–55
evil-needle stories, 139, 142, 147–55. *See also* needles (hypodermic) in Chinese culture
evolutionary theory, 116–18
expansion medicine (*kaitogu igaku*), 12

Faber, Ernst, 63
Fang Bao, 53
fangyi (epidemic control), 17–20, 136–39
Fan Yanqiu, 164
Farm Colonization Program, Manchuko-era, 136
Farmer, Paul, 261
Farrar, Reginald, 95
Fayrer, Joseph, 115–16
feidianxing feiyan (atypical pneumonia), 239
Feng Heling, 216
Fidler, David, 256
First Opium War (1839–42), 110
Fracastoro, Girolamo, 27
Framing Disease (Rosenberg), 75
Fryer, John, 114
Fu Daiwei, 168

Gamsa, Mark, 144
garbage collection, 10, 53, 56–58, 63. *See also* night soil and waste treatment
Ge Hong, 29
geographical determinism, 249
germ *chong* (vermin), 9
germ theory: acceptance of, 9, 27, 45, 136, 242; *chuanran* and, 45, 99, 239; eight infectious diseases identified by, 99; integration of contagion, 249; introduction overview, 9; Kitasato's contribution to, 12–13; public health movements and, 17, 27–28; role in containing plague, 75, 81, 86
Giddens, Anthony, 256, 270
Ginzburg, Carlo, 152–53
Global Conference on SARS (WHO), 257
global infectious disease control, 256–65
Global Malaria Eradication Program, 183, 190–91
global medicine, 277
Gong Tingxian, 38
Gordon, Charles Alexander, 122
Gotō Kioshi, 160
Greater East Asia Co-Prosperity Sphere, 12
Great Jia'nan Irrigation System, 188
Great Leap Forward, 205, 215
Guangdong Provincial Hospital of TCM, 231, 233, 238, 243
Guangdong sores, 39–40
Guanghua (Kwong Wah) Hospital, 235
Guangzhou College of TCM, 231, 233, 238, 243
Guangzhou College of TCM Hospital, 233, 243
Guns, Steel, and Germs (Diamond), 249

Haining County, schistosomiasis in. *See* schistosomiasis
Handy recipes for urgent uses (*Zhou-hou beiji fang*), 29
Hang-Ki (Heng Qi), 112–13
Harbin Plague Hospital, 81
Harrison, Mark, 117, 124
Heaton, Charles, 114–15

heat-wind epidemics, 238, 240–41
He Lianchen, 100–101
Henderson, James, 112
hereditary transmission of disease, 35–36, 38, 40
Heymann, David, 264, 270
Hinrichs, T. J., 104n65
Hirst, Fabian, 75, 79, 88
history of medicine, 273
hokō system, 200n16
Home Quarantine Order (HQO), 265
Hong Kong, SARS in, 234, 261, 266. *See also* bubonic plague, Hong Kong (1894)
Hong Kong Baptist University, 234
Hong Kong Hospital, 234
Hong Mai, 35
Hoping Hospital, 267
household registration system, Taiwan, 13
Huang Shaohong, 204
Huang Zunxian, 65
human body: the contagious, 27, 35–38, 43–44; microclimate of, 242, 244–46
human excrement. *See* night soil, commoditization of; night soil and waste treatment; night soil use in agriculture
Hunt, Nancy Rose, 140
Huo Yuanjia, 142, 148, 154
hygienic modernity. *See* Japan, colonial project of hygienic modernity; *weisheng*
hygienic practices: advice literature about, 121; diet and, 109, 112–16, 119–22, 126; in identity formation, 124, 155; personal, 7; of settlers in Manchuria, 135–36

identity: Chinese, modern, 4–5, 135; climate and, 115; colonial China, 5; colonial India, 5, 124–25; diet and, 110; elites within the empire and, 155; hygienic practices in formation of, 124, 155; medical training and professional, 16; racial character and, 116–19

Iijima Wataru, 12, 135, 148
immunity to disease, 117–18
imperialism, 115, 117, 124–25, 154, 249,
    274–75
India: climate of, 112; colonial identity in,
    5, 124–25; colonial medicine and public
    health in, 4, 14, 16; malaria control in,
    187
Indian mutiny (1857), 125
Indochina, colonial culture in, 124
industrialization, 121, 174–75, 199
infant mortality, Taiwan, 176
infection, root meaning, 28
infection vs. *chuanran*, 239
infectious disease (*chuanranbing*). *See*
    chuanranbing (infectious disease)
*Influence of Tropical Climates on European
    Constitutions, The* (Martin), 112
Institute of Infectious Diseases, 12
integrative medicine, 8–10, 231–32, 244,
    246–48, 250
International Plague Conference, 88, 95,
    98, 146
International Sanitary Conference, 95–96
International Sanitary Convention,
    102n22
International Settlement of Shanghai:
    plague containment in, 94; urban
    sanitation, 10–12, 58–64
Internet, 261
Isaburō, Miyauchi, 52–53
Ishii Shirō, 141
isolation vs. quarantine, 269

Jamieson, Robert Alexander, 111, 113
Japan: infectious disease regulation in,
    96; as model of medical modernity,
    134, 161; modern sanitary movement
    (*eisei*) in, 7, 133–37, 148–51; plague
    opportunity for expansion, 77–78;
    public health system in, 65; sanitary
    practices in, 10–11, 52, 64–65; Western
    medicine in, adoption of, 12
Japan, colonial project of hygienic moder-
    nity: ethnic distinctions in disease
    treatment in, 137, 188–89; images of

doctors in, 133, 139; overview of, 12–15;
    rural China, 12–13, 149–51, 210–12;
    vaccination campaigns, 14, 137, 143.
    See also specific countries
Japanese imperialism, 154, 275
Japanese midwives, 172
jianran (dye by immersion), 29–31
jianyi. See quarantine (*jianyi*)
Jiaxing County, schistosomiasis in. *See*
    schistosomiasis
Jiaxing Hospital, 212
Jingwu Athletic Association (Jingwu Tiyu
    Hui), 142
Jin Yuehua, 216
Johnson, James, 112
Joint Commission for Rural Reconstruc-
    tion (JCRR), 189–90
Jones, Margaret, 179n57

Kangxi, Emperor of China, 53
Kitasato Shibasaburo, 12–13, 78–80, 93,
    95, 98
Kleinman, Arthur, 274, 276
Koch, Robert, 12, 97, 186
Kuang-Chi Liang, 191
Kumar, Deepak, 5
Kuomintang (KMT): midwives in Taiwan,
    169, 178n44; schistosomiasis control,
    210–13

labor migration, 174–75
Laderman, Carol, 163
Leibig, Justus von, 126
Leopold II, 140
leprosy (*mafeng*), 8–9, 36, 38–39, 40, 44
Leslie, Charles, 273
Liang Qichao, 98
Liaodong Peninsula, Japan's investment
    in, 134
lifestyle and disease, 121
Li Shizhen, 39
Li Tengyue (Ri Tōgaku), 167
Liu Shiyong, 154
Liu Tingchun, 65
livestock and disease control, 207
Livingstone, David, 117

Livingstone, Frank, 185
Li Youping, 247
London School of Tropical Medicine, 116
Loong, Lee Hsien, 268
Lu Shizhong, 35

Mackay, George Leslie, 172
Mackay, Mary Helen, 172
mafeng (leprosy), 8–9, 36, 38–40, 44
Magara Masanao, 160, 172
malaria, 184–85; contributors to epi-
    demics of, 198–99; diagnosing, 186–87,
    194; immunity to, 118; mortality rate
    from, 186–87, 199; prevalence statistics
    of, Taiwan, 195–96; risk and illness
    statistics, 183, 186, 189–90, 196; treat-
    ment programs for, 194
malaria control: education programs
    about, 187–88; global efforts in, 183,
    190; human factor in, 184–85; in India,
    187
malaria control, Taiwan: DDT-spraying
    operation in, 190–94, 196; history of,
    183; Japanese colonial state, 183,
    185–89, 197; JCRR programs, 189–90;
    narratives on, 189; overview of, 13, 15,
    17–20; post–Second World War, 189,
    197–98; total eradication, elements of,
    194, 196–97
malarial anemia, 118
Malaysia, colonial, 163
Manchuko (Changchun), 134–35
Manchuria: expansion medicine in foster-
    ing Japanese settlement in, 12; Japa-
    nese concept of, 133–35; medical
    ecology of, 150; as plagueland, 134–36,
    147. *See also* bubonic plague; pneu-
    monic plague
Manchuria, colonial policies of hygienic
    modernity: agricultural resettlement,
    hygienic challenges of, 135–36; defini-
    tion of, 133; epidemic control (*fangyi*),
    136–39; evil-needle stories embodying,
    139, 142, 147–56; legacy of, 14; over-
    view of, 12–14; remote medical care,
    149–51; resistance to, 155; scientific

infrastructure and governance in, 135.
    See also pneumonic plague, Manchuria
    (1910–11)
Manchuria Medical School, 149, 155
Manchurian plague. *See* pneumonic
    plague, Manchuria
Mandel, Simon, 247
Manson, Patrick, 112, 116–19, 120, 122,
    276
Mantetsu, 135
Mao Zedong, 11, 211–14, 222, 232, 275
Mararia (malaria) (film), 197
Mardel, Simon Nicholas, 236–37
Martin, James Ronald, 112, 115–16
Masanao, Magara, 160
Ma Xiaonan, 237–39, 243
May Fourth movement, 4
medical atrocities, 140–42, 155
medical ecology, 146–47, 149–50, 154–55
medical modernity, 83, 134, 161. *See also*
    weishing
medical professionals: diet in tropics,
    views of, 112–24; evil associated with,
    139–40; evil Japanese physician, 139,
    142–43, 147–55; Japanese, images of,
    133, 139; qualifications for British,
    127n2; training of, 16, 212, 216
medicine, historical comprehension of,
    273
Mengmen quanshu (Xiao), 40
Mesny, Gérald, 79–80
miasma and theories of, 8, 27–28, 126
miasmatic *qi*, 40–41
microscope, 74–75, 77–82, 85–86, 99,
    239
midwifery reform, colonial Taiwan: ban-
    ning of lay midwives during, 163–64;
    certification in, 162, 172; education
    programs and, 172, 179n54, 179nn56–
    57; overview of, 13, 15; research
    methodology and, 162–63; state strate-
    gies, 171
midwives: Japanese, 172; lay, KMT Taiwan,
    169, 178n44; modern, colonial Taiwan,
    172–75; social networks of, 172–75. *See
    also* childbirth

midwives (lay), colonial Taiwan: biomedicine incorporated by, 170; diversity in,
164–65; industrialization and, 174–75;
infant mortality with, 166–69, 175;
male devaluation of, 175
migration, rural to urban, 174–75
Military Medical Unit 731, 14, 133, 141–43,
155
Ming-cheng Lo, 155, 176
Ming dynasty, 37–43
missionary dietary habits, 113–14
Mitchell, Timothy, 185
Mitter, Rana, 155
mobile medical care, 149–50
modernity: China's path to, 5; contributors
to building, 176; ironies of, 155; medical, 83, 134, 161. *See also weishing*
modernity-scientific achievement association, PRC, 5
Moore, W. J., 115
moral cause of disease, 36, 38, 40
moral economy of health, 115–16, 121,
123–24
moral economy of risk, 19, 256
mosquitoes, U.S. war on, 183. *See also*
malaria control
mothering and motherhood, scientific,
161–62, 171
Mozi, 29
Mr. Science, 4
Müller, Dr., 112
mutual contamination (*xiangran*), 31

Nanjing Treaty, 110
Nathan, Carl, 77
National Public Health Conferences, 232
natural selection, 116–18
Needham, Joseph, 3, 5
needles (hypodermic) in Chinese culture,
148–49, 151. *See also* evil-needle
stories
Nelkin, Dorothy, 269
Nelson, T., 110
New York Times, SARS coverage by, 229–
31
nicotine use, 114–15

night soil, commoditization of, 10, 54–56,
60, 220
night soil and waste treatment: International Settlement of Shanghai, 58–64;
in late Imperial period, 65–67; overview of, 10–11; in premodern China,
52–58; summary overview, 67–68. *See
also* urban sanitation
night soil use in agriculture, 51, 54, 206–8,
220
North Manchurian Plague Prevention
Service, 96, 146
notifiable infectious disease, 93–97, 99,
106n100
Notter, J. Lane, 114, 115

On epidemics due to the warm weather
(*Wenyi lun*) (Wu), 88
On the three causes of diseases (*San yin
fang*), 36
Ooi Eng Eong, 233
On the origins and symptoms of all dis-
eases (*Zhubing yuan hou lun*) (Chao
Yuanfang), 30–35
the other: climate in defining, 111–13;
hygienic regimes in distancing, 124;
rumors, stories, and fears creating, 153.
See also borders

pathogenic *qi*, 31, 37. *See also* environment
Patriotic Hygiene Movement, 215
Pelling, Margaret, 27, 90
People's Republic of China (PRC):
Chinese-Western medicine integration
mandate, 8, 10, 244, 250; healthcare
policy of, 232; modernity-scientific
achievement association and, 5;
schistosomiasis control, 205, 210–18,
221–22; Unit 731 and, exposure by, 155.
See also China
Perrins, Robert, 136–37
person-to-person disease transmission,
31–39. *See also chuanran*
Pettenkofer, Max Josef von, 27
Ping-chen Hsiung, 167
plague: Chinese identification as *yi* or

wenyi, 25; medical ecology of, 146–47; outbreaks of, frequency of, 135, 138, 149; transforming the identity of, 75–76. *See also* antiplague measures; bubonic plague; pneumonic plague

Plague Fighter, The (Wu), 78

pneumonic plague: in 1935 Kerqin grasslands, 151; bubonic plague compared to, 78, 80, 85–87; in Manchuria (1921), 81–82, 145

pneumonic plague, Manchuria (1910–11): *chuanran*, belief in possibility of, 25–26, 45, 74, 88–93; death statistics from, 86–87, 134; diagnosing, 81–82, 85–86; mortality rate of, 87, 98; overview of, 9–10, 17–20; photographs of, 144, 154; retrospective sanitary regulations during, 95; scientific investigation post-, 146–47; social characteristics of, 97–98

pneumonic plague, Manchuria (1910–11), antiplague measures: autopsies as, 144–45, 154–55; blocking network of infection, 92–93; brutal nature of, 82–84, 144; Chinese medicine, challenges from, 84–88; cremation as, 83, 145, 146; detention as, 81–84; gauze masks as, 79–81; inspections as, 151; police enforcement of, 78–80, 84, 102n28; quarantine as, 81–84; railway traffic restrictions, 81, 145; resistance to, 79–80, 87; rumors, stories, and fears, 139, 145, 147–52; vaccination as, 151

pneumonic plague, Manchuria (1910–11), containing: achievement of, 73, 96; germ theory in, 75, 77–82; historical context for, 75–76; primary difficulties of, 74; Qing State sovereignty and, 77–78, 83–85, 99, 124; traditional vs. modern beliefs affecting, 91–92

pollution-generating epidemic, 8, 29, 41–42

postcolonial studies, 4–5

Prout, William, 126

public health: modern beliefs about, duality in, 155; risk assessment politics in, 255–56; as a social good, 16

public health campaigns, 17–20

Public Health Department, 59, 61

public health policy and infrastructure: beginnings of, 59; in China, catalyst for, 97, 99, 274; International Plague Conference recommendations for, 96; during late Imperial period, 64–67; modern, introduction of, 63; overview of, 17–20; Shanghai, 59, 61

Puyi, Emperor of China, 142

qi (breath, energy): epidemic, 8, 25, 29, 41–42; pathogenic, 31, 37; vicious, 37

Qing dynasty: disease-transmission developments of, 37–43; medical practices of, 168; plague containment and sovereignty of, 77–78, 83–85, 99, 134; Plague Prevention Service created during, 96; schistosomiasis in, 204

quarantine (*jianyi*): as antiplague measure, 45, 81–84, 139; Asian immigrant communities, 229; isolation vs., 269; SARS prevention through, 257, 258–59, 265–69

racial determinism, 116–19, 122–26

railways: medical care in remote areas, 149–50; in plague control efforts, 138–39; in plague transmission, 77, 81, 145

ran (contamination), early connotations of, 28–31, 33, 36

ranyi (exchange by dyeing), 31–33, 38

Record of Yijian (*Yijian zhi*) (Hong), 35

Records of the deities (*Ji shen lu*), 35

Reid, A. G., 111

Rennie, David F., 112–13

Research Institute of Warm Diseases (*wenbing*), 237–41

risk classification, 257–59, 263–65, 269–70

risk communication, 255, 261, 268–70

risk society, 256, 270–71

rivers, refuse in, 57

road maintenance, 63

Rosenberg, Charles, 75, 97, 267
Rosenthal, Elisabeth, 230
rural hygiene, 12, 149–51, 210–12
Russia, 77–78

safety-danger framework, 258, 264, 270,
    272n21
Sakai Kiyoshi, 171
San Francisco plague (1900), 100
San Guo zhi (History of the three king-
    doms), 29
sanitary movement, modern (eisei), 7,
    133–37, 148–51. See also weisheng
sanitary police: clean-street enforcement,
    52, 61–62, 102n28; enforcing anti-
    plague measures, 78–80, 84, 102n28,
    139; malaria control, Taiwan, 186;
    Nationalist government, 210; in
    regimes of hygienic modernity, 11, 13
sanitary practices: International Settle-
    ment of Shanghai, 10–12, 58–64;
    Japan, 10–11, 52, 64–65. See also urban
    sanitation
SARS (Severe Acute Respiratory Syn-
    drome): biomedical characteristics of,
    255; global spread of, 256–65; TCM
    interpretations of, 242, 245–46
SARS epidemic (2003): overview of,
    17–20; TCM interpretations of, 42; TCM
    practitioners in, roles of, 233–34; WHO
    and, 18, 229–30, 235–37, 246–47, 256,
    259–65
SARS epidemic (2003), media coverage:
    conceptual blind spot of, 234–35;
    economics of, 229–30; outside vs.
    inside China, 228; TCM treatment of,
    230–31; in Western media, 229–31
SARS prevention: borders for, 256–59;
    Chinese herbs for, 9, 230, 253n41;
    economics of, 263; lessons learned for,
    269–70; political framework of, 267–
    68, 270; quarantine for, 257–59, 265–
    69; racial discrimination in, 229–30;
    risk classification, 257–59; in Singa-
    pore, 265–67; in Taiwan, 256–59,
    265–69

SARS treatment: biomedical model eclips-
    ing, 234–35; Chinese herbal medicine
    for, 9, 243–44, 248; climate factor in,
    244–46; data, 235–36; effectiveness
    evaluations, 235–37, 243–48; in Hong
    Kong, 234; integrated approach to,
    9–10, 231–33, 246–48; media coverage
    of, 228, 230–31; outside China, 234;
    wenbing (four-level) approach, 9–10,
    243–44, 246
scabies (dafeng lai disorder), 36, 38
Scheid, Volker, 250
schistosomiasis: 1950–60s infection rates,
    204; the environment and, 206–10;
    human factor in, 206, 208; infection
    rates of, 216; medical professional
    training programs on, 212, 216;
    occupation-infection rate relation,
    209; treatment of, 212–13, 216–19
schistosomiasis control: 1948–1955 (KMT
    to PRC), 205, 210–13; 1956–58 (PRC di-
    rective), 213–18, 221–22; 1959–69 set-
    backs, 222; introduction overview of,
    17–20; post–Cultural Revolution suc-
    cess, 222; resistance to, 219–21; snail
    removal projects, 215, 221; traditional
    vs. modern beliefs affecting, 218–21
Science and Civilisation series
    (Needham), 3
science and technology studies (STS), 3,
    162, 213
scientific medicine, 273
scientific racism, 125
Scientific Research Advisory Committee
    on Severe Acute Respiratory Syndrome
    (SARS) (WHO), 236
Scientific Research on Nationally Pro-
    duced Drugs, 232
Scotland, 123
seasonal epidemics, 41–42
Second Opium War (1856–60), 110
Second World War, 190
Secret record of rotten sores (Meichuang
    milu) (Chen), 39
sewage treatment plants, 10–11, 52. See
    also night soil and waste treatment

sexual intercourse in disease transmission, 34, 36, 38–40, 43, 48n40, 49n57
Shanghai Hygiene (Henderson), 112
Shanghai International Settlement, 11–12
Shanghai Municipal Council, 59–61
Shanghan lun, 34
Shang shu, 29
Shao Rong, 55
Shen Bao, 63, 83
Shengji zonglu (imperial medical encyclopedia), 36
Shen Junru, 213
Shen Qingfa, 237–40, 243–44
Shenshi nongshu, 55
Shi Youquan, 220
Shi Zhaoji, 77–78, 80
Simond, Paul-Louis, 79
Simpson, Ruth, 258, 264, 270, 272n21
Singapore, SARS prevention in, 265–67
Sino-Japanese War, 11, 64, 143, 204–5
smallpox, 44, 96–97, 159n51
snails and schistosomiasis, 206–8, 215, 221
social discrimination, disease and, 268–69
Somerville, J. R., 114–15
Soper, Fred, 191
Sota Nagamune, 160
southern medicine (*nanho igaku*), 12
South Manchuria Railway Company (Mantetsu), 14, 77, 134–35, 136, 138, 148
South Manchuria Railway Company hospital, 134, 136
Spielman, Andrew, 194
Stoler, Ann, 115, 124
street cleaning, 52, 55, 57, 59–67, 102n28
Strickmann, Michel, 35–36
Studies on Warm Diseases (*Wenbing xue*) (Shen), 238
Su Delong, 213–14
Sun Simiao, 31, 33
syphilis, 39

Taijin Treaty, 127n6
Taipei Hospital, 172
Taiwan: death in, leading causes of, 199;

SARS prevention in, 256–59, 265–69. *See also* malaria control, Taiwan
Taiwan, colonial occupation: birth statistics in, 172; death in, leading causes of, 186; education for girls during, 172; *hokō* system, 200n16; industrialization and, 174–75, 188, 199; infant mortality and, 166–69, 176
Taiwan, colonial policies of hygienic modernity: ethnic distinctions in disease treatment in, 188–89; JCRR programs, post-WW II, 190; malaria control and, 183, 185–89; overview of, 12–13, 15–16; public health and, support for, 16; public health and infrastructure, 164. *See also* midwifery reform, colonial Taiwan
Taiwan, KMT rule, midwives in, 169, 178n44
Taiwanese women: birth statistics of, 172; childbirth narratives of, 163–66, 168–69, 172–74; education for, 172; Japanese elites deficiency model, 160–61
Taiwanese women, as midwives, colonial Taiwan: biomedicine incorporated by, 170; certification of, 172; diversity in, 164–65; industrialization and, 174–75; infant mortality with, 166–69, 175; male devaluation of, 175; social networks of, 172–75
Taiwan Provincial Malaria Research Institute, 189–92
tarbagan research, 146
TCM. *See* Chinese medicine, traditional (TCM)
technology: microscope and plague, 74–75, 77–82, 85–86, 99, 239; women and, 162
Temkin, Owsei, 273, 276–77
ter Haar, Barend, 153
Tianjin Treaty, 110
Tissot, Auguste A. D., 121
toilet habits, 219–20
toilets, flush, 11, 61
toilets, public: cleaning for disease prevention, 219–21; economics of, 220; Inter-

toilets (*cont'd*)
national Settlement of Shanghai, 59,
62; late Imperial period, 52–54
Treatise on cold damage (*Shanghan lun*),
36
tropical hygiene: diet, effect on health of,
109–16, 119–22; elements comprising,
124
tropical medicine, 249
the tropics, as a concept, 111–15, 124
Trotter, Thomas, 120–21
tuberculosis (*xulao*), 8–9
typhoid fever, 159n51

Unit 731, 14, 133, 141–43, 155
University of California, Berkeley, 229–30
urban aesthetics, 61, 63, 65
urbanization, 174–75, 188, 199
urban sanitation: late Imperial period, 53,
65–67; overview of, 9–10; premodern
China, 57–58; street cleaning, 52, 55,
57, 59–67, 102n28; traditional lifestyles, impact on, 67. *See also* night soil
and waste treatment

vaccination: bubonic plague, 138–39,
148–49; Chinese responses to, 14, 148,
152; pneumonic plague, 151; rural
China and, 150–51; smallpox, 44, 150;
statistics, 151, 159n51; trends in use of,
154
vaccination campaigns, 14, 137, 143
vampires, 133, 140–43
variolation. *See* vaccination
vicious *qi*, 37
victimization, *bazimamoto* stories of, 154
Volkmar, Barbara, 28, 104n65

Wade, Thomas, 112–13
Wagner, Wilhelm, 56
Wallace, Alfred Russel, 113
Wang Ang, 168
Wang Tao, 32
warm disease. *See wenbing* (warm
disease)
war memory, constructions of, 155

waste management. *See* night soil and
waste treatment
Watson, James, 122–23, 125
weisheng: Chinese vs. British concept of,
126–27; dual nature of, 156; experienced as *fangyi* (epidemic control),
137; meanings of, 132–33; overview of,
7–8. *See also eisei* (modern sanitary
movement, Japan)
wenbing (warm disease): climates and
constitutions in, 8; Cold Damage
(*shanghan*) vs., 240; four-level approach to treating, 9–10, 243–44, 246;
literature on, 240; recipes for stopping,
29; SARS and, 9, 237–41, 246; sexual
intercourse in, 36; two-stage process of
contamination, 31
wenyi (epidemics): avoiding (*biyi*), 91–92;
chuanran contamination as factor in,
25–26, 40–42, 45, 88–93; diseases
becoming, 240; Manchurian plague
challenging traditional understanding
of, 25–26, 74; seasonal change role in,
240–41, 242
West Africa, malaria in, 185
West China Hospital of Sichuan University, 247–48
Western medicine: Chinese medicine vs.,
234–35, 241–43; cosmopolitan medicine vs., 177n2, 273; Meiji Japan, 12.
See also biomedicine
Western medicine–Chinese medicine
integration, 8–10, 231–32, 244, 246–48,
250
White, Luise, 140, 154
Williams, Perry, 75
women, technology and, 162. *See also*
midwives; midwives (lay), colonial
Taiwan
World Health Organization (WHO):
malaria-control efforts of, 15, 183,
190–91, 194, 198; SARS and, 18, 229–
30, 235–37, 246–47, 256, 259–65
Wu Lien-teh (Wu Liande): Manchurian
plague containment role of, 9, 14,
75–76, 78–81, 83–84, 91, 98–99; on

open-air autopsies, 144–45; plague-prevention research of, 146–47; public health construction claims of, 96; quarantine concept of, 45, 46
Wushantou Dam, 188
Wu Yi, 231
Wu Yingen, 237, 240
Wu Youxing, 41, 45, 88

xiangran (mutual contamination), 31
Xiao Xiaoting, 40
Xie Zhaozhe, 52, 54
Xi Liang: on antiplague measures, 82; *chuanran* term used by, 27; on *chunran* role in epidemics, 25, 45, 88, 90–91; emphasis on role of microscope of, 75; report on controlling plague by, 74; sanitary regulations issued by, 95; on shift from *wenyi* to *chuanranbing*, 76
Xu Bihui, 212
Xue, Yong, 51
Xu Jianguo, 236
Xu Xuan, 35

Yang cui, 164
Yao Hubao, 220
yi (epidemics). *See wenyi* (epidemics)
yi (exchange), 34
Yin Haiguang, 197
yin-yang binary, 245
yinyang yi, 34, 36, 38
Yu Botao, 91
Yu Yue, 91

Zerubavel, Evitar, 258
Zhang Deyi, 64
Zhang Gao, 36
Zhang Ji, 31, 240
Zhang Lu, 41
Zhang Xiaorui, 236
Zhong xi yifang huitong (Ding), 93
Zhou-hou beiji fang (Handy recipes for urgent uses) (Ge Hong), 29
Zhou Yangjun, 41
zhu (pouring), 32–33
Zhu Xi, 37
zhuyi (exchange by pouring), 31–34, 38

Angela Ki Che Leung is a research fellow at the Institute of
History and Philosophy of the Academia Sinica, and a professor
of history at the Chinese University of Hong Kong.

Charlotte Furth is professor emerita of history, University of
Southern California.

Library of Congress Cataloging-in-Publication Data

Health and hygiene in Chinese East Asia: policies and publics
in the long twentieth century / edited by Angela Ki Che Leung
and Charlotte Furth.
p.   cm.
Includes bibliographical references and index.
ISBN 978-0-8223-4815-3 (cloth: alk. paper)
ISBN 978-0-8223-4826-9 (pbk.: alk. paper)
1. Public health—China—History—20th century.
2. Public health—Taiwan—History—20th century.
3. Sanitation—China—History—20th century.
4. Sanitation—Taiwan—History—20th century.
I. Liang, Qizi. II. Furth, Charlotte.
RA527.H428 2010
362.10951—dc22
2010024246